THE CANCER DIRECTORY

DR ROSY DANIEL

How to make the integrated
cancer medicine revolution
work for you

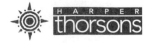
HARPER
thorsons

HarperThorsons
An Imprint of HarperCollins*Publishers*
77–85 Fulham Palace Road,
Hammersmith, London W6 8JB

The website address is: www.thorsonselement.com

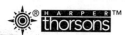

and *HarperThorsons* are trademarks
of HarperCollins*Publishers* Ltd

First published 2005

10 9 8 7 6 5 4 3 2

© Dr Rosy Daniel 2005

Dr Rosy Daniel asserts the moral right to
be identified as the author of this work

A catalogue record of this book
is available from the British Library

ISBN-13   978-0-00-715427-2
ISBN-10   0-00-715427-5

Printed and bound in Great Britain by
Martins-The-Printers Ltd, Berwick Upon Tweed

Contents

Acknowledgements

The writing of this book is the culmination of 20 years of work in integrated cancer medicine and I am hugely grateful to my wonderful editor, Wanda Whiteley of Thorsons, for giving me the opportunity to commit what I have learned to paper in *The Cancer Directory*.

For my learning I am most deeply indebted to all those who have guided me along this fascinating path of discovery. Without doubt, I have learned most from the thousands of people with cancer and their families with whom I have shared the pain and triumph of their cancer experience. I wish to acknowledge and thank each and every one of you for the enormous privilege of sharing your intimate and profound realities and insights with me.

As rich as this has been the learning and sharing that has taken place with my amazing colleagues both at the Bristol Cancer Help Centre, where I worked for 15 years, and in the wider holistic health community of Great Britain. In particular, I am most indebted to the founders of the Bristol Cancer Help Centre, Pat Pilkington MBE and the late Penny Brohn, who gave so many of us the opportunity to develop a unique new model of integrated cancer medicine which has been of such great value to those who have experienced it as patients or practitioners. They have undoubtedly created a total revolution in medical thinking and practice since they started their pioneering work in 1989 and have demonstrated, against much early resistance, the great power of the individual in caring for their own health. They have also brought the emotional and spiritual experience of illness and healing into clear focus, and we are all hugely enriched by the wonderful combination of their deep, loving concern and stoic persistence, their elegant perception of the spiritual nature of living and dying and their immense and riveting creative intelligence. My very special thanks go also to the team leaders with whom I worked when I was Medical Director at Bristol – namely Barbara Siddall who led the group therapy and counselling, Janet Swan who led the healers, Ute Brookman who led the nutritional therapists, Helen Cooke who led the nurses, Jane Sen who created the most sensational healthy food and Andy Fagg and Thea Bailey who led the body work. All of you made a most inspiring contribution to my understanding of true multi-disciplinary integrated medicine, along with your wonderful teams, our coordinators and my fellow holistic doctors.

Most important in the orthodox side of cancer medicine has been the help of the extremely supportive Professor Karol Sikora. He was the first oncologist to recognize the value of the 'Bristol Approach', integrating holistic supportive care into his own unit at the Hammersmith Hospital in the 1980s. He has been a wonderful mentor and friend and has provided excellent medical guidance in this Directory, along with the wonderfully helpful cancer nurse, Patricia Peat, who runs Cancer Options. I would also like to thank chemist Andrew Panton for his invaluable help in researching the alternative cancer treatments referred to in this Directory. And of course I am thrilled with the wonderful foreword that was written for the Directory by Bernice Miller, who, 12 years after her diagnosis of cancer, is such a shining and joyful reminder to me of what can happen if you just refuse to have cancer! Bernice also assisted me with researching and shaping the book initially, which was terrifically helpful. Your contributions have widened the scope and depth of the work greatly, and I cannot thank you enough for your hard work and dedication to getting it right.

The other major contributor was Patricia Hassam, who voluntarily checked the entire Resources Directory for accuracy. If ever there was a labour of love this was it and I thank you and commend you unreservedly for this most generous gift of your time and energy. I have also received countless hours of back up from my Personal Assistants, Niki Dunnett and Emma Dennis, my Health Creation team in compiling the Resources Directory initially, and fantastic attention to detail from the Thorsons editorial, design and production team: Wanda Whiteley, Susanna Abbott, Simon Gerratt, Kathy Dyke, Jacqui Caulton, Natasha Tait and Kay Carroll. You have all been wonderful. Thank you so much for your kindness and patience in pulling all the work together.

But the real heroes have been my extraordinarily supportive husband Mike, children Sophie and Elouise and my dear friends and family, who have been patience and kindness personified. It is impossible to produce this much work without it dominating one's home and social life for many years, and yet they have all truly understood and honoured the need for this work to be completed without a single complaint or grumble. I thank you with all my heart, my darling family, and promise you that the celebration will now begin!

About the Author and Contributors

Dr Rosy Daniel is an internationally-renowned Integrated Medicine Consultant who has worked as an holistic doctor (and later Medical Director) at the Bristol Cancer Help Centre between 1985 and 1999, and then as an Integrated Medicine Consultant at the Harley Street Cancer Centre in London and at Health Creation in Bristol. She now practises at the Apthorp Centre in Weston, Bath.

She is the author of:

- *The Cancer Lifeline Kit* (Health Creation, 2003), which includes The Cancer Lifeline Programme, The Health Creation Programme, The Carer's Guide, The Message of Hope video and The Cancer Lifeline Recipe Cards by Jane Sen
- *Eat to Beat Cancer with* (with Jane Sen, Thorsons, 2003)
- *The Cancer Prevention Book* (Simon & Schuster, 2001)
- *Living with Cancer* (Robinson, 2000)
- *Healing Foods* (Thorsons, 1996)
- *Loving Medicine* (Gateway Books, 1986).

She has also produced and features on *The Holistic Approach to Health* video for the Bristol Cancer Help Centre that forms part of their introductory pack.

Dr Daniel now teaches and broadcasts nationally and internationally on subjects such as the integrated approach to health, psychoneuroimmunology, mind–body medicine, the integrated medicine approach to the treatment and prevention of cancer, and cancer nutrition.

Her 1999 research *Meeting the Needs of People with Cancer for Support and Self-Management* confirmed her awareness of the acute need of people with cancer and their carers to have the best, most empowering support and the most up-to-date information about what is available in cancer care to allow them to take an active part in the journey back to health. Research is now in progress on her new Cancer Lifeline Kit to assess its health and cost benefits for widespread use in integrated cancer medicine of the future.

She aims, through her organization Health Creation, to be able to make a major impact on the incidence of heart disease and cancer through the application of the Health Creation Programme and supporting Mentor Service in businesses, schools and community settings. Throughout 2005 she is piloting Health Creation in Business with a view to launching a Health Creation Award for Investors in Health, which she hopes will become an important organizational standard towards which participating groups can work. In this way Dr Daniel intends, over time, to help shift the focus within society from that of passive healthcare to active health creation, thereby helping to prove wrong the gloomy prognostications that cancer incidence will treble over the next 20 years!

The Contributors

Professor Karol Sikora has been a leading cancer specialist for nearly 20 years. He is Professor of Cancer Medicine at The Hammersmith Hospital, part of the Imperial College School of Medicine in London. He is also currently advising an international hospital group on the creation of a novel cancer centre in London, transcending the NHS–private medicine interface. He believes passionately in bringing together the best from both the orthodox and complementary worlds to create truly integrated holistic care for people with cancer. He has contributed to Chapter 4 of this book.

Patricia Peat is a cancer nurse who runs an information service for people with cancer called Cancer Options. Through this service, individuals with cancer can obtain a tailor-made report of all treatments – orthodox, complementary and alternative – worldwide that are relevant to their specific condition and stage of illness. She has also contributed to Chapter 4 of this book.

Andrew Panton is a Member of the Royal Society of Chemistry, holding a BSc in chemistry and an MSc in analytical chemistry. Andrew has a special interest in nutritional medicine, and in the toxic and carcinogenic effects of chemical ingredients in cosmetics and in personal care and household products. He has contributed to Chapter 5 of this book.

Bernice Miller, who has also written the Foreword for this work, is a most remarkable force of nature. She used her diagnosis of breast cancer in 1989 to drop her stressful business lifestyle in favour of extreme physical fitness and a totally effervescent *joie de vivre*. Fifteen years on, she remains dedicated to her health, happiness and creative lifestyle, and I am quite sure that nobody who laughs and loves as much as Bernice will ever die of cancer! Bernice has also helped with the compiling of the Resources Directory.

Foreword by Bernice Miller

The Cancer Directory is a state-of-the-art guide to the best in integrated cancer treatment available today, incorporating the latest orthodox, complementary, alternative and mind-body treatments with the immense power of becoming active in one's own defence through self-help approaches and lifestyle changes. The aim of this volume is to provide the vital information you need to obtain a comprehensive overview of the many and diverse approaches to cancer. This will enable you to make informed decisions as to your optimal combination of treatment, support and self-help that should prove most effective and right for you.

Huge strides are being made in all fields of cancer care. Holistic support and complementary therapies are finally becoming accepted into mainstream orthodox medicine; the powerful mind–body connection has at last been substantiated scientifically; numerous new technologies and developments in genetics and immunology are pointing to entirely new approaches to cures within the orthodox model; alternative medical treatments in pioneering clinics throughout the world are producing exciting results. The time is coming when the worlds of orthodox and alternative medical science will meet on such ground as vaccines and dendritic-cell therapies, which are now being given in both mainstream hospitals and alternative clinics.

But what is absolutely clear is that the best results are no longer to be found by choosing either one path or another, but by integrating as much knowledge and practice as possible for a result that will be far greater than the sum of the parts in both human and medical terms.

Until now, there has been no single reliable source providing patients and practitioners with a comprehensive overview of this brave new world of integrated cancer care and treatment, and reliable information or guidance within mainstream healthcare is scant. But there is a constant barrage of partial and often misleading information on new breakthroughs and discoveries: just enough to put new and ongoing cancer patients in fear of missing out on something that could save their lives.

As one of England's foremost Integrated Medical Consultants, and 15 years as a doctor at and then Medical Director of the world-famous Bristol Cancer Help Centre, Dr Rosy Daniel is uniquely qualified to produce this authoritative and up-to-the-minute guide. She has helped over 20,000 cancer patients get the best combination of orthodox and complementary treatment, and this book will save those with cancer and their families hours of research and worry by bringing the most crucial professional information and experience of what has worked for others directly into their hands.

For over 20 years, Dr Daniel has developed her own highly valued approach to integrated cancer treatment, and she is now viewed as a truly reliable bridge between the worlds of orthodox and complementary medicine. Described by Professor Karol Sikora, one of the UK's leading oncologists, as 'the sane end of the alternative cancer world', she is constantly being consulted by cancer healthcare professionals and by those providing cancer services for her advice on how to set up the ideal integrated cancer care of the future.

First, and above all, her approach involves a high degree of emotional and spiritual empowerment for the patient. This is followed by a sensitive eliciting of the state, needs, problems and values of each person she sees before a personalized action plan is created together with the patient. The plan has three phases: preparation to enable the best experience of and outcome from treatment; working to strengthen the body and repair the immune system; and changing the lifestyle of the individual to achieve optimal health in the long term.

In Part 1 of this book, Dr Daniel aims to embrace and comfort the reader, preparing him or her for the journey ahead and providing guidance on how and when to use the information in the Resources Directory. Dr Daniel's extensive experience has taught her that almost more important than the medicines themselves is to set the right psychological foundations for getting the best treatment outcomes and recovering health. Scientific research has now established beyond doubt that the mind–body connection is one of the most powerful elements in the conquering of 'dis-ease' in the body, but this knowledge is scarcely applied in the orthodox approach to health and far from fully applied in many alternative models. *The Cancer Directory* contains the most up-to-date thinking in this field, and sets out the steps that readers can take to get themselves into the optimal state of mind to facilitate their recovery and get back into the driving seat fully in control of their lives, with a positive plan, hope and peace of mind.

The next most crucial step for those with cancer is to make the right treatment decisions in terms of the most effective treatment that will also be the least damaging in the short and long term. It is also vital that the course of action taken feels right to the individual involved, and is congruent with their personal life and healthcare values. Great emphasis is therefore placed upon help with information gathering, getting the best of all approaches, deciding on treatments, forming a plan, and working positively with doctors and practitioners to achieve the very best treatment outcomes. This is very hard for the recently diagnosed, who are still in shock and emotional turmoil. The objective is to set out guidelines to facilitate this process, and offer as much guidance as possible on when and how to make what types of decisions.

The current best practices in the most advanced orthodox medical treatment centres are outlined, giving the reader a bench-mark against which to measure the treatment they are being offered locally. Information is also given on what is going on at the frontiers of medicine around the world to enable the reader to check out the very best resources, research trials and treatments available for their individual problem, with advice on how to obtain second and third opinions as and when necessary.

Also described are the latest developments in alternative medicine in the fields of:

- **herbal medicine, such as carctol, catechins, indole-3-carbinol and turmeric**
- **immunotherapy, such as immune boosters, dendritic-cell therapy and vaccines**
- **metabolic therapy, such as essential sugars, essential fatty acids, pH balancing, enzymes and antioxidant vitamins**
- **mind–body medicine, such as the 'Journey' process by Brandon Bays, and the transformational approach of the Bristol Cancer Help Centre**
- **physical therapies, such as hyperthermia, light therapy and oxygen therapy**
- **nutritional therapies, such as the Gerson diet and the Nutrition Trust.**

The valuable role of complementary medicine as symptomatic relief and supportive care is described, using illustrations where recent research has shown maximum synergy. Information is provided as to how and when to build these into a treatment programme to minimize the symptoms of illness and side-effects of treatment. *The Cancer Directory* looks at the newest developments within these therapies, and their applications in pioneering hospitals and hospices.

Perhaps most important of all for a long-term sustained recovery is the section on pro-active holistic health creation. New research continues to confirm the importance of incorporating the basic principles of promoting positive health and healthy lifestyle changes into any healing regime. Dr Daniel says, 'After putting out the fire with cancer medicine, it is time to rebuild the house with holistic health creation.' Long-term survival is most dependent of all, she feels, on this continuing work to achieve high levels of energy, immune function and happiness. She also considers the opportunity created by serious illness for a complete life reorientation, describing her unique new Health Creation Programme, which highlights and focuses the individual on where they are currently vulnerable, exactly what needs to change and how to change to maximize the potential for long-term sustainable health.

Once readers have identified their values and choices, they will be able to find the appropriate resources to get the help they need in Part 2 of the book, which contains the Cancer Resources Directory. This will provide the reader with a comprehensive set of resources in the areas of:

- frontier orthodox cancer medicine
- pioneering hospitals offering integrated cancer care
- alternative cancer medicines
- nutritional organizations
- alternative cancer doctors
- alternative cancer clinics
- integrated medicine doctors and services
- complementary medicines organizations (to find therapists)
- psychological and spiritual support services for people with cancer and their carers
- retreats, spiritual development and holistic holidays
- cancer information services
- cancer care and practical help with nursing, social needs, financial help and insurance
- cancer prevention
- product suppliers for natural medicines and supplements.

There is also a Bibliography containing a comprehensive collection of the most useful reading material, a section containing all of the scientific references for the research supporting the use of an integrated approach to cancer care, a Glossary of the terms used in this book and in the field of integrated medicine, and an Index for easy navigation through this book.

The Cancer Directory is essential reading material for anyone newly diagnosed with cancer and for the healthcare professionals who help them. Only by understanding the full range of needs and healthcare choices available to those with cancer will the very best choices be offered, the chances of survival be most enhanced and the most loving, compassionate care be given.

Only by fully empowering those with cancer during their treatment and recovery process will the innate creative intelligence and inner strength of each person be brought to bear in the quest to heal physically and spiritually through the crisis of illness.

Integrated cancer medicine is the medicine of the future, and Dr Rosy Daniel is undoubtedly leading the way.

This book is essential reading for everyone affected by cancer. Information is empowerment, and this volume contains all you need to know about cancer from both the orthodox and complementary worlds of medicine. This is simply the best guide to integrated cancer medicine there is!

PROFESSOR KAROL SIKORA

Introduction: how to use this book by Dr Rosy Daniel

If you are reading this book, it is likely that you, or someone very close to you, have received a diagnosis of cancer.

My heart goes out to you at this painful, confusing and frightening time. Nothing prepares us in life for the shattering blow of a life-threatening diagnosis. Almost all of us live our lives feeling immortal – as if bad things only happen to other people. But, from time to time, we are pulled in on the fishing line of life and brought face to face with our mortality – and forced to face the completely fragile nature of life. The more perfect and settled our life has been, the harsher the blow and the more imperative it is that both you and those around you treat you with the utmost gentleness, care and sensitivity as you come to terms with what is happening to you. You will need time and very good support to find ways to make sense of the crisis and, most important of all, to bring all possible creative intelligence to bear in finding the most effective healthcare solutions for you.

My own understanding of both the pain and possibilities within the experience of cancer came from my intense relationship with the remarkable Penny Brohn, co-founder of the Bristol Cancer Help Centre. Penny was diagnosed with breast cancer at age 38, with three children aged under 10. Both of her parents had died within the previous two years, and her marriage was so shaky that, at the point of diagnosis, her world collapsed completely. But, after a few weeks of abject misery, grief and despair, the combination of her own native cunning and the immense unconditional love of her great friend Pat Pilkington enabled her to pick herself up, dust herself off, and find the complementary, alternative and self-help approaches that enabled her to turn a five-year prognosis of survival into 21 years of a glorious and adventurous life.

Her journey took her all over the world – from the alternative clinics of Dr Issles in Bavaria and Dr Contreras in Mexico to monasteries deep in Wales and mind–body medical centres in London. This journey also took her into the depths of her own psyche and spirit with counselling and spiritual healing, and towards the gentle restorative energy medicines of acupuncture, homoeopathy and craniosacral therapy. She learned how to nourish her body properly with healthy food, metabolic supplements and immune stimulants, and how to meet her emotional needs with the love of women friends instead of focusing only on the love of her husband. She lifted her spirit by becoming a writer, painter, mosaic artist and gardener, and fulfilled her life purpose by setting up the pioneering Bristol Cancer Help Centre, thereby changing the face of medicine for ever.

Penny was very frightened but she was also an extraordinarily brave person. She had no idea where to start and what would work. Every step of her journey was an exploration, a negotiation with herself, her carers and her medical team. The only guiding star she had on her journey was her profound feminine intuition and the counsel she received from those whom she called her 'gentle giants' – the doctors, nurses, therapists and healers who had also been brave enough to step outside of the rigid box of medical thinking in an attempt to understand the big questions: What role does an individual's lifestyle have in the development of cancer? What are the person's needs during the illness and its treatment? Most important of all, what power could a person bring to bear to affect the health of his or her body and the chances of recovery?

As a spiritual woman, Penny was also constantly aware of the power of prayer and the immense benefits that could be available through spiritual healing and seeking spiritual guidance.

Penny's amazingly comprehensive view of the nature of illness and healing sparked a revolution in cancer care. At first, it was explosive, as doctors feared that alternative doctors and practitioners would harm patients, taking them away from potentially effective medical treatment while fleecing them financially. Later, during the 1980s and 1990s, a truce was declared as many practitioners positioned themselves and their approaches as being complementary to medicine rather than alternative. But since the late 1990s, a new medical movement has emerged, led by His Royal Highness The Prince of Wales and his Foundation for Integrated Health, to help pull down the walls dividing care for the body from care for the mind and spirit, and help remove the conflict for patients between choosing between orthodox, complementary or alternative medicines. The aim has been to foster a climate in which people with cancer and their carers can be helped to obtain the best of all worlds – individually tailored treatment to meet their needs at all the different stages of cancer and its treatment.

This is vital, as one thing is certain – your needs will change. Sometimes you will feel strong, independent and entirely in control through the use of your self-help approaches. At other times you may feel ill, vulnerable and tempted to become dependent on the professional help of others. This was another of Penny's great teachings for her doctors – to recognize the changes in her state and needs so that they were able to perform a complicated but perfect tango with her as she explored her options, defined her needs, made her negotiations, and flowed between fear and certainty.

To help you make sense of your reactions, needs and choices, you will find three main types of information in the pages that follow. The first type is emotionally based to help you recognize your state, define your needs and determine the kind of support you will need before embarking upon your healing journey. The second type of information is descriptive, giving you an overview of the kinds of approaches available so that you can define your healthcare values, and make your own choices as to what approach, or blend of approaches, is right for you. These two levels of information are found in Part 1 of this volume. The third type of information is factual, and is contained in Part 2. Once you have defined your needs and values, and made your choices, this *Directory* will help you to find the best resources that you need.

My goal in writing this book has been to share with you my understanding of the emotional map of the cancer experience for both those with cancer and their carers, which has come as a result of more than 20 years of working with people with cancer. I have also wanted to convey the theory, practice and benefits of each dimension of the integrated medicine model. Finally, I have wanted to act like a truffle hound, rooting out the treasures buried within the immensely complex terrain of alternative, complementary and self-help approaches to cancer to guide you directly to what I believe works.

Many people with cancer have said to me that they felt like they had to get a PhD in the subject within six weeks of their diagnosis. They have had to learn about their disease, the treatments and all the possible alternatives in a very short period of time to make their choices. In many cases, the Internet made things worse as the array of options has become so mind-boggling. So, the intention of this *Directory* is to share with you the pearls of wisdom I have gained over many years of sorting the wheat from the chaff, learning from the experience of the 20,000 or so people I have worked with. These individuals, like Penny, have by trial and error found their own way to fight cancer and heal themselves effectively, and their hope and mine is that you will be able with this book to 'cut to the chase', and avoid weeks of research and worry. I hope that, in the pages of this book, you will find everything you need but, if you do not, then both I and my team of Health Creation Mentors are available for consultation to coach you through getting the best treatments, the best treatment outcomes and getting yourself fully established on the road to recovery. I am available personally to help you through my Bath clinic (tel: 01225 423333) and through my interactive Cancer Lifeline Kit and supportive Health Creation Mentor Service, with backup from my three Health Creation doctor partners (contact the Health Creation Helpline on 0845 009 3366).

Most important of all, please be reassured that there are people living today who have survived every single kind of cancer. It is clear that the ones who do best are those who truly face their situation, go through their feelings, and then set about taking a positive course of action to become proactive in their own defence.

My love and very best wishes go with you as you embark upon your road to recovery, and I hope that this *Directory* will guide you to many exciting and fulfilling sources of invaluable help. Meanwhile, please be aware that this is a living document. I would be extremely grateful for your feedback, input, ideas and corrections. All possible efforts have been made to make this *Cancer Directory* as comprehensive and accurate as possible, but your help in improving it further for future readers will be much appreciated.

Please send your ideas and feedback to:

Dr Rosy Daniel,
Health Creation,
77a Alma Road,
Clifton,
Bristol BS8 2DP

PART ONE

The keys to success: transforming health crisis into health creation

CHAPTER 1

How to make the integrated cancer medicine revolution work for you

Right now, if you are newly diagnosed or have been re-diagnosed with cancer, you may be feeling dispirited, frightened and confused. It is vital that you consider the following encouraging facts:

One   Cancer is a two-way process – it can grow but it can also shrink or go into remission.

Two   People have recovered from every kind of possible cancer and are still alive to tell the tale.

Three   A healthy body has detection and repair mechanisms specifically for cancer cells. The integrated medicine approach works to repair and boost these natural anti-cancer processes in the body.

Four   There are many factors in addition to orthodox medicine, over which you have primary control, and which can positively affect your health and well-being.

Five   Your personal response to your cancer can make a huge difference to both your quality of life and chances of survival.

Six   You are unique and the average medical statistics do not always apply to individuals.

Seven   Your conventional treatment is only one component of your approach to fighting cancer.

Eight   It is vital that you do not rely too much on the effectiveness of medical treatment alone to 'cure' you of cancer. Give up the passive patient role and join forces with your doctors, and become as pro-active as you can about recovering your health.

Nine   It is you and not your doctors who are in overall charge of your situation.

Ten   Astonishingly, many of those who have embarked upon the integrated-medicine approach to cancer have ended up admitting that they are actually glad they had cancer because they now feel so much happier, healthier and more alive than ever before.

Continue re-reading this list of facts until the message sinks in!

Go forward in the knowledge that you are a very powerful person in your anti-cancer team. There is a great deal of help available to strengthen, support and guide you in your treatment and self-help programme. It is possible to stabilize and live with cancer (rather than dying from it), and even to go into remission from cancer altogether.

A cancer diagnosis can start a profound and exciting journey of healing and self-development, giving you the push and permission to change what has been making you ill or unhappy for years. This book will help you to understand and discover every type of help that is available to empower you in both your fight against cancer and your personal healing journey.

What Is Integrated Cancer Medicine?

Integrated cancer medicine is the most powerful medicine available to those with cancer because it draws together every possible form of help that is available for you to fight cancer and heal yourself. Since the 1960s, there has been a revolution in medical thinking and science, and it is now clear that our health and chances of recovery from illness depend both on what the medical profession can do for us and what we can do for ourselves. Many of the factors that affect our health and well-being are within our own control, and involve us becoming stronger physically, mentally and spiritually to deal with and overcome illness. This means that, when serious illness strikes, we must seek to understand how the illness has developed, what our needs in going through the illness and its treatment are and, most crucially of all, how to use the help available at all levels of mind, body and spirit to get ourselves well again.

In practical terms for each person with cancer, this means opening up a treasure chest of possibilities to find the right type of help to crack the healing code. As mutually respectful partners on this detective mission, those with cancer, their doctors, therapists and supporters can draw from orthodox, complementary and alternative medicine the psychological, spiritual and self-help approaches necessary, as well as look longer term into the role of nutrition, lifestyle reorientation and environmental factors, all of which may play key roles in overcoming the disease and becoming a part of the winning statistics.

Historically, those who become ill have really only had the medical model to rely upon. In such a model, a person with cancer is completely dependent on the knowledge and skill of doctors and nurses, and the current level of scientific understanding of the disease. This puts the ill person in an entirely passive role – which is all very well if the doctors have the ability to fix the problem. But if the power of medicine is limited, as in most cases of cancer, this leaves the patient with nowhere to go, feeling as if he or she has gone over the edge of a precipice. Another weakness of the medical model is that it leaves you powerless, with nothing to contribute to your own recovery process and chances of survival.

In stark contrast, the integrated medicine model puts the person with cancer at the very centre of the recovery process, as the therapeutic team:

- seeks to understand your needs, values and insights in relation to the illness
- supports and empowers you to get the very best treatment options that best suit your values and needs
- helps prepare you psychologically and physically for your treatment
- helps you explore the meaning of the illness, the self-help path and how you can transform the crisis of illness into the opportunity for health creation.

In the integrated medicine model, illness is not seen as a random occurrence, but as a logical result of factors that have created a chink in your armour. Our job is to try to understand how the illness has developed, and use this message from the body to work creatively to get your health and life onto a stronger, happier footing than before.

Within the integrated approach, you will find loving care and recognition of the trauma and stress that diagnosis, illness and treatment may be causing you. You will find hope that a creative way can be found to overcome your illness. You will find empowerment and the vital help you need to become mighty in your own defence. You will find respect for your personal needs, values and insights, and you will find the opportunity to transform the total misery and threat of illness and its treatment into an opportunity for a profound re-engagement in living the life you love.

To make the integrated medicine revolution work for you, you will need to find your way to exactly the right resources nationally and locally. This means that you will have a map or overview of what is available, and what forms of help might be useful and when. So, in the pages that follow, you will find help to:

- understand the different types of help available
- understand when to use what type of help
- understand your reactions to illness
- understand the best state of mind to promote recovery
- set up your own support network
- get the information you need to make the very best treatment decisions, whether orthodox or alternative
- make informed treatment decisions that are right for you
- be well prepared for your treatment psychologically, physically and practically

- get the best treatment outcomes with support from complementary medicine
- convalesce properly after treatment
- get yourself on the road to recovery with positive health creation.

What Types of Integrated Medicine Are Available?

There are seven kinds of help available in integrated cancer medicine:

1. Orthodox cancer medicine
2. Alternative cancer medicine
3. Complementary supportive care
4. Psychological approaches
5. Spiritual help
6. Self-help approaches
7. Healthy lifestyle reorientation

1. Orthodox cancer medicine

This is the medicine provided by mainstream cancer doctors and nurses, and is written about in detail in Chapter 4. Within orthodox medicine, you will find help to obtain:

- an accurate diagnosis of your condition
- if desired, a prognosis for your condition (knowing the average outcome statistically for those with your condition)
- the conventional cancer treatments of surgery, chemotherapy, radiotherapy and possibly adjuvant treatments such as hormone therapies
- where available, the opportunity to be entered into a research trial in which the most up-to-date treatment is being tested
- where available, treatment with newly emerging technologies such as laser, cryotherapy and highly specialized radiotherapeutic techniques
- if appropriate, palliative care (treatment to control cancer symptoms) and residential respite care in a hospice
- where available, supportive care within orthodox settings from counsellors, psychologists, specialist nurses, chaplains, social workers and health visitors. Some enlightened units also offer complementary supportive care such as aromatherapy, massage, relaxation, visualization and group-therapy sessions.

2. Alternative cancer medicine

Alternative cancer medicines are those that may be used as an alternative to orthodox cancer treatment. These are written about in detail in Chapter 5 (The alternative frontier: getting the best alternative treatment), and fall into the areas of:

- anti-cancer nutrients that are taken by mouth to help combat cancer directly or to stimulate the body's immune and tissue-healing systems
- herbal medicines that are believed to have direct anti-cancer properties or indirectly inhibit cancer growth
- intravenous metabolic cancer therapies that provide high-dose nutrients or herbal extracts for the body designed to exert a cytotoxic (cancer cell-killing) anti-cancer effect
- immunotherapy aimed at repairing or boosting immune function to get the body fighting cancer naturally
- neuroendocrine therapies aimed at rebalancing the body's hormones and neurotransmitters to inhibit cancer growth
- physical therapies in which heat, light or oxygen is used to treat cancer
- nutritional therapies where strict diets are used to combat cancer
- mind–body medicine, where mind–body approaches are used to restore immune function and direct tissue-healing.

3. Complementary supportive care

Complementary cancer medicine involves the use of natural medicines or therapies that can be used in a supportive context alongside orthodox treatment for physical, emotional and energy support. These are written about in detail in Chapter 7; their role in symptom control is covered in Chapter 8. These are usually accessed in the community from complementary therapists practising in complementary therapy centres or from their homes, but are becoming increasingly available in hospitals and hospices (from nurses or complementary therapists). These include:

- touch therapies such as massage, aromatherapy, osteopathy, craniosacral therapy, shiatsu, acupressure and reflexology
- energy therapies such as acupuncture, reiki healing, spiritual healing and Johrei
- natural remedies such as herbal medicines, including European, Chinese and Indian Ayurvedic herbs, and homoeopathic remedies
- mind–body symptom control through hypnotherapy, visualization, relaxation, guided imagery and affirmation
- nutritional and immune support.

4. Psychological approaches

The psychological approach to cancer is covered in Chapter 2 and includes:

- providing sympathetic counselling to help in the recovery from the shock and trauma of diagnosis and re-diagnosis, and in facing the pain and loss
- ongoing support to rise to the challenge of the illness and its treatment
- using psychological approaches to increase the chances of recovery through:
  - a positive coping style
  - getting out of depression
  - finding the meaning or message of the illness
  - using illness to change to a far more fulfilling lifestyle
  - using positive mind–body approaches such as visualization, affirmation and hypnotherapy suggestion (where mind–body medicine is used as a form of alternative medicine).

5. Spiritual help

Spiritual help is needed by those facing a life-threatening illness as, almost immediately, the really big questions of the meaning of life and death are raised. The role of spiritual advisors as part of the support network is written about towards the end of this chapter. Another type of spiritual help is spiritual healing, included in Chapters 7 and 8. The broader aspects of the role of our spiritual health in long-term recovery are discussed in Chapter 9.

Spiritual help is available from:

- spiritual advisors or religious guides, who help you to examine your beliefs and give spiritual support
- spiritual healers, who can help to provide energy support, spiritual uplift, relief of pain and symptoms and, sometimes, physical healing of disease
- transpersonal counsellors, psychosynthesis counsellors and Health Creation Mentors who can all help you to focus on creating spiritual health and fulfilment.

6. Self-help approaches

Self-help approaches, described in Chapters 7 and 8, can help you achieve the best outcomes from treatment and symptom control. They can also contribute to long-term health creation, as discussed in Chapter 9.

Self-help techniques to prepare for treatment and reduce symptoms include:

- relaxation, visualization, breathing techniques, affirmations and self-hypnosis.

Self-help techniques for long-term health creation include:

- healthy eating
- regular exercise, including aerobic exercise such as swimming, walking, running, a gym workout, dancing or tennis, as well as the more holistic types of exercise such as yoga, tai chi or chi gong
- spiritual practices such as meditation.

7. Healthy lifestyle reorientation

Healthy lifestyle reorientation, covered in Chapter 9, includes the key areas for creating long-term sustainable health, such as:

- stress reduction – both external stress and self-stressing tendencies
- establishing the correct work/play balance
- establishing healthy, loving relationships
- experiencing a sense of belonging
- becoming fulfilled and able to express oneself creatively
- feeling well nourished at all levels of the body, mind and spirit
- ensuring that your environment is healthy and free from negative influences.

Timing Is All: The Four Phases of Recovery

The healing journey from here, diagnosis, to there, recovery and a healthy, fresh new lifestyle, is, in the words of Penny Brohn, co-founder of the Bristol Cancer Help Centre, 'a process and not an event!'

How dearly we all wish that there were a quick way to get rid of the uncomfortable feelings and symptoms of illness, get through our treatments, and back into a secure 'normal' life. But, unfortunately, the treatment and healing process does take time, and there are challenges associated with each step of the treatment and healing process. It is therefore important that you get the big picture, understand what you will have to go through, pace yourself appropriately and map out which aspects of the integrated approach will be right for which stage of the healing journey.

The main tendency is for everyone affected by cancer to get into a terrible panicky rush. The medical profession often sets the hurried pace, making it appear imperative that you receive treatment within hours or days of diagnosis. This is very unhelpful as it leaves you with no time to recover from the initial shock, to prepare for treatment and, most important of all, to take the necessary time to consider the treatment options on offer (while getting your head around the short- and possible long-term side-effects).

As for integrated approaches, people with cancer often confuse the more short-term use of supportive complementary help and symptom control with the longer-term health creation measures necessary for a sustainable improvement in health and, hopefully, prognosis. The worst pitfall would be to rush into making major life changes while in the middle of treatment!

Sometimes, having got the message that illness can follow long periods of stress or unhappiness, people become very motivated to change, but run into problems when they try to make big changes when they are weak and vulnerable. If illness has made you realize that you need to change your job, confront difficulties in your relationships or move house, do wait until you are well and physically strong enough, through your treatment and convalescence, before making such big life changes.

To help you identify the process of recovery, it is wise to see it in four distinct phases:

Phase 1 Getting through diagnosis and treatment positively
Phase 2 Dealing creatively with the problems of illness
Phase 3 Health revival: the state shift to get the body and mind strong again
Phase 4 Life revival: getting into a healthy, happy and fulfilling lifestyle.

Phase 1 Getting through diagnosis and treatment positively
- Take the time to go through your reactions to the diagnosis
- Set up your support network
- Make appropriate adjustments to your working and social commitments
- Obtain full and clear information on all of your treatment options
- Make a truly informed decision regarding treatment
- Prepare well for treatment psychologically, physically and practically
- Convalesce properly from treatment.

Phase 2 Dealing creatively with the problems of illness
It may be that the cancer itself, or the treatments you receive for it, creates some residual health problems or troublesome symptoms. Often, creative solutions are available for these problems from complementary and mind–body medicine. There are also specialized support organizations that can provide individually tailored help for specific cancers and the problems or disabilities associated with such cancers or their treatment so, in this phase, attention is given to:

- symptom control with natural medicines
- the mind–body approach to symptom relief
- complementary therapies for symptom relief
- complementary therapies for the side-effects of treatment
- help with specific cancers
- help with specific disabilities
- help with specific cancer-related issues.

Phase 3 Health revival: the state shift to get the body and mind strong again

This starts with good old-fashioned convalescence after illness and treatment – a sadly forgotten concept in the modern lifestyle! Often, people do not even stop work for their treatment, let alone take the time to recover properly. Yet, this phase is absolutely essential for the overall recovery process as cancer treatments are usually extremely taxing on the body and its resources. An intensive detox and health-revival period is needed to compensate for this.

But even more important for overall recovery is the need to change the underlying state and chemistry of the body and mind, so that it is no longer a hospitable place for a recurrence of cancer.

Creating a state shift in the health of the body and mind involves changing from being:

- low energy
- poorly oxygenated, unfit with sluggish circulation
- poorly nourished
- acidic
- under par or damaged in terms of immune function
- full of excess sugar, toxins and fat
- stressed, fearful and anxious

to being:

- high energy
- well oxygenated
- lean and well nourished
- fresh

- alkaline
- fit and supple
- calm, happy and positive.

To achieve this state shift, you need to focus on:

- excellent nutrition
- a low-acid diet
- detoxification of the body
- re-energization of the body
- physical fitness, stretching and oxygenation
- healthy breathing patterns
- relaxation and rest
- immune stimulation
- freeing the body and mind from the grip of fear, stress and tension.

Phase 4 Life renewal: getting into a healthy, happy and fulfilling lifestyle

In Chapter 9 you will find that the most important determinant of long-term health and survival is the state of our spirit. This means having a strong will to live, a clear purpose in living and a joyful spirit, with genuine sources of pleasure, personal fulfilment and spiritual uplift.

So, in this phase of the recovery process, we are doing the 'earthworks' to help bring ourselves fully alive into a lifestyle that totally expresses, inspires and energizes us.

This involves:

- changing your priorities in life to focus on that which is really important to you
- removing any destructive influences from your life
- replacing that which drains you with that which nourishes you
- taking time to enjoy yourself
- putting yourself first
- learning how to nurture yourself properly
- reconnecting with that which gives you true joy and excitement.

The Importance of You: Letting Go of the Medical Model

Most of us brought up in the developed countries are hard-wired into the medical model. This has taught us that, when we are ill, the doctor is in charge. He or she has all the knowledge and expertise, and we must do as we're told and be good, compliant patients.

There may well be times in your recovery process where you will need to put your complete trust in your doctors, and their expert knowledge and skills. However, the medical profession is far from having the answer to cancer, and it is likely that your contribution to your recovery process will make as much of a difference, if not more, than the cancer medicine you are taking.

It is very hard to hear and believe this when you are first diagnosed with cancer, as we all believe that there is a great big medical safety net underneath us that will catch us if we fall. But, sadly, this is often not the case with cancer and, to make matters worse, doctors often (understandably) oversell the potency of cancer medicines. While it is important to empower the medicines and treatments that we are having, it is not advisable to be lulled into a false sense of security when doctors say you are all clear after cancer treatment.

Indeed, doctors may well have succeeded in removing all detectable cancer from the body, but what medical cancer treatment has not done is changed the underlying conditions in the body in which the cancer developed in the first place. In fact, medical treatments will have made the body more toxic and weakened the immune system. Moreover, it is not possible to detect the microdeposits of cancer that may cause recurrences in the future. So, as uncomfortable as it may be, it is important to wake up early to the potential threat of recurrence, and become fully active in your own defence from the time of the first diagnosis of a primary cancer, rather than waiting until a second or third recurrence before taking action.

Cancer is a lifestyle disease in which the main causes are poor nutrition and toxicity in the body due to chemicals, radiation, viruses, alcohol, smoking and lack of exercise. It is possible to revive your body's ability to detect and heal cancer but, to do this, you must let go of your dependency on the medical model and belief that cancer medicine alone will cure you. Put yourself firmly in the driving seat and in control as the most important member of your integrated medical team.

This will mean from day one addressing the really big nitty-gritty issues of whether or not you really do have a genuine reason for living and whether you are therefore sufficiently motivated to put in the effort required for your recovery.

If you find that your will to live is shaky for any reason – perhaps because of loneliness, heartbreak, disappointment, grief or frustration – take heart. It is possible to obtain good-quality therapeutic help to revive the state of your spirit and will to live. The next chapter tells you how to find this sort of help, and how to make sure that you are primed in exactly the right frame of mind to maximize your chances of survival.

CHAPTER 2

The psychological foundation for health

Scientific research has now established beyond doubt that the mind–body connection is one of the most powerful elements in the conquering of disease in the body. But this knowledge is scarcely applied in the orthodox approach to health, and far from fully applied in many alternative models. This chapter sets out the most up-to-date thinking in this field, and outlines the steps you can take to get yourself into the best possible state of mind to facilitate your recovery.

When you are given a diagnosis of cancer, you have two main problems: first, of course, there is the physical illness itself; and second, there is the terrible emotional turmoil you are thrown into by the diagnosis, along with all the fear and upset that it creates in you and those close to you. Many people with cancer have said that their physical problem has been manageable, but that it is their peace of mind that has been completely shattered. Your emotional needs and state of mind are just as important as your medical treatment, and it is vital that you receive the support and encouragement that you need. It is also important for you to identify and change the negative beliefs you have about cancer, so that you don't risk buying into these beliefs and giving up before you even start.

Facing the Demons

You are up against three things straightaway. The first is your own negative beliefs about cancer. You may have heard upsetting stories, or have a view of cancer that is entirely based on the collective fear we all have about cancer in our Western society. Second, you have to face the reactions of those close to you, and all the upset and fears that they may be experiencing in relation to your diagnosis. Third, you may have gathered some statistics from your consultant on the *average* survival times with your particular kind of cancer. He may even have given you a prognosis in terms of the number of months or years that this 'average person' with your condition might be expected to live, based on the medical treatments available when the research was done – often many years earlier.

However, statistics never apply to individuals, and the course of your illness is unique to you. There are over 200 types of cancer and the way it develops or regresses is different in everyone who has it. Challenge your negative beliefs. Make sure you have really taken on board the encouraging information presented at the beginning of Chapter 1, and keep repeating it to yourself until you truly believe it! People do actually survive with every sort of cancer, and there is no reason why that should not include you.

Getting into the Right Frame of Mind

It has now been shown that there is a major survival advantage associated with getting yourself into a good state of mind, using positive coping strategies and learning how to use effective mind–body approaches that can reactivate your immune system and your body's ability to fight back against cancer.

The way you react to a diagnosis of cancer comes down to four crucial factors:

- the beliefs you and others who influence you have about cancer
- the way you feel about your life
- how frightened you are about death and dying
- whether you believe in your own power to affect your health.

The hardest place from which to deal with your diagnosis and illness is where you are depressed, ambivalent about your life, fearful of dying, fearful of cancer and feeling impotent in terms of changing your state of health. But, I assure you, if you are prepared to look at and work with these things head on, with the right support, you can turn the situation around completely. The diagnosis of cancer inevitably throws you into a process of asking yourself and others the big questions about the meaning of life, the purpose of your life and what it is like to die. Certainly, if well facilitated, thinking about your relationship to living and dying can completely alter your ability to cope with your diagnosis and even turn it into a positive experience.

When you become aware of the many things you can do to enhance your chances of survival with cancer, your fear of cancer will start to diminish. You will begin to feel bigger and more powerful than the disease. You might even think of the diagnosis as a much needed wake-up call to enable you to go through a complete health and life revival, moving you step by step towards a life that really excites and fulfils you. As you do this, your attitude towards life will change and you will feel happier, spiritually stronger and more uplifted. The best thing is to see the illness as a message from your body that all is not well, and to use the illness as an opportunity to get your health and lifestyle onto a better footing.

By developing inner strength and thinking deeply about the true nature of life and death, it is likely that you will change your attitude towards dying, too. I do not say this lightly. It is said on the basis of having watched thousands of people with cancer go through the process of using this crisis of illness to completely transform their health and lifestyle. Strangely, a combination of becoming far happier and fulfilled in life, developing inner peace through self-help practices and looking at the question of death head-on almost always results in individuals being freed from their fear of dying. Often, with this release comes a profound new love of life and the realization that, previously, a great deal of life energy was being lost through a deep and somewhat unconscious fear of dying.

However, while you are going through your reaction to the news, it is very important to be aware of how you really feel and to find the support you need to express your emotions; then, as the shock subsides, you can work out how you are reacting and coping (or not) with the diagnosis. Your reaction can make a big difference to your prognosis, and some reactions will be helpful while others will not. There are also some underlying states of mind that can either boost or impair immune function. There is help available to change the way you are coping and to lift negative states of mind so that you can get into the best frame of mind for recovery.

The Psychological Basis for Remarkable Recovery

Caryle Hirschberg: The Role of Belief

In 1995, Caryle Hirschberg, a medical researcher, and Mark Barasch, a journalist who had cancer, published the findings of their Remission Project at the Institute of Noetic Sciences in America. Their book *Remarkable Recovery* was the first-ever publication on what it is that survivors of cancer have in common (rather than those who get cancer)!

In the questionnaire she sent to these survivors, they were asked which they felt were the most important of 30 self-help practices that had made them well. The practices ticked with the greatest frequency (by over 50 per cent of the participants) were:

Prayer	68%
Meditation	64%
Exercise	64%
Guided imagery	59%
Walking	52%
Music and singing	50%
Stress reduction	50%

They were also asked which they felt were the most important psychospiritual factors in their recovery. Of the 26 items on the list, those reported with the most frequency (over 50 per cent) were:

Belief in a positive outcome	75%
Having a fighting spirit	71%
Acceptance of the disease	71%
Seeing the disease as a challenge	71%
Taking responsibility for the disease and its outcome	68%
Renewed desire and will to live	64%
Positive emotions	64%
Faith in a higher power to heal them	61%
New sense of purpose	61%
Changing unhealthy habits and behaviour	61%
Having a sense of control	59%
Lifestyle changes	59%
Self-nurturing	57%
Good social support	50%

The reason I love Caryle's data so much is because these are not the theories of a scientist, but the reported beliefs and feelings of a group of people who have actually achieved the scientifically unachievable – recovery from a serious cancer. What is striking about these findings is the importance of belief – whether it be in one's own power to heal through self-help, or belief in a higher power to heal, or in the power of prayer or believing that one is going to live and recover fully.

This is what I have witnessed again and again in my 20 years of working with over 20,000 people to recover their health after cancer. From often very sceptical beginnings, two things most frequently ended up astonishing those who apply themselves to the holistic integrated healthcare approach: the first is just how much help is available through prayer and spiritual healing; the second is just how powerful a person can be once he or she begins to use and harness the power of his own mind.

This can be achieved through pure belief, hypnotherapy or the use of your own creative will through visualization and affirmation. In these practices, you literally see in your mind's eye or choose in words the reality you want for your future. This is another reason it is so important not to remain passive, waiting for either orthodox or alternative medicine to cure you, but to instead get yourself firmly in the driving seat, choosing that the illness will go from the body and visualizing yourself going on into the future, growing old disgracefully!

It also suggests that, if you are currently closed to or sceptical of the power of your own mind or of the help that is available through spiritual healing or prayer, it would be wise to suspend disbelief and at least try to explore such forms of help before dismissing them. They could ultimately provide the vital key to your healing, as has been discovered by so many former sceptics I have worked with.

So, the keys are:

- cultivate a strong belief in your own power to self-heal
- cultivate a strong belief in the power of your doctors and their treatments to cure you
- open yourself to the possibility of healing through spiritual healing and prayer
- use hypnotherapy, visualization and affirmation to choose health and recovery, seeing yourself healed, free of disease and well and happy in the future.

Dr Stephen Greer: The Role of a Fighting Spirit and Alleviating Depression

Before Caryle and Ian's work, back in the mid-80s, psychosocial oncologist Stephen Greer published his work showing how the very different survival times among women with breast cancer depended on the coping style they adopted within a week of the initial diagnosis. The coping styles he defined were:

- a fighting spirit – taking an active stand against your cancer and believing fully that you can affect your survival
- denial – pretending to yourself and others that nothing is seriously wrong
- stoicism or fatalism – leading to becoming resigned to what is happening
- helplessness and hopelessness – becoming anxiously preoccupied, or collapsing.

His findings showed that those with a fighting spirit fared far better than those in the other three categories both in terms of quality of life and overall survival. Those in denial did next best whereas those who were resigned, depressed and anxiously preoccupied did least well of all. At the 13-year point, 80 per cent of those who had started with a fighting spirit were still alive versus only 20 per cent of those who had collapsed into helplessness. Worse, those who had psychologically collapsed had died quickly, within two years of diagnosis. This means that the average survival rate of 60 per cent for breast cancer at five years masks a huge difference between those who do very much better than expected because of a positive belief in themselves compared with those who do very much worse because they do not.

As this difference in survival rate is bigger than that seen with any medical treatment for breast cancer, Dr Greer realized it was very important to identify those who reacted negatively to their diagnosis and help them to change psychologically so that they could begin to believe in themselves more and become less depressed. Through the use of cognitive behavioural techniques, such patients gained self-esteem and confidence, and began to believe they could survive. Lo and behold, his later studies on the survival rates among these women showed great improvement.

The lessons here are:

- It is vital to feel empowered and believe in your ability to heal yourself
- It is vital to lift your depression
- It is vital for healthcare professionals to provide extra psychological help to improve the coping styles of those who have responded by becoming helpless and anxiously preoccupied by their illness.

Dr Candace Pert: The Scientific Basis for the Mind–Body Connection and the Need to Express Emotion

While both Hirschberg and Greer were gathering their data, huge breakthroughs were being made in the laboratory as the science of PNI, or psychoneuroimmunology, was rapidly expanding through the pioneering work of Dr Candace Pert. She studied the connection between our states of mind, the nervous system, the neuroendocrine system, and the function of the immune system and other healing tissues of the body. It all started with her discovery of the receptor for an opiate secreted in the brain. This naturally occurring opiate was later discovered and identified as endorphin (known as enkephalin in the US). This was a breakthrough, as endorphin was a new kind of messenger molecule different from the kind of neurotransmitters we had known about before. Endorphin was the first molecule to be identified as a neuropeptide or informational substance, and further informational substances were found to be present in all tissues of the body.

This finding started an avalanche of discovery so that, by the mid-1990s, a further 200 of these substances had been identified, secreted in response to different feelings and thoughts, and able to radically affect our tissue functioning. As the PNI findings began to link up with the medical studies, it became clear that those who are chronically stressed or lonely had depressed immune function – with both lower numbers and far lower activity levels in the immune cells. Similar findings were made in those with low self-esteem and those who chronically repressed their feelings. It was even found that the blood cells in depressed people actually carried less oxygen than those who are happy. Dr Pert had discovered that unexpressed emotions can become lodged in the body's tissues in the form of 'molecules of emotion' inhibiting organ function.

The lesson here is:

• Stress over which we have no control, loneliness, grief and unexpressed feelings can inhibit both our immune function and tissue-healing capacity. Conversely, becoming happy and self-expressive can revive our tissue functioning.

Dr Susan Kobasa: The Role of Emotional Patterning

Things became even more interesting when it was found that the immune system has a memory, and that painful memories or repeats of past experiences in which a person has failed or been defeated, can also trigger immune collapse. Researcher Dr Susan Kobasa had described a psychological syndrome she termed 'learned helplessness', when those who had experienced failure earlier in life tended to keep repeating the pattern. Now science was showing that this result was mirrored in the immune system. On the other hand, she had also found that a 'personality hardiness' in those who respond to stress as a stimulating challenge resulted in a similarly healthy immune response. Here, at last, was a reason why earlier researchers could not make a direct link between stress and cancer – it depended not on stress *per se*, but on how the individual *responds* to stress.

The lesson here is:

• It is very important to provide psychological support to those who are not coping well and who see themselves as losers in order to change this underlying negative belief and replace it with strong, positive coping skills and experience of success.

Dr Leslie Walker: The Role of Empowering Cancer Treatment
The final piece of the jigsaw appeared more recently from UK researcher Professor Leslie Walker, who has worked for more than 20 years on the connection between mind–body approaches and improved survival in women with breast cancer. His recent study showed a staggering 17.5 per cent increase in survival 13 years after treatment in women who were taught relaxation techniques and, through hypnosis, to believe that their chemotherapy would cure them. In this case, the benefit of the treatment itself was 15 per cent, so the effect of the mind was greater than that of the medicine! Most interesting of all was the fact that the women who achieved this huge rise in survival rate were those whom Walker called 'women who were too nice'. The medical description was 'women with a high level of social conformity' who tended to look after everyone else and bottle-up their own feelings. He also found an increase in immune function after relaxation and hypnotherapy, so once again it appears that a positive belief in cure and recovery is vital.

The lessons here are:

- It is vital to use visualization, affirmations or hypnotherapy to empower your treatments and to develop belief in their ability to cure you.
- It is important to identify and help those who are too 'other-focused' and to help them learn how to put themselves first.

Professors Spiegel and Fawzy: The Role of Support
This all fits with earlier studies done in the US, looking at the effects of psychological support on survival in those with breast cancer and melanoma. Professor David Spiegel showed a doubling of the average breast cancer survival time in those who had weekly support; Professor Fawzy showed a drop in the melanoma death rate from 10 per cent to 2 per cent in those who received weekly support, and confirmed an improvement in immune function, too. The emphasis in both interventions was on the expression of feelings (rather than being positive).

The lessons here are that:

- It is vital to receive support in expressing your feelings rather than bottling them up.
- Being positive does not mean hiding your grief or anger.

Blowing the Myth of Positive Thinking

If, while reading this, you have been feeling upset and emotional, please know that those who have a fighting spirit are almost always those who also have strong emotions and a big reaction to their diagnosis. It is absolutely normal to feel shocked and grief-stricken after receiving a diagnosis of a serious illness. Having a fighting spirit does not mean being permanently positive about having cancer and a fixed, determined grin on your face!

Some readers may misinterpret the information above, believing that it is harmful to become emotional or feel despondent at times about what is going on. This could not be further from the truth. According to PNI, a good cry or outburst of anger are just as good for boosting immune function as having a good laugh. It is repressing your feelings and becoming depressed that flatten the immune response. In fact, 'fighters' are defined by their ability to face reality, expressing the appropriate emotional response and 'bottoming out' with their feelings, and THEN to set about gathering the information and support they need to mount a realistic, proactive response to their situation.

Working Out How You Are Dealing With Your Diagnosis

Do you think you are reacting with a fighting spirit and believe in your power to heal yourself?

If you think you are reacting with anything other than a fighting spirit and want to change this, it important that you find help and support to deal with your diagnosis differently. Please go to the Resources Directory (pages 255–417) to find help in contacting a counsellor or psychologist trained in cognitive behavioural therapy to help you learn a more positive coping style. Your oncology department may also have a clinical psychologist who can help you, especially if your pattern is to give up and collapse in the face of difficulty.

Do you believe in the power of your cancer treatments to cure you?

You may choose to work with a hypnotherapist to develop powerful positive associations with your treatments, or you could use the relaxation and visualization exercises given in *Cope Positively with Cancer Treatment*, a CD available from Health Creation (call the Helpline on 0845 009 3366), to empower your treatments.

Do you need help from prayer or spiritual healing?
Contact the local prayer group associated with your church or religious group. Find a healer through the National Federation of Spiritual Healers (helpline: 0845 123 2767). They also do distant healing through prayer for those who are unable to get to a healer. Some of their healers will visit the home or hospital if necessary.

Have you got enough psychological support to express your feelings fully?
Find out about local support groups and counsellors from your GP, the hospital or the Resources Directory (pages 255–417).

So, far from pretending you feel all right if you do not, with support, try to face what is really happening to you, express your feelings, and then create an action plan based on your *true* situation and needs. Once you have done this, you will feel genuinely positive that you have a working plan and are back in control again.

Underlying States of Mind that May Need to Change

As well as the states of mind that arise in reaction to the diagnosis, there is the question of what was going on for you emotionally before you were diagnosed. As you move into your healing journey, it is important to look at the big issues of:

- improving your will to live
- decreasing your stress levels
- learning to express your feelings in everyday life
- letting go of loneliness and depression
- healing emotional wounds from the past
- identifying and changing the 'limiting beliefs' by which you live your life.

Looking at your will to live

The nitty-gritty issue for anyone facing a life-threatening diagnosis is the question of how strong is your will to live? This is a highly confrontational question, but a vital one to nail if you are going to succeed in fighting cancer. Carl Jung realized many years ago that all of us have an equal and opposite urge towards life (*eros*) and towards death (*thanetos*). When the eros side is strong, we feel powerful and passionate towards life. But when thanetos is dominant, death can seem very seductive.

So, do not feel that you are alone if the diagnosis of cancer has in some way excited you or felt like a good way out of the stress and distress of living. Ultimately, of course, we all have to die. Dying is a totally natural part of living. But it is awfully sad and wrong to give up and allow yourself to die because your spirit has been crushed by loneliness, grief, disappointment or a broken heart.

I have often witnessed incredible healing when someone has genuinely turned the corner and chosen life. For you, perhaps the diagnosis of cancer can be a real turning point and an opportunity to say 'yes' again to finding joy in living. This may happen quite naturally because often the diagnosis of cancer itself throws into sharp focus all that is precious about your life. But if you feel ambivalent about living, the best help you can get is to work with a transpersonal or psychosynthesis counsellor who will work with you gently and creatively to rekindle your zest for life. This is explored more fully in Chapter 9.

The problem of stress

A little bit of stress is healthy and often brings out the best in us. But prolonged stress, particularly stress over that which we feel we have no control over is a major depressant of our immune function. It may be hard to accept but, usually, the stress we are experiencing is of our own making. This is either because we get ourselves into or tolerate ridiculously stressful situations or because we have innate self-stressing tendencies, pushing ourselves to unrealistic limits. It really comes down to deciding that your health and happiness is more important than the goals for which you strive. The diagnosis of cancer can be the most perfect excuse to pull out of anything that is causing you stress.

Expressing your feelings

The next new trick you may need to learn is how to express your feelings in everyday life (not only in relation to the diagnosis). You have already discovered how those who are too nice have suppressed immune function. It is good to copy the Europeans and let rip with your feelings! Remember, anger is as good at improving white blood cell activity as laughter.

Getting out of isolation and loneliness

Another problem for our immune system is isolation and loneliness. So, do everything you can to get back into connection with people. This can be through belonging to groups who support and value you – whether that is a regular class, or a support, community or religious group. Nowadays, there are a huge number of growth and development classes you can join, and there are many support groups that either relate specifically to cancer or are less specific, such as women's or men's groups.

Getting out of depression, fear and anxiety

Perhaps you have more serious problems mentally and realize that you are actually depressed. Here again, you are not alone! It is estimated that up to 77 per cent of people with cancer are measurably depressed and it is really little wonder with all the uncertainty and trauma that are experienced. Most cancer units have a clinical psychologist whose job it is to help people come out of cancer-related depression or anxiety, so this route might be worth investigating if you feel really down. But a combination of support from a support group, counselling and spiritual healing can be equally good to lift depression. If you consider yourself to be a fearful or anxious person, this is another state of mind that it would be good to change. The best way of cracking fear and anxiety is by learning to relax and, better still, to meditate or to have a soothing massage or aromatherapy.

Freeing ourselves of limiting beliefs

Most of us allow ourselves to be governed by the limiting beliefs we have picked up during our childhood as to what we are able to achieve or not. This means that, if we have learned that we don't ever succeed, or that we are not loveable or that good things never happen to us, then this is what happens to us. It is like we have been programmed with faulty software, which will always stop us from reaching our potential and achieving what we want. But through the integrated medicine revolution, a huge number of effective ways of changing our state of mind have surfaced, including developing self-esteem and confidence, and replacing negative beliefs with positive ones. If you recognize that you are being run by your limiting beliefs, then NLP (neurolinguistic programming) can be a powerful tool to change this.

Getting the Help You Need

Counselling

The first step is usually finding someone who will listen really well to what you are going through. This is usually found in a counselling relationship and, again, I would recommend transpersonal or psychosynthesis counselling, where the state of the spirit is given attention along with help to change our feelings, beliefs and behaviour in positive ways.

The counselling relationship is often believed to be only about helping you to accept what is happening to you, grieving appropriately and becoming adapted to the change. However, in transpersonal or psychosynthesis counselling, the relationship is more about trying to find out what is right about your life and only needs your focused attention to flourish. Help can be given to try to see the message in the crisis and to grow positively from the experience, rather than just learning to accept what is happening.

This is a far more positive and creative form of counselling that fits well with the integrated medicine model. Yes, you may need some straightforward compassionate counselling at first, to help you deal with the shock and your reactions but, later on, you need a counsellor who can help you reframe the crisis as an opportunity for healing and growth. A counsellor of this kind may also help you look at the benefits you may be gaining from illness, helping you learn how to get these benefits without having to be ill. A good counsellor will help you change from being passive in your life to taking an active role in the creation of your ideal lifestyle. He can help you rekindle your will to live and reconnect with that which really turns you on.

Often, a transpersonal or psychosynthesis counsellor will also be able to help you develop a positive mental focus through developing visualization or affirmations with you to help you strengthen your belief in yourself and in your healing. Your counsellor, or a spiritual advisor, can also help you in your spiritual explorations, perhaps helping you to open up to the possibility of healing from a higher source.

The important thing is not to see a counselling relationship as being only about helping you when you are in extreme distress or seeing it as meaning that there must be something wrong with you. Having regular counselling throughout your recovery process can completely transform a potential nightmare into a true blessing, helping you to grow and even benefit in the long term.

Preparing for the Worst, Working for the Best

Another helpful role of the counsellor is to help you, if you feel you need to, face and plan for the worst-case scenario that could happen. You can then spend much less time worrying and fantasizing about it, and get on with creating a different, much more positive reality. This may mean that you choose to use some of your early sessions with your counsellor thinking about how you would feel, and what would need to happen if everything went really badly.

If you do this, the level of detail that you go into is up to you, but it could involve thinking right through the practicalities of whether you have made a will, what financial resources are available for your dependants, who would care for them if you were unable to, and how you would like to be cared for if you become disabled and dependent. You can even go into the details of where you would like to die and what kind of funeral you would like to have. This will inevitably force you to face your feelings and beliefs about death, so you may also need the help of a spiritual advisor. This may sound extremely grim, but most people who have employed this head-on approach have found it tremendously liberating. Paradoxically, any step you take in the direction of both healing old wounds and preparing to let go of life will enable you to live all the more fully. This, in turn, will enhance your energy, vitality and health and, consequently, the chances of stabilizing your disease.

Healing Your Emotional Wounds

Another thing that might emerge from this process is the urge to complete unfinished emotional business with anyone against whom you are holding a grudge, or by whom you feel you have been aggrieved or hurt. It may not be necessary to go anywhere near these people to do this work – it may be quite possible to make your peace with others during your counselling sessions. This often has very surprising results, as the dynamics of these old and difficult situations and relationships can often change dramatically once you have shifted *your* position.

Attending to these background emotional issues will be part of your long-term Health Creation Programme (see Chapter 9) and be best addressed after you have been through your treatment.

Facing the Cancer Diagnosis: Understanding Your Reactions and Identifying Your Needs

Now that we have looked at the psychological foundation for recovery, let us take a look into the question of how you are feeling now. It is very possible that, having recently had a diagnosis, you are still in a state of shock. It is important to understand the effects of shock and how to deal with it.

Dealing with shock

The diagnosis (or re-diagnosis) of cancer can put you into severe emotional and physical shock. Extreme shock is an odd thing. You may feel that you are able to cope but, in fact, your thinking and reaction times may be severely impaired. If you do receive bad news when you are not expecting it, it is safer to wait at the hospital or surgery until someone can come and pick you up. It is certainly better not to attempt to drive or go out onto public transport while you are in such a state and feeling so vulnerable.

It is estimated that in a state of shock, less than one-tenth of what you are told is retained. Because of this, the most important thing to remember is to never make important decisions while you are in a state of shock! Yet, medical personnel may rush straight from telling you your diagnosis and prognosis to explaining your treatment options.

The sense of urgency created by doctors at the time of diagnosis is usually exaggerated. Yes, it is a good idea to move ahead with appropriate treatment for cancer as soon as possible after diagnosis, but the treatment will be far harder to cope with – and may even be less effective – if you are in a state of shock and fear, and feeling out of control. There is clear evidence that being well prepared psychologically, with a positive attitude towards treatment, conveys not only psychological and quality-of-life benefits, but also a distinct survival advantage.

It is therefore highly advisable to take the time you need to:

- **go through your emotional reaction to the diagnosis**
- **think about what seems the best treatment option for you (and this may even be having no treatment)**
- **prepare yourself mentally, physically and practically for treatment, before it starts.**

Possible emotional reactions to expect

Everyone is different. Initial reactions to a diagnosis of cancer can range from extremely strong emotions to total numbness, and any degree in between. Your state can also vary profoundly from one hour to the next, so that you may find yourself suddenly in a highly emotional state, unexpectedly feeling out of control.

If you need to withdraw, withdraw. If you need to scream, shout and rage, then scream, shout and rage. If you need to weep, please allow yourself to let go completely and grieve over your situation. There is no need to keep up a brave face. This will not ultimately serve you, and will definitely delay the process of your being able to get your feet back on the ground, able to make clearly thought-out decisions about the way forward. Take all the time you need to go through your reactions. Do not be afraid to cancel work and social engagements if you need to. You have effectively been bereaved, and everything will go much better if you allow yourself the proper space and time to begin to come to terms with what you are experiencing.

There is often a sense of intense disbelief and the recurring question of 'Why me?'. Many people go straight into fear, or even terror, and this can be felt both mentally and physically. Such extreme fear can cause a racing heart, sweatiness, a feeling of weakness and sometimes diarrhoea. The mental anguish can make it impossible to concentrate, perform normal tasks, keep up a social front or sleep properly. Over time, this all-pervasive fear can become focused into more specific fears, such as fear of pain, disability, disfigurement, hospitals and doctors. But underneath it all, it is usually the having to come face to face with one's fear of death and the deep uncertainty caused by the diagnosis that causes such a strong reaction.

Often, the next feeling experienced is grief. This may be grief at the thought that you might die and leave others behind, or grief for yourself and the loss of your sense of a certain future. Often, relatives, too, will go into anticipatory grief. This can sometimes be so extreme that you find people treating you as if you had gone already! Combined with the withdrawal of friends or colleagues who are too embarrassed to talk to you about what is happening, you may be left feeling abandoned and isolated – as if you have passed through an invisible glass wall and are no longer part of the ordinary world around you.

You may find yourself experiencing a mixture of feelings, such as jealousy, resentment or even anger, towards those who are still healthy. You may dread the thought of becoming dependent on people with whom you do not wish to have that degree of intimacy, or even feel guilt at the thought of not being able to fulfil your ordinary functions. Of course, this will be tempered by the enormous love, closeness and gratitude you will feel towards those who stick with you through this crisis, with whom your relationship will deepen and grow immeasurably.

There can then be the other side of the story. You may, as already mentioned, have been expecting something like this to come along. You may even welcome the illness, feeling that the whistle has finally been blown on what has been an unhappy or unproductive state of affairs in your life. You may even find yourself feeling excited by the challenge of cancer, experiencing it as a much-needed wake-up call. Some may even welcome the possible imminence of death.

Do not think it is odd if you feel this way. Many people feel this way, especially if life has been really tough.

You may have beliefs or even a deep 'soul memory' that dying is not so much an ending as a transition into a far freer state of being and, thus, actually look forward to making the transition. Or it may be that life has been so hard for you that dying seems like a blessed relief. But, on a more pragmatic level, it could be that the diagnosis and possibility of death make every moment of life seem extremely precious and exciting and that, in one fell swoop, any sense of boredom or depression with life evaporates.

There is also another phenomenon that people often experience – which is a sense of being almost unnaturally calm. It is as if you are at the still point, within the 'eye' of a hurricane. While relatives and friends are being thrown into chaos by the new development, you may find yourself strangely quiet and 'present' with the ultimate truth and reality of your situation. It is as if there is a spiritual acceptance of the truth of what is happening to you and, from somewhere deep inside, you are being given the inner strength to deal with it.

If you have received bad news, take all the time and space you need to go through your reaction before making treatment decisions.

Ask yourself:
- What am I feeling now about my diagnosis?
- How am I reacting to my diagnosis?
- What help do I need at this time?

Getting immediate help

Find out what support resources are available at the hospital where you have been diagnosed, or at your regional cancer centre, which may be larger and better equipped. Next, find out what help there is from your GP, community nurses or local hospice, then find out if there are any local or national support groups or local private counsellors who can help you. Do not be afraid to ask for the help you need, and use it for as long as you need it. Getting good support for your emotional state will greatly help you both in the decision-making process to follow and in getting you the best outcome from your treatment.

It may be that your GP, community nurses or health visitor could be called to the house to give you immediate support, or that a local support group could provide someone to keep a close eye on you for the first week after diagnosis. Certainly, if you avail yourself of the services of a Health Creation Mentor, they will be particularly vigilant in this initial time, helping you to access the best possible support available in your area (tel: 0845 009 3366).

It is very likely that you will need crisis counselling at this time to help you get through your initial reaction. This kind of counselling is beneficial and rather different from the kind of counselling you will need later on to help you get well again. This may also be the time you may wish to reach for the help of spiritual guidance from where you usually worship, or for a spiritual healer. There may be many questions you wish to ask, but the main role of these spiritual helpers will be to try to help bring you into your still, calm centre, where you may find peace and inner strength during the difficult times.

Finding Support
- Your local cancer unit or regional cancer centre
- Specialist nurses such as Macmillan, Marie Curie or practice nurses
- Your local hospice (which are not only for the seriously ill)
- Your GP
- Support groups (see the Resources Directory, pages 384–404)
- Counsellors (private or through your GP surgery)
- Spiritual advisors or healers (see the Resources Directory, pages 372, 404–6).

Also, find out what support is available from:

- Your family
- Your partner
- Your friends
- Your colleagues or occupational health department
- Your local church or relevant religious community.

Use the Resources Directory to see what specific help may be available from support groups or charities dealing with your kind of cancer or resulting disabilities, and any problems you may have arising from the treatment. Help may also be available to deal with the financial, legal or social problems due to your diagnosis.

Find out what help is available nationally from:

- Illness-specific support groups
- Disability-specific support groups
- National charities
- Legal services
- Social Services
- Citizens' Advice Bureaux.

Telling other people

When you first become ill, especially if there is a health crisis or serious operation to go through, telling kind enquirers over and over again about what is happening can be very upsetting and draining, both for you and those close to you. Sometimes, it can help to delegate this task to a supporter who will be the message bearer, only putting through those you have placed on a special list.

As you emerge from the shock of the initial impact, it will be time to think about telling other people. You may initially feel like hiding what you are going through. A common reaction is to try to keep life as normal as possible, keeping what you are going through private. This is your choice and can be effective, but it can also be a stressful, lonely way to go about things, leaving you compromised at crucial moments when you may need help.

It is better, if possible, to enlist the help of friends and colleagues. Everything will be a lot easier if you can confide in those you work with so that they give you the best of their support now and in the future, and excuse from duties at short notice, if necessary. Of course, if you don't want them to keep asking how you are, you can make this clear at the beginning. If you are asked something like this, be honest as it helps them know what to do.

The other big consideration is what you tell your family, particularly aged parents and children. Often, people do not tell their elderly parents what they are going through – partly to spare them the upset, and partly to spare themselves from having to deal with their reaction. Of course, everybody has to be the judge of their own situation but, if a parent is not given this information, you may be depriving yourself of a great deal of extra love and closeness that could come your way. Often, as hard as it may seem, giving somebody the opportunity to help you can be extremely important for them, helping them to feel valuable, and reassess their own values and priorities, too. It may even help an older person feel less depressed or sorry for themselves, putting their own worries into perspective and giving them a meaningful focus in terms of helping to care for you. This new closeness can sometimes be very healing for parent-child relationships that have gone awry in the past. Also, the older generation may have more experience and understanding to deal with illness and the concerns it creates. So, in the main, unless the individual concerned is very frail or the relationship is very conflicted, it is much better to be truthful about what is going on.

Deciding Whom to Tell

Whom do you need or want to tell?

Whom do you *not* want to tell?

What do you want to tell them about your situation, and how do you want them to be with you?

What 'ground rules' do you wish to set regarding confidentiality or the way you want them to interact with you?

Whose help will you enlist to tell others?

Who will tell them, what and when?

It is also good to be as honest as possible with your children. They will know that something is wrong even if you try to hide it from them. Being real with your children is probably the best education, gift and preparation for life you can ever give them. Children often have a better ability than adults to live in the present. This means that they tend to focus more on the way you are day by day rather than continuously looking at possible futures, which is what adults tend to do. However, what makes interactions with children easier is if you have managed to express your emotions and fears with your counsellor or close supporters before telling them. This will leave you in much more receptive state to allow them to express their feelings to you.

Asking for Help

Developing a personal support network

As well as needing immediate help to cope with your reaction to diagnosis, it is likely that you are going to need longer-term help both to support you through your treatment and to support you through your recovery programme. An effective strategy can be to form a support group of friends around you. This involves actively recruiting a group of friends that you can call on if the going gets tough. The need for this will depend on the seriousness of your situation and your own emotional state. But it is a mistake to assume that, because you have a close partner or family, you have a support network.

Those closest to you will be going through their own reactions and, quite often, distress ricochets around families like a ball in a pinball machine. You may feel you are able to offload your feelings, but find, later on in the day or week, that they come bouncing back to you in the form of a marital row or a sick child. It is therefore good to form a group of six to eight friends who are 'signed up' members of your personal support group who can pledge to be there for you in times of need. You may wish to have your support group meet once a month at your home to hear about what you are up to and what your needs will be in the forthcoming month. This will help them as well as you.

At first, this might feel like an embarrassing thing to do – to concentrate so much focus and attention on yourself. However, you are giving people an opportunity to express their care and love, and it is likely that they will find this very rewarding. You will also find that being clear and articulating your needs gets easier as time goes by. In so doing, you will be providing a tremendously healthy model for your friends and family to follow in their own lives. It doesn't all have to be a one-way street either. You may choose to structure the support group so that everyone in it has a chance to express their feelings and ask for the support they need from the group each month. You will probably find this empowering as, although there may be some areas in which you are very vulnerable and needy, there will be others in which you are strong and able to give good-quality support to others.

Veronica's Story

Before you become concerned about 'being a burden', read Veronica's story below. In the 1980s, she changed her 'three months to live' with liver cancer secondary to a melanoma into more than nine years, living to see her children leave school. When she realized that her friends avoided telephoning her in the weeks following her diagnosis, perhaps through embarrassment or a lack of knowing how to help, she sent out this 'round-robin' letter:

Dear Friend,

Yes, I have cancer.

Yes, I have been told I have only three months left to live – but actually I AM STILL HERE and I need help!

If you would like to help me, the things I need or would really like are:

1. Flowers every week to cheer me up
2. My organic vegetables picked up each week
3. Money for my holistic therapy
4. Any information any of you can find out about alternative treatment for cancer, anywhere in the world
5. My children taken out while I meditate and visualize
6. A holiday in the Bahamas . . .

and on to a total of 20 wishes.

All 20 of Veronica's needs and wishes were met, and she received letters filled with love and gratitude – such as:

Thank God you told us what you needed. We really wanted to help, but we had no idea what to do for the best.

Perhaps there are many people around you in your family, social and work circles who feel just like Veronica's friends did, and who would be relieved if you would let them know how they could best help you! Let the people who care about you know exactly what help you need. Be specific about your needs, but do not get upset if they say no this time.

Mapping Out Your Personal Support Network

Think now about the family members, friends and colleagues who may be able to help support you now and in the future.

Setting Up Your Personal Support Group
- Ask yourself whether you want (or want supporters) to set up a personal support group.
- If the answer is yes, think about which of your friends you would like to invite to be part of this support group.
- Contact these friends and invite them to join the group.

Suggested guidelines for a personal support group

Below is a set of guidelines on which you could run your support group. Read out or send a copy of these guidelines to all the members of your personal support group.

A Framework for Setting Up a Personal Support Group

A personal support group is being set up by _____.

I have cancer, and need ongoing emotional support and a ready source of practical help at times of crisis. I will also be very happy to provide support for other group members when I am able to do so, but this may not be possible all the time, and will depend on the demands of this illness and its treatment. I would like to invite you to join the group. Please think about the following suggestions for how the group will be run before saying 'yes' to joining. Perhaps you will want to make some suggestions of your own, too? I believe that:

- The group should ideally comprise a minimum of six people besides me, who are not themselves seriously ill at this time. It can include family members, but there should be as many or more non-family members if possible.
- The group members should be able to spare at least two hours every month to come to a group meeting, and have some extra time free each month to provide some care or practical help as needed.
- Ideally, none of this group should be involved with me professionally so that there is no risk of breaking confidentiality or compromising their professionalism.
- At each meeting, it is recommended that each person in the group take 10 minutes – entirely uninterrupted – to tell the others first how they feel, what they are having to deal with and then the support they would ideally like in the following month. The voicing of the support required is not necessarily an active request so much as an opportunity for each person to formulate and voice their needs.
- The time taken by each group member can be lengthened or shortened, depending on the time available and the group members wishes – even three minutes each can be highly effective.

- If possible, members should try hard not to jump in and try to 'fix' the way someone is feeling with practical solutions or advice, as this may shut them down emotionally, stopping them from having a good cry or rant. A great deal of the value of the group will be in supporting each other to express our feelings, and its effectiveness will depend greatly on the ability of the group to sit and bear witness to the others' distress without trying to make them feel better immediately. It is important to think about whether this is possible for you.
- It will be important to keep the group to time. It can be helpful to pass a watch around to be held by the person talking, or for one person to keep time and gently ring a small cymbal or bell when the time is up.
- After the initial go around the group (which will take about an hour for six people), we can then move into practical mode, looking at the practical possibilities for the group to offer each other help in the forthcoming month.

As you prepare for and go through treatment, and then embark upon your recovery process, your wider support network will then also include the holistic therapists you take on to help you.

Your support network will give you great security as the days go by and, even if not needed all the time, will give you a tremendous resource to call upon if things get difficult at any point.

Finding a cancer 'buddy'

Sometimes the most helpful thing may be to find someone else to talk to who is going through the same thing as you are. This is often referred to as having a cancer 'buddy'. You can then compare notes about the treatments you are being offered and share support as you go through them. If you feel this would be helpful, you could ask your consultant, local cancer healthcare personnel or support group network for help to find a 'buddy' for you.

Preparing for the moment of 'peak vulnerability'

People with cancer always say that the moments of peak vulnerability are when they:

- visit their doctor
- wait for test results
- receive bad news
- go through cancer treatment
- stop the cancer treatment.

It is important to arrange to have special support available to you at these times. Take people with you to your appointments. Ask your medical team to get results to you as quickly as possible. Protect yourself at times of receiving bad news, cancelling social and work commitments as needed so that you can take the time to work out what it means to you before having to deal with everyone else's feelings.

Longer term, have a good proactive Health Creation strategy in place for when the treatment stops. Find out about alternative medicine routes, too, in case there is no medical treatment available for your condition, or for times when the medical profession can offer no help.

In Summary

In this chapter, you have been advised to:

- Have support when you receive the news of your diagnosis, taking action to find the results yourself if you have been waiting for more than a week for results.
- Be aware of the powerful effects of shock and be very protective of yourself.
- Avoid having treatment or making big decisions while still in shock, asking for more time to consider your treatment options.
- Seek help from counsellors or other support services before you tell the news to others. You'll need to express your emotions.
- Take advantage of the support available. You are not alone!
- Develop a strong belief in your treatments, your self-healing ability and the power of spiritual healing.
- Gather a strong emotional-support network behind you comprising friends, therapists and a support group.
- Use hypnotherapy, visualization and affirmation to empower your treatments and recovery.
- Find counselling help to enable you to express your feelings, decrease your stress, heal past emotional wounds, and start living a lifestyle that is truly fulfilling and exciting.
- Bring yourself out of isolation, depression, stress, fear and anxiety by changing negative beliefs and coping styles for positive ones, getting professional therapeutic help until you are strong and positive.

CHAPTER 3

Getting the right treatment for you

Becoming clear about what you are dealing with and the choices you have is hard when only recently diagnosed and when you are still in shock and emotional turmoil. The aim of this chapter is to facilitate the process, and to offer as much guidance as possible on when and how to make what types of decisions.

Getting the right treatment depends on:

- getting a clear diagnosis
- working well with your doctors
- information gathering to find out what treatment is available
- weighing up your options from all aspects of integrated medicine, and being clear as to what benefits are actually on offer
- making treatment decisions and having a plan that integrates the best of all treatment approaches.

Remember that an important part of the Hippocratic Oath, taken by all doctors, is a pledge first to do no harm. Bear this in mind when deciding what cancer treatments to undergo. Try not to use medical treatment just to treat your fear, or that of your supporters or doctors. There are much better ways to deal with fear, such as through healing, counselling, relaxation, meditation and loving support. Only subject yourself to harsh medical treatment if the result will be a definite improvement in your physical state and prognosis. Watch out for being over-sold on the benefits of medical treatment especially if your cancer has been resistant to earlier treatment. Often, people say their doctor has given them a 35 per cent chance of the treatment working – but this may actually mean a 35 per cent increase in disease-free time (the time till symptoms reappear compared with having no treatment) and not a 35 per cent chance of cure. While it is understandable for doctors unaware of alternative routes to put pressure on patients to have medical treatment, sometimes this pressure is out of proportion to the true benefits and personal costs of receiving such treatment.

Getting a Clear Diagnosis

A great many of us, when looking at a possible symptom of cancer or cancer recurrence, simply cannot face going to the doctor to hear the diagnosis, and just sit in a kind of limbo hoping it will go away. Some people in this situation will seek out alternative cancer treatments or embark on a holistic health regime to be on the safe side.

While the fear of having and facing a cancer diagnosis (or re-diagnosis) is entirely understandable, not getting a proper diagnosis means that you may live for years thinking you have cancer or a recurrence – and even treating it – when you do not. Alternatively, it may mean that you can lose the opportunity to treat what could be cancer or pre-cancer in its early, potentially curable, stages.

However you choose to deal with the diagnosis once you have one, getting the support you need to go through the diagnostic tests is very important. Having an accurate diagnosis and staging of your illness means you can then make an informed decision about what you are going to do. This puts *you* back in control.

Early symptoms of cancer

The symptoms to look out for which could be cancer include:

- a new or unusual lump anywhere on the body or in the abdomen
- a change in the appearance of a mole
- a sore on the skin or in the mouth that won't heal
- persistent coughing, hoarseness or blood in the sputum/spit
- prolonged constipation or diarrhoea, or blood in the stool
- difficulty in passing urine or blood in the urine
- unexplained weight loss
- unexplained fatigue
- difficulty swallowing and unexplained nausea
- severe headaches and odd neurological symptoms (such as weakness or numbness)
- unexplained abdominal swelling
- vaginal bleeding between periods and any vaginal bleeding after the menopause.

Of course, all of these symptoms can also result from much less serious conditions than cancer and, more often than not, a doctor will be able to reassure you that nothing is seriously wrong. However, it is important to wait until all of the appropriate diagnostic tests have been done. Too often, GPs give reassurance on the basis of a clinical examination in their surgery, only to be proved wrong at a later date. GPs expect patients to come back if symptoms persist, so it is important to trust yourself and keep going back if you think something is not right. Although most people are sent for tests immediately, far too many visit their GP over and over again before they are sent for the appropriate X-rays, blood tests or other investigations. They can then discover in the end that their intuition was right – that something is seriously wrong and that a cancer that could have been treated easily as a primary has now spread to other parts of the body. So, please be alert to whatever messages your body is giving you.

If you are really concerned that a GP is not responding to you appropriately, get a second opinion from another GP or even arrange to have investigations done privately or through an integrated medicine doctor.

Ask yourself what support you need to get through the diagnostic process.

Visiting your GP

Once you have overcome your fears and are able to actively seek a diagnosis, make an appointment with your GP. If you wish to, take a friend or partner with you. Clearly explain your symptoms and your concerns about having cancer or a recurrence of cancer. This is important so that the GP takes your situation seriously and so that, if you do not have cancer, you can be properly reassured.

Receiving good news

Once the tests have been done, it is often possible for doctors to give you reassurances that all is well. This is particularly common for those who have had a primary cancer and who understandably then suspect every headache or twinge of being a recurrence. What is important here is your peace of mind, and the doctors should help you to get the reassurance you need until you feel better and settled again.

But even if the news is good, you may perhaps wish to treat the incident as a 'wake-up call', and embark upon a Health Creation Programme as an insurance policy to avoid your ever having a scare like this again.

Receiving bad news

Regrettably, 270,000 people per year in the UK do receive a diagnosis of primary cancer, and an equal number have a diagnosis of secondary spreading. A cancer diagnosis is something we all dread. If you are sitting in the horrible hot seat at this moment and have just got the news, be reassured that a great deal of help is at hand!

Despite the high rates of cancer in the developed countries (four in every 10 of us will develop a cancer during our lifetime), most of us live our lives feeling immortal, believing that these things only happen to other people. The news of a life-threatening diagnosis can be like a bomb going off in the centre of our lives, completely shattering our security and our sense of the life we expected to have.

Nevertheless, there are people reading this who can say, 'No, I actually expected my diagnosis of cancer. I knew that my life and health were seriously out of kilter and that it was only really a matter of time before I got seriously ill.'

Most probably, if you are reading this book, you have already been through the initial impact of receiving a diagnosis of cancer. However, if you are waiting for test results, it is important that you are protected at that moment of greatest vulnerability. Try to take someone with you, and ask for the privacy and time you need with the doctor to enable yourself to take on board fully the information you are being given.

Getting support while waiting for test results

If you are waiting for test results, what support do you need to help you through this tense time?

- A talk with my GP
- A talk with my practice nurse, health visitor, social worker or practice counsellor
- A talk with the consultant or hospital support team
- A talk with a private counsellor
- A talk with a spiritual guide
- Being able to confide in a friend or family member
- Being able to tell colleagues at work and arrange to be excused from normal duties
- Being able to take time off to go into 'retreat'.

If you have you been waiting more than a week for test results, it is reasonable to seek help to find out what has happened to your results. You could try telephoning your GP, the practice nurse or your consultant's secretary. Ask them to chase your results for you. Make it absolutely clear that you wish to receive your results over the telephone or face to face from one of your medical team.

The moment of truth

The time will come for you to get your test results. If you are expecting bad news, it may be helpful to find out before your appointment with the consultant what kind of assistance is available from a member of the support team (if there is one) or a specialist nurse at the hospital. This is particularly relevant if you live alone, have no close partner or confidante and nobody around to look after you and see you through your vulnerable period after you get home. You may also wish to find out what support is available from the GP's surgery, the local community nurses or hospices, counsellors, skilled volunteers, support groups, chaplains, spiritual helpers or psychologists. Quite often, resources are to hand which busy doctors and nurses forget to tell you about. So, it is advisable to do some homework in advance if you are at all worried.

Finding Out What Support Is Available at the Hospital

This information is available from the clinical staff (nurses and clerks) where you go to see the consultant, from the cancer or unit information centres (if they have these), and from those in charge of the surgical wards, and chemo-/radiotherapy treatment units.

Getting Support When You Receive Your Results

Ask yourself whether you prefer to be alone to get your test results or with a supporter. If you do take a supporter, who will you ask to accompany you?

If you prefer to go alone or have no choice, who can be at the end of a phone to support you or stay with you overnight if the news is bad? Is this arrangement confirmed? You can celebrate with them, too, if the news is good.

If you want someone to be with you after the appointment, let him know the time of your appointment and arrange where you can meet when you are finished. Ideally, arrange to have him pick you up if you need support.

Working with Your Doctors

Establishing the best relationship with your doctors – whether that is your GP, surgeon, oncologist or radiotherapist – will be very important for your ongoing security and peace of mind. You may be lucky and find an enlightened doctor who will help you obtain the best integrated medicine, but you may find yourself in a position where you need to gently, but firmly, inform those who are caring for you as to your values and needs. It is hard to have to do this at the point when you are so vulnerable, and would like and expect the care you get to be completely appropriate. However, as with any new relationship, unless you make your needs and feelings clearly known, it will be difficult for others to arrive at any appropriate responses.

It is important to remember that doctors are there to serve you and not the other way round! You have a right to the proper time, attention and care from your doctors and, if for any reason you do not feel comfortable with the consultant you have been referred to, you should go back to your GP and ask to be referred to someone else. We now live in a time when healthcare services are supposed to be patient-centred, so it is essential that you are satisfied with the service you are getting. If not, you need to register this with the cancer services manager in your area or hospital – otherwise, things will never improve.

Right from the start, it is important that your consultant treats you as an equal partner in your healthcare management. If you have taken on board what has been said at the very beginning of this book, you will have already realized that you are a vital member of your cancer management team. This view is backed up by leading UK oncologist Professor Karol Sikora and by the scientific evidence showing how strong a survival advantage is experienced by those who are active in their own defence.

You want to be treated as an individual, so it is useful to let the doctor know:

- how you are viewing your situation and the way you are choosing to deal with it
- how much information you want to be given
- how hard you want to fight your cancer and to what lengths you are prepared to go medically
- if you prefer not to have medical treatment or to stop the treatment you are having
- how you are reacting emotionally to your situation and how well you are coping (or not)
- which treatments (if any) you are not prepared to have
- whether you are ready emotionally and physically to start treatment.

It is important that you:

- take full charge of your situation, never allowing yourself to be railroaded into any treatment decision
- let the doctor know your current situation, values, needs or desires which may affect your treatment decisions

- ask for understanding, flexibility and help if at any time you feel too vulnerable to have treatment
- ask for the support you need
- explain (or seek professional help to explain) to your doctor the science and theory underpinning any approaches you may be using as a complement or alternative to medical treatment
- ask your doctor to be tolerant of and support the choices you are making with regards to your healthcare.

It may cheer you to know that there is an American study that proves that 'difficult' patients do best and survive longer. One support group even had T-shirts printed saying 'I am a difficult patient' to wear on hospital visits to wake up the medical team. I've even heard of a woman who always attended her outpatient appointments in a ballet tutu so she would be remembered and treated as an individual!

This may be too drastic a step for you, but it is a good idea to try to establish a personal rapport with the team looking after you – even if it is because you are always the one asking the searching questions or making your needs known. Humour is, of course, always the best way, and the combination of wit, cunning, being well prepared, assertive and funny is irresistible.

Your aim is to:

- **obtain all the appropriate information about your situation**
- **be given the time to digest and react to this**
- **make informed consent to treatment only when you have truly understood what the treatment entails, and its potential benefits and side-effects compared with other treatments on offer**
- **prepare yourself well for treatment, building up your belief in the power of the treatment with visualization and affirmation**
- **embark upon your treatment feeling fully confident that you have picked the very best course of action for you.**

Remember, too, that if you are not happy with your consultant or his opinion, you have the right to ask for a second opinion.

Information Gathering to Find Out What Treatment Options Are Available

Knowing the right questions to ask

To get the information you want, you need to ask the right questions. Knowing what these questions are is difficult unless you have a basic understanding of cancer as a disease. A full explanation of cancer and its treatment is given in Chapter 4 for those who desire the full details. In essence, the information you need in order to ask the right questions is as follows:

- There are as many different types of cancer as there are types of cells in the body. Cancer arises from a single cell in which genetic material has been damaged. The damage allows the cell to replicate and spread out of control. As these 'wild' cells continue to grow, a lump or tumour is formed – this is known as a **primary cancer**. If the cell that started to grow out of control originated from breast tissue, this will be a breast cancer; if it was a bone cell, it will be a bone cancer, and so on.
- As the tumour grows, it may begin to invade the local blood and lymphatic vessels. At this point, cells may break off from the main tumour and travel to nearby lymph nodes, which may also become swollen because of the cancerous tissue that starts to grow in them. From there, the cancer may travel even further afield through the bloodstream or lymphatic vessels to distant sites in the body. There are certain preferred sites where these cells will become lodged, leading to a possible **secondary cancer**, or **metastases**, to start growing – for example, breast cancer secondaries can show up in the bones, lungs, liver or brain.

When a doctor is initially assessing the cancer, he will try to establish:

- the **histology** or type of the tumour – the cell type of origin of the cancer
- the **grade** or degree of aggressiveness of the tumour
- the **stage** of the disease – whether the tumour is still at its primary site or whether it has spread locally from the tissue of origin to nearby lymph nodes or even further afield to form secondaries or metastases
- whether there are any special **markers** (such as blood tests) by which its progress can be measured, or unique characteristics, such as being **hormone-positive**.

For most tumours, **stage one** means there is a primary only; **stage two** means the primary has begun to invade the blood vessels locally; **stage three** means that the tumour has spread to nearby lymph nodes; and **stage four** means that it has metastasized throughout the body. These stagings will differ somewhat from one type of cancer to another.

To diagnose and grade the tumour, the specialist will take a sample of the tumour tissue, usually by taking a **biopsy**. The tissue sample is then studied under the microscope to determine just how aggressive the cells are, and the results will appear on a histology, pathology or histopathology report. Cancer cells are described as **well differentiated** if they still closely resemble the cell of origin – in other words, a well-differentiated cancer of the breast will contain cells easily recognized as having originally arisen from breast tissue. Because the cells are also still similar in nature to normal breast tissue cells, the tumour would also be described as **slow-growing** and **low-grade**.

At the other extreme, the tumour cells may be barely recognizable as breast tissue cells because they had become 'wild'. Such cells would then be described as **poorly differentiated**, and the tumour as **fast-growing** or **aggressive** and **high-grade**. Again, the grading system varies with different types of cancer, but most tumours will be graded on a scale of one to four.

Staging the tumour means having further **screening tests** done after a positive biopsy. These may be blood tests, X-rays and/or ultrasound, CT (computed tomography) or MRI (magnetic resonance imaging) scans of the parts of the body to which the cancer may have spread. How much you wish to know will also affect how much screening you allow your doctors to do. Some consultants, on discovering a primary tumour, will leave no stone unturned in looking for possible secondaries. Other consultants take a much more passive view, waiting until there are symptoms before looking for the presence of metastases.

Generally speaking, there is not much point in undergoing extensive screening unless it will potentially change the treatment being offered. For example, if the chemotherapy for a primary cancer is the same as for a similar cancer that has already spread, your consultant may not think it necessary to carry out widescale screening. But you may wish to know if there are secondaries, as this may significantly change your approach to the cancer and your life choices. So, you will need to be clear with your doctor as to just how far you want him to go with this process and how much information you wish to be given.

To get a clear picture of what you are dealing with, you need to find out:

- the **type** of cancer you have or its **histology**
- the **stage** of the cancer or how far it has spread
- the **grade** of the tumour or how aggressive it is

- the **markers** of your tumour by which the effectiveness of treatment or progress of the disease can be measured
- if the tumour is **hormone-positive**.

Once you have this information, you will then be armed, if you so choose, to go away and read about the cancer you have and discover the possible treatment options for your cancer type, stage and grade.

The exception is in the case of tumours of the blood cells. These are the **leukaemias**, in which there is no solid tumour because the cell that has grown out of control is one of the various types of white blood cells. The way this sort of tumour is diagnosed is by performing blood counts or looking at bone marrow. These tests might reveal that one cell type is growing very fast at the expense of other blood cells, the levels of which may be lower than normal. With leukaemias, classification is in terms of whether the illness is **chronic** (slow-growing) or **acute** (fast-growing).

Depending on how much information you wish to be given, you might ask your doctor for answers to some or all of the following questions:
IF YOU DO NOT WANT TO KNOW THE ANSWERS TO THESE QUESTIONS, TELL THE CONSULTANT AND GP WHAT YOU DO and DO NOT WANT TO KNOW.

- What type of primary cancer do I have (or what is the histology of the tumour)?
- How large is the primary site?
- Has it spread to the lymph nodes draining the site from which it has arisen?
- Has it spread elsewhere in the body, and what is its stage (1, 2, 3 or 4) (or how far has the tumour spread)?
- What is the 'grade' or degree of aggressiveness of the tumour?
- Are there other prognostic indications from the pathologist?
- Is the cancer hormone-receptor-positive? If so, to what hormones is the tumour sensitive?
- Are there any blood markers by which the growth or shrinkage of the tumour can be measured?
- To which parts of my body might this type of tumour spread?
- Would it be advisable for me to be screened thoroughly for secondary cancer?
- If secondary cancers were found on screening, how would this affect the choice of treatment I am being offered?

- In the case of leukaemia, is it acute or chronic?
- Left untreated, what is the usual course of events with this type of cancer?
- What is the prognosis (or average survival time) with this cancer if medically treated?

Finding out more about your cancer

When you have found out the type, stage and grade of your cancer from your consultant or GP, you may wish to gather more information before making any decisions about medical, complementary and alternative medicine approaches to treatment.

It is best to think a bit about how and where you should look before you embark on this process. Information about cancer is divided into two main categories – what has been written for people with cancer; and what has been written for doctors, nurses or other healthcare professionals.

In the former, the medical and scientific jargon will have been translated into plain English and (hopefully) it will have been written with consideration of your feelings. In contrast, the latter information will have been written for those with an understanding of science who only need to know the facts – and is likely to be very blunt.

It is important now that you do not become overwhelmed with information and, even more essential, that you do not become overly depressed by what you read. Your approach will therefore depend on your personality, and how much information you can take and in what form. A helpful source of information on cancer for those who have cancer is CancerBACUP. As well as a full range of informative leaflets about every type of cancer, they also have a nurse 'phone-in' service to answer your specific questions about your situation. For medical and scientific information, there is the Internet and medical libraries. However, people often complain that the Internet can lead to information overload, and that the information gleaned from medical libraries is often non-user friendly.

Other sources of information are the big cancer-research institutes such as:

- Cancer Research UK
- National Cancer Institute USA
- The American Cancer Society
- The Royal Marsden Hospital, London
- Memorial Sloane-Kettering Cancer Hospital, New York
- University of Texas MD Anderson Cancer Center, Houston.

Going to the Frontier with the Internet
Useful websites for more information about orthodox cancer medicine include:

---

www.cancerbacup.org.uk: The best UK information site on all aspects of cancer with good links to other sites

www.cancer.gov: The largest cancer website in the world, belonging to the US National Cancer Institute in Washington

www.oncolink.org: The excellent site of the University of Pennsylvania Cancer Center with good links to other US sites

www.oncology.com: The website of the American Society of Clinical Oncology, where treatment protocols and drugs are well explained

www.cancerhelp.org.uk: Smaller, manageable site from the University of Birmingham

www.cancerresearchuk.org.uk: Britain's cancer research charities site

www.macmillan.org.uk: Site of the Macmillan Fund, with useful contacts especially for support groups and palliative care

www.cancereurope.com: The European School of Oncology site, with good links to other cancer sites in the EU.

Look in Chapter 4 for more cancer-treatment information, and in Part 2 of this Directory for useful websites and contact details of those offering helpful cancer information.

If you would like to speak to a doctor in more detail about your cancer, you may be able to get help from the pathology department of the hospital that diagnosed your tissue samples. Pathology departments have doctors called 'pathologists', whose job it is to understand the course that specific diseases tend to follow. Because pathologists do not see many patients, they usually have quite a lot of patience. You may find that one of these doctors is willing to come to the phone, if you ring the pathology department, and tell you in detail about the nature of your tumour and its likely behaviour in the future. Of course, it is possible that all this information will simply raise more questions than it answers, so it is perfectly appropriate that, having gathered your information, you go back to your consultant and/or GP to ask your next round of questions.

If you would like a broader integrated medicine perspective, this may also be the time to seek the advice and help of an integrated medicine doctor (see the Resources Directory).

Knowing when to stop

It is important to know when to stop with this process of seeking information about your cancer so that you do not become overly preoccupied with reading more and more about your condition. As soon as you feel satisfied that you have a reasonable grasp of the situation, it is time to move on to making your treatment decisions.

Understanding the medical approach to cancer

Once you know about your cancer and have assessed your situation and the level of risk, you can consider the treatment options.

Generally speaking, the aim of cancer doctors is to attempt to remove the primary tumour before it has spread, then to destroy any stray cells around the site of the primary with radiotherapy, or more distantly spread cells with chemotherapy. With blood cancers, attempts are made to destroy the cancer cells in the blood with chemotherapy and then to remove the abnormal parent cancer cells from the bone marrow, replacing them with healthy cells. This involves bone marrow grafts, which use healthy new marrow from a donor after the patient's unhealthy bone marrow is destroyed.

Nowadays, cancer treatments tend to be more aggressive, offering the whole gamut of surgery, radiotherapy and chemotherapy right from the start of the treatment process. In the 1970s and 1980s, it was more usual to treat the primary tumour only, saving radio- and chemotherapy for recurrences. However, the thinking these days is that it is better to go for complete eradication or cure from the outset rather than allowing the cancer to become established in the body.

Because doctors want to 'nip cancer in the bud' as soon as it has been diagnosed, there is often an enormous sense of rush and panic at the time of diagnosis. And being on the receiving end of this can be traumatic. While you are still reeling from the news and going through an emotional reaction, those around you are busy trying to get on with starting your treatment. So again, it should be stressed how important it is that you slow them down until you have made the right choice for you and are ready to undergo your well-considered treatment.

On occasions, you may be advised to have chemotherapy first to shrink and contain the primary tumour before attempting to remove it surgically. Sometimes, the primary or secondary tumours may be deemed inoperable – in which case, the treatment offered is usually chemotherapy. If the tumour is widespread throughout the body, the treatment given may be palliative – intended to deal with the symptoms rather than cure the disease. This usually amounts to shrinking the tumour with radio- or chemotherapy to buy vital time for you to get your own integrated health creation programme together.

When thinking about treatment, the following are the questions you need to ask:
- What treatments are suggested for my cancer and why?
- What are the chances of the tumour being cured?
- What are the side-effects of treatment in the short and long term?
- What are the risks of treatment?
- Do I trust my cancer consultant or do I need to seek a second opinion?
- Is my hospital able to give me access to the most up-to-date treatment for my type of cancer, or should I be looking further afield?
- Which are the centres of excellence for my particular kind of cancer nationally and internationally?
- Are there treatment research trials going on for my kind of cancer and, if so, would I like to be entered into one of those trials?
- Do I want to go straight into medical treatment of my cancer or do I need time to prepare myself mentally, physically and practically first?
- If the results with conventional medical treatment are not likely to be good, do I want to keep medical treatment on hold as an option while I work entirely on improving my health with alternative cancer treatments and holistic health promotion?
- If I wish to defer treatment while trying to work with natural methods, am I sure that I am not putting myself at undue risk in doing so?
- You may also wish to ask: If the tumour cannot be cured, what is the likely progression of the disease and my life expectancy?

Specialists who look after people with cancer

There are four different types of specialists who look after people with cancer:

- surgeons, who are usually the first to be consulted if there are primary or secondary tumours that are removable (but who are not necessarily cancer specialists)
- medical oncologists, who specialize in the treatment of cancer with chemotherapy and/or radiotherapy
- palliative care physicians, whose role is to help manage your symptoms, and arrange for your support and care
- anaesthetists, who can offer specialist help if there is a problem with severe, ongoing pain.

It varies from place to place whether you see an oncologist or surgeon first, but it is wise to make sure you do see an oncologist at some point because they are specialists in cancer and its treatment. Ask your GP whether there are any other relevant specialists who may be able to help you.

Getting more details

When your specialists tell you about your treatment options, it is important to establish the details of the proposed treatment so that you can make an informed decision.

As you focus on a particular treatment as the most likely one for you, make sure to ask the following questions:

- What will the treatment involve?
- When and where will it take place?
- Who will be responsible for my treatment?
- How long will it continue for?
- How will it make me feel?
- How long should I take off work for treatment and convalescence afterwards?
- What side-effects can it cause?
- How long will it take me to get over these side-effects?
- Will these side-effects be permanent or temporary?
- What are the benefits of the treatment in terms of prolonged survival, symptom improvement or disease-free interval (the time you can expect to enjoy with no problems from the cancer)?
- Are there any extra (**adjuvant**) treatments that might further improve my well-being or chances of survival while having this treatment?
- Does the doctor see any problem with my taking vitamin/mineral supplements alongside the treatment (making sure his or her opinion is a well-informed one)?
- Does the doctor know of any promising 'medical frontier' treatments or trials that might offer a better chance of prolonged survival than the treatment I am being offered and, if so, where are these treatments available and at what cost?

Once you are in possession of this information, you will be able to decide whether the side-effects (temporary and permanent) of the treatment outweigh the possible benefits you may receive in terms of symptom improvement and life expectation.

You may find this in-depth questioning of your doctors too difficult to go through. Some people do not want to know exactly where cancer is in their bodies if it is not causing problems nor do they want to pin their doctors down to telling them the exact facts about the effectiveness of the treatments being offered, as this may inhibit their being able to put 100 per cent of their faith in the treatment.

However, I would strongly recommend that, at the very least, you get a clear diagnosis of the primary tumour so that you are certain that you do have cancer, and get some indication of how serious your situation may be. In this way, you can make an informed decision about whether to go ahead with conventional treatment or not with an assessment of the risks involved if you do not feel able to undergo medical treatment.

Thinking about Timing

Next, think about the timing of your treatment. Ask yourself:

- **Do I want to go straight into medical treatment for my cancer, or do I need a little time to prepare myself mentally, physically and practically first?**

Take the time you need to get yourself in the right frame of mind for treatment. Preparing properly for treatment is covered in detail in Chapter 7.

Understanding the treatment offered

Before you commit to a particular treatment, be sure you understand both the benefits and side-effects that you may experience.

Quite often, because people are so anxious about what the treatment will do in the short term, they do not really hear or take on board what is being said about long-term side-effects. For example, a woman asking about chemotherapy treatment may be thinking about its effects on her hair, nails and energy levels, and whether she will be able to work and look after her children. She may completely miss the fact that, in the longer term, the chemo could cause infertility, depression or nerve damage.

While thinking about the possibility that tamoxifen treatment for breast cancer may cause weight gain, a woman may miss the point that it also carries a 5–10 per cent risk of causing endometrial cancer. Clearly, doctors and other healthcare professionals do not like to dwell on the downsides of treatment but, as mentioned earlier, it is better to be aware of and prepared for the worst-case scenario than having it sprung on you at a later date, facing you with a new set of losses and fears. It may be worthwhile having two separate discussions with your doctors or nurses – one about the short-term effects of the treatment and a blow-by-blow account of receiving the treatment; and another about the possible or likely long-term side-effects of the treatment.

A useful source of information about drug treatments is the drug information centre found in most big hospitals. This is usually staffed by helpful pharmacists, who will take the time to answer your questions or send you printed material about the medicines you are being offered. Pharmacists are far more knowledgeable about drugs and treatments than doctors and other healthcare professionals, and will have detailed information sheets and research data for each medicine being offered at their fingertips. If you do not have access to a big hospital, you can still speak to the pharmacist responsible for the oncology ward who will often be only too pleased to share his or her knowledge and experience with you.

Learning more about the proposed treatment

Make sure that you are asking the right person about the nature of the treatment – the consultant or nurses involved with each aspect of your treatment – and about any relevant details, be it surgery, chemotherapy, radiotherapy or hormone therapy (or any other forms of treatment on offer).

It is then wise to ask yourself if you are satisfied with the information that you have been given, or do you feel the need to seek a second opinion?

Reviewing Your Options

When reviewing your options for treatment and before you make your treatment decision, make sure you have collected together all the relevant information by going through the checklist below.

- Options on offer at the hospital in your area
- Range of options on offer at the leading centre of excellence for your particular cancer
- Options that might be available in other parts of the world
- Research trial alternatives
- Alternative cancer medicine choices
- Your integrated medicine complementary and self-help options.

Hopefully, all this information has given you clear guidance on how to find what options are available at your hospital, including getting the opinions of the different specialists mentioned, where appropriate.

If you would like an opinion from a centre of excellence, you need a referral from your GP or consultant. In the UK, it is usually possible to get such an opinion on the NHS if it is clear that the services offered by such a centre are more comprehensive than what is available in your own area. If you have health insurance, check first that your policy covers you for second or third opinions. Treatments in another country are unlikely to be covered by your health insurance, and you should check costs carefully before embarking on this route.

Sometimes, doctors in foreign medical centres are prepared to give an initial opinion of what they can offer you on the strength of letters from your consultants, and having seen your X-rays and/or scans. Because of major advances in digital technology, it is now also possible to send scans to distant locations via e-mail (not to mention by post or courier).

This form of consultation, while lacking the personal touch, can save costly and exhausting trips abroad unless there is likely to be a significant benefit.

How far you wish to go with this process of getting a 'world picture' is entirely up to you. For some, this may feel like far too great a burden whereas, for others, it will be a source of great comfort to know that no stone has been left unturned.

Reviewing your **alternative cancer treatment** options is covered in Chapter 5. A great number of alternative cancer remedies are on offer around the world, with variable levels of information as to their effectiveness. In Chapter 5, you will find:

- basic information on how to use the most well-known alternative cancer medicines
- the approximate cost of their use
- the current level of scientific information about them
- whether you can self-administer them or not (i.e. are they available for sale, by prescription only or clinic-based?).

Reviewing what the **complementary medicine** and **self-help approaches** have to offer is the subject of Chapters 7 and 8.

Making Treatment Decisions and Creating an Integrated Medicine Plan

Chapters 4 and 5 will tell you about the treatment choices that are available, and Chapter 6 offers a checklist to go through to make sure you are ready to make your final decision. Chapters 7 and 8 will help you to prepare for your treatment and find the relevant, effective complementary supportive care during treatment.

Once you are clear as to the choices you wish to make, it is wise to draw up your plan of action so that you remain crystal-clear about what you are going to do, how you are going to do it and with what support. If you need help in doing this, or a short cut, then seek specific guidance from an integrated medicine doctor (see the Resources Directory) to devise a medically supervised programme that is tailor-made for you and your needs.

If you choose to receive neither orthodox nor alternative medicine, you should proceed straight to Chapter 9 on the long-term health creation approach to recovery.

Meanwhile, if you are looking for creative solutions to help with troublesome symptoms, they can be found in Chapter 8.

CHAPTER 4

The medical frontier:
getting the best orthodox treatment

The oncologist's perspective by Professor Karol Sikora with cancer nurse Patricia Peat

This chapter covers the current best practices available at the most advanced treatment centres, giving you a benchmark against which to measure the treatment you are being offered locally. This information will enable you to check worldwide for the very best resources and treatments available for your individual situation. Advice will be given on how to obtain second and third opinions as and when necessary.

In the last 20 years, there have been dramatic strides in our understanding of what cancer is and how best to treat it. Some cancers that were almost uniformly fatal in the past, such as Hodgkin's disease and testicular cancer, are now mostly curable, thanks to chemotherapy. We are more open about the diagnosis of cancer in society and there is much media interest in cancer stories – good and bad. We are also living longer, which means that, as cancer is more common in older people (due to the declining effectiveness of the immune system, and longer exposure to poor dietary habits and environmental pollutants), the incidence of the disease is increasing.

Above all, we have managed to break some of the taboos that surround cancer so that the diagnosis is now usually acknowledged between doctor and patient, family and friends. This new frankness means that the need for information has never been greater.

Consumerism is hitting healthcare in a big way and, if used correctly, can change for better the way in which we obtain care. But, to avoid tilting at windmills, it is essential that you arm yourself with facts. To this end, we offer you here an unbiased guide to the world of cancer and its treatment to help you find the combination of orthodox and complementary medicine that will provide you with the best springboard to deal with your situation.

Nevertheless, on a cautionary note, please remember that with all forms of research the end results cannot be guaranteed. So, some of the areas being currently researched or developed and included in this chapter may not ultimately become available treatments. To confirm what really is available now, the major cancer information services listed in the Resources Directory (pages 257–63) can give you up-to-date information on all orthodox treatments, surgical procedures and clinical-trial availability to help you assess the potential effectiveness of any treatments you have been offered.

But first, let us go back to the beginning of the story and think more about the nature of cancer so that the modes of treatment can be better understood.

What Is Cancer?

The cancer cell

To understand cancer, we need to think about the construction of the body. About one thousand billion cells are needed to make a person. Each cell carries information on how to function from the time it is developed till the time it is supposed to die. Depending on where it is situated in the body, the cells of different tissues are specialized to have different functions. A muscle cell has tiny molecular ropes that allow it to contract, so pulling other structures to cause a movement. A skin cell has a tough waterproof coat to protect us from the environment, while a liver cell is a chemical refinery that is continuously clearing the blood of potential poisons.

All organisms, including man, grow from a single cell that splits into two in a process called 'mitosis'. In health, the two new cells are identical to the one they came from. These two daughter cells then divide to form four cells, then eight, and so on. In most people, the cells work in perfect harmony, but sometimes they go wrong. If a cell dies, then one of its many identical kin takes over its job.

But if a cell starts to grow and divide in an abnormal way, problems may arise. The information carried in the cell's DNA, the thread of life, becomes altered, forming an abnormal cell with abnormal growth patterns. This is called 'malignant transformation' and is the first change towards cancer. The abnormal cell continues to grow, but does not mature properly, and has characteristics that differ from its healthy parent cell. As this cell reproduces, over time, each new generation of cells becomes a little less like the cell it originated from and, thus, less effective at performing its designated tasks. Cancer cells can develop because the DNA in the cell nucleus has been damaged by either radiation, chemical toxins or viral infection. This is more likely to happen in tissues that are inflamed and poorly nourished due to a low blood and oxygen supply.

Characteristics that distinguish a normal cell from a cancer cell

Cell Recognition

A normal cell recognizes its borders. It sees other cells next to it, but knows it is not supposed to invade and spread into their territory. A cancer cell lacks this information and will invade the surrounding tissues.

Immune Attack

In health, when a cell becomes abnormal due to infection or cancer, the immune system recognizes its abnormality and destroys it. When cancer develops, the ability of immune cells to recognize the abnormality is lost, thereby allowing the abnormal cells to carry on growing unchecked.

Staying in Place

A normal cell knows where it should be, and stays there until it dies, when another cell takes its place. It does this by sticking to the cells surrounding it. A cancer cell loses this 'stickiness' and breaks away from its surroundings to be transported via various body systems to other organs, where it takes up residence and starts to divide and grow into a new tumour. This is known as 'metastatic spread', or the development of a secondary cancer.

Metastatic spread

With different types of cancer, there are differences in how quickly metastatic spread can take place. But it also depends on the individual who has it (more about this later).

There are two types of tumour – benign or malignant. Benign tumours are usually localized and do not spread. They are often enclosed in a clear capsule – a rim of normal tissue – which demarcates the limits of the abnormal cells. These tumours may be detected because, as they grow, they press on other structures in the body such as blood vessels or the intestines. In contrast, malignant tumours are virtually never encapsulated, but erode adjacent tissues by extending crab-like infiltrations in the body in all directions.

Most cancers do not spread completely haphazardly – certain tumours have favoured sites of metastases. Prostate cancer, for example, tends to spread to the bones, often the spine or pelvis. Breast cancer usually goes first to the lymph nodes, but then favours the liver, bones and lungs. Colon cancer spreads first to the liver, following the blood flow from the colon to the liver.

Cancer cells produce chemical factors that enable them to grow as a group, and we are only just beginning to understand the growth factors involved in sustaining cancer cell growth. In future, we may be able to devise anti-cancer drugs that can block these growth factors.

Classifying cancer

Cancer can strike any organ of the body, each with its own pattern of behaviour. There are currently 208 classifiable sites at which cancers arise, and many of these are broken down into further subtypes. This reflects the many different cell types that make up the human body, many of which can grow out of control.

Tumours are named according to the site at which they originate, not by the organs they spread to. For example, a patient with breast cancer that has spread through the bloodstream to the liver is said to have metastatic breast cancer. If it then spreads to the bone, it is still breast cancer, but metastasized to bone. On the other hand, it is possible to have a primary bone or liver cancer, which has arisen in these tissues and metastasized elsewhere. This may cause confusion because of poor communication in rushed clinics.

Tumours are also named to reflect the type of structure from which they have come. A carcinoma, for example, comes from cells lining body cavities called 'epithelial cells'. Such cells are found in the lungs, colon, breast and prostate gland. Carcinomas are by far the most common type of cancer. Tumours derived from the body's structural tissues, muscles, tendons, bones and cartilage are called 'sarcomas'. Those arising from the lymphatic system are called 'lymphomas', and cancers of the white blood cells and bone marrow are known as 'leukaemias'.

If you ever hear any terms used to refer to your particular cancer which you do not understand, ask for an explanation. Cancer classification is complicated, and there are often several words that mean much the same thing. If you don't understand a term, don't go away feeling too embarrassed to ask what it means – check it out and save yourself unnecessary stress.

Diagnosing Cancer

How is a cancer diagnosis usually made?

The only way to diagnose cancer definitively is to test a sample of abnormal cells from the site of the tumour. The usual way of doing this is to obtain a biopsy, or a small tissue sample, under either a local or general anaesthetic, depending on the site of the tumour.

Cancer has no specific symptoms – it depends on where the tumour is, how big it is, which structure it is invading and whether it has spread to other parts of the body. A patient with lung cancer, for example, may have a cough with or without blood or phlegm, or a persistent chest infection that does not respond to antibiotics. The usual symptom of breast cancer is a lump in the breast, although it may well have spread by the time it can be detected this way. If it has spread, then its symptoms will depend on the site of the metastases – in the lungs, it may mimic a lung tumour; in the liver, a liver tumour, and so on.

Because cancer produces so many different types of symptoms which can be mistaken for minor illnesses, there may be a period of several weeks with repeated visits to the GP before the symptoms are taken seriously. The best rule of thumb is that any progressing symptom that does not disappear after two to four weeks should be further investigated. Usually, this involves being referred to a hospital where the investigations can be done rapidly.

If cancer is suspected, there are two important requirements: to do a biopsy to find out exactly what type of cells have gone wrong and, therefore, how best to treat them; and to 'stage' the disease to find out how far the disease has spread as this, too, dramatically affects not only the optimal treatment, but also the likely outcome.

The tests to determine the site and stage of the cancer include:

- Biopsy, to study a piece of tissue thought to be cancerous – the definitive way to make the diagnosis
- Blood tests, to check for anaemia, bone-marrow function, liver and kidney function, and search for tumour markers – substances produced by cancer cells and detectable in the blood, thereby alerting doctors to the presence or spread of cancer
- Plain X-rays, to provide information about various parts of the body
- Contrast X-rays, injecting or ingesting a radiopaque substance to increase what can be seen on the X-ray
- CT (computed tomography) scans, to provide detailed information about the structure of various internal organs
- MRI (magnetic resonance imaging), a powerful imaging technique based on magnetic field shifts in the body
- Bone and liver scans, to show areas of dysfunction in the bone and the liver that may be due to the spread of a cancer.

Staging

Determining how far a cancer has spread is a critical starting point before deciding on treatment. There are several systems available and this often causes confusion, even among doctors.

One of the most commonly used staging systems is the TNM system, developed by a committee of the International Union Against Cancer. Here, the letter T stands for 'tumour', with T_1 referring to a small tumour and T_4 referring to a very large one.

The N stands for 'nodes', the lymph nodes draining the organ in which the tumour is found. Enlarged nodes containing growing tumours are classified as N_1 or N_2 depending on their site and number.

The M stands for 'metastasis' (spread) and is either present (M_1) or absent (M_0).

Other staging systems are often simpler. Early-stage disease may be called stage 1 whereas late-stage disease, or more advanced cancer, is then stage 4. Different criteria may be used for cancer at different sites of the body, so ask your consultant to explain exactly what the staging means for your type of cancer. A person with disease that has not spread is likely to have a better outcome than a patient whose disease has already left its primary site. This is because a localized tumour is more likely to be cured or removed altogether by either surgery or radiotherapy.

Grading

The grade of a cancer, determined by the pathologist by looking at the cancer cells through a microscope, is also useful in predicting the outcome of a cancer. A high-grade tumour contains very abnormal cells, which have mutated greatly, grown rapidly and often spread throughout the body. This is also referred to as 'poorly differentiated'. At the other end of the spectrum are low-grade tumours, which can look similar to the tissue from which they have been derived and are referred to as 'well differentiated'. Such tumours grow more slowly and are less likely to spread quickly. The outlook is usually better for low-grade tumours, but there is a paradox. High-grade aggressive tumours are often more sensitive to chemotherapy as the chemicals work best against the most rapidly dividing cells in the body. Unfortunately though, rapidly growing cells can continue to evolve and can become resistant to specific drugs rather rapidly, too.

It is also possible to have varying opinions as to the grade of a tumour among pathologists. So, if you are in any doubt, or the pathology seems uncertain, ask for a second opinion from another pathologist.

Secondary cancer

Cancer that develops in the body away from the site of the original tumour is called a 'secondary cancer' or a metastasis. These may be found at the time of diagnosis or they may develop later on. If secondaries appear, it can often be a more severe blow than the original diagnosis.

Cancer can spread around the body by:

- invading local tissues
- entering the lymphatic system and lymph nodes
- entering the bloodstream and travelling to distant sites
- direct infiltration of a neighbouring organ.

Some cancers have a predictable route of spread and favour certain organs for secondaries whereas others are more unpredictable.

Assessing your situation

Working out the chances of your treatment being successful is difficult because the response to treatment varies considerably from one person to another. However, the three essentials that guide your outcome are the:

- primary site of the tumour
- stage of the tumour
- grade of the tumour.

Another important piece of information is how you respond to treatment. There are four types of response and you will hear the following terms being used:

- A 'complete response' is where the tumour has disappeared completely
- A 'partial response' is where it has shrunk to half its size, as visualized by X-rays or some other quantifiable measure
- 'Stable disease' means that the disease is not growing
- 'Progressive disease' means that growth is continuing despite treatment.

Following surgery, if the primary tumour has been completely removed, then technically the patient has had a complete response. With chemotherapy, it is vital to assess response early on in the course of treatment to make sure there will be benefit and that it is worthwhile to continue the treatment.

Choosing Your Cancer Treatment

Cancer statistics

The best way to assess the cure rate for a particular type of cancer is to look at survival curves compared with those who do not have cancer. If 100 patients with lung cancer are treated and we look at their survival curve, it will be clear that they do less well than those of the same age without lung cancer. The definition of 'cure' means that the survival rate of a treated group of patients is the same as those of similar age and gender who did not have cancer.

Getting information about your cancer

As already discussed in previous chapters, people with cancer vary greatly in the amount of information they wish to receive about their illness. Most doctors have come to respect their patients' preferences, and most cancer specialists try to answer questions as honestly as they can. Because people differ greatly in their needs, the oncology team will generally be tentative as to how much information to impart to you until they get to know you, and what your needs and preferences are. This is to avoid giving information to those who don't want it.

You therefore need to make sure that you let them know exactly how much you want to know, and initiate discussions about any aspects they may not be covering. The team will take their cues from you. As you encourage good communication, you will find they will do their best to meet your needs. This is not easy at a stressful time, so having somebody with you and a list of questions you need to have answered will be helpful.

To get the information you want, you have to know what to ask. This is a major problem especially at a time when you are feeling emotionally vulnerable. Many people are unfamiliar with the workings of a car, but are quite happy to nod wisely while the mechanic explains in technical terms what is wrong. But with cancer, you cannot just do that. Having a reasonable understanding of your options makes good sense, and getting information often requires tenacity and persistence. Some doctors and clinics just won't seem to tell you anything – partly because there is often never enough time. Giving information takes time, especially if it is a genuine dialogue between the doctor and patient. However, it is your life we are talking about, so arming yourself with information is an important way to empower yourself and get yourself back in control.

Living as we do in a consumer age, you have a right to expect high-quality information that allows you to explore different avenues. So, to get to grips with your situation, see the Resources Directory for recommended websites, and other resources for the information you need to guide you to integrated medicine doctors who can help you review your options.

Alternatively, use the Cancer Options team (see the Resources Directory) and have specialist cancer nurses do the research for you, break down the information into clear, readable formats and provide background explanations to the treatments. They can also advise you on how to discuss the treatments with your doctors, how to go about getting a second opinion and how to get into clinical trials. They can then provide you with a report and work through it with you until you feel happy and confident that you have received all the information you need to decide on your best treatment plan.

Another useful method is networking. People diagnosed with cancer often feel they are alone. Yet, once they start discussing their situation with others, they are often surprised to find how many other people known to them or their families are also dealing with cancer. So, find out from them where they are getting their information. They may be using the Internet or specific cancer charities and support groups. However, it is always worth remembering that everyone's cancer is unique to some degree, and treatments and progress cannot be compared specifically.

Chapter 5 on alternative cancer medicines will provide access to further information with which to arm yourself as you make your treatment choices.

A cancer question checklist

Comprehensive lists of questions to ask your doctors are given in Chapter 3 and cover:

- your cancer
- your treatment options
- the nature of your treatment once you have chosen.

Nowadays, most cancer doctors tend to avoid giving estimates of survival time as individuals are very different, and there is a risk that a time given by 'the voice of authority' may become a self-fulfilling prophecy. Rather than having a timescale ticking away in the background, focusing on your recovery is essential.

Getting a second opinion

Doctors often disagree, which may seem surprising, but medicine is still in many ways an art rather than science. There are several ways in which the same result can be achieved, and cancer medicine is no exception. Many large centres have case conferences where individual patients are discussed and treatment options reviewed. There is regular disagreement on even the simplest decisions, such as whether to recommend radiotherapy after an operation or how many doses of chemotherapy should be given. Where doctors don't yet have the knowledge, clinical trials are set up to try and determine the best way to treat a certain type of cancer. Doctors have to come up with the best treatment plan for each person, with constantly moving goalposts as treatment techniques and drugs are continuously evolving.

Variations in treatments are offered by different NHS doctors, and you may also choose to get your treatment privately. Treatment approaches vary around the world and you may feel you would like to look further afield to:

- check that the treatment being offered to you is considered the best regime available
- establish if any other countries have any new developments or technology not yet available in your country
- look at other treatments to see what fits best into your personal approach and value system.

To find out what other options are available to you, you can:

- explain your preferences to your doctor and ask him to find you other options to be looked into
- use your own resources and information to research what is available and discuss it with your team
- use the UK Cancer Options team to do your research and work through the choices with your doctors.

There are several issues to consider when looking at your options:

- Would you be prepared to have treatment in another part of the country?
- Would you be prepared to have treatment abroad?
- Do you have any financial resources that can be used to increase your options?

No doctor of any standing will be offended if you ask for a second opinion in your own country. We all realize the complexity of modern medicine and that no one is infallible. If you are not happy with what is being proposed, ask for a second opinion. It will save time and money to take all your test results and a letter with your complete medical summary about your condition with you.

You can either leave the choice of who you see for a second opinion to your doctor, or you can use the websites in the Resources Directory or the Cancer Options team to find top specialists for your kind of cancer, then request a referral from your GP to the doctor of your choice.

Taking your time

After researching and gathering the information you need, making your decisions will take time. It may take you a few weeks to gather all the details you need to work out the best treatment plan for you. Unfortunately, this often conflicts with the natural urge and pressure from others to take quick and decisive action, and begin your treatment as soon as possible. Nevertheless, remember that many people have done this and, later on when they have looked around and have a greater understanding of cancer, wished they had taken more time to look at the pros and cons of each treatment option. The fact that you are reading this book shows that you are already taking a careful and measured approach to choosing your treatments.

If you have only just been diagnosed, taking the time to consider the future implications of your treatment and your own personal philosophy of how you want to deal with your cancer, and devising a treatment plan that suits you may be the most valuable time you spend to ensure your longer-term well-being.

However, especially when first diagnosed, you may feel unsure if it will be detrimental for you not to start treatment immediately. It would be worthwhile checking how much time you can take safely with your own doctor or an integrated medicine consultant (see the Resources Directory pages 351–3).

Explain that you wish to consider all the options available and ask them the following questions:

- How aggressive is my tumour and how fast is it growing?
- How long would you estimate my cancer has been there?
- Do you feel it would be detrimental to postpone action for a few weeks while I look at all the options? (If the answer is yes, ask why. What do they think will happen to your cancer during the delay?)

If you are considering treatments that are beyond your doctor's field of expertise, such as immunotherapy or intravenous metabolic treatment, you may find that some doctors will not consider them a worthy alternative, and will try to influence you into looking only at more conventional treatments. You need to be sure that you are getting a balanced and reasoned opinion. Sadly, it is not unusual for a doctor to write off a treatment approach while having absolutely no knowledge of what it's about. Conversely, some alternative doctors may be overly dismissive of the value of conventional medical treatment. In this case, arrange to speak to an integrated medicine doctor who is genuinely committed to getting you the very best of both worlds – orthodox and alternative.

Discussing complementary and alternative options

While your doctor may be happy to discuss various orthodox treatments, a frequently different reaction may appear when you bring up the subject of integrating alternative treatments with what he has to offer.

Ideally, your doctor will be receptive and open to what you want to consider. If he has no knowledge of a particular treatment or approach, he should welcome any information you can supply him and study it. He can then consider whether there are any contraindications to using it alongside orthodox treatments, and he can engage in an informed discussion with you about formulating a treatment plan which best meets all of your needs.

However, this scenario is not typical of what happens to the majority of people who try to discuss integrating their cancer treatments with their doctors. You may encounter a number of reactions, ranging from dismissal to an outright declaration that what you are considering is rubbish and a waste of money. So, you need to be prepared with the right attitude to achieve the best possible working relationship on this matter.

Attend the appointment armed with as much information and research evidence about the treatments you are considering as possible. If your doctor dismisses the treatments out of hand, ask him:

- How much does he actually know about the treatment?
- On what evidence is he basing his opinion?

If your doctor has little knowledge of the treatment, offer him the information so that he can give you an informed opinion. If he offers you a sound reason why he considers your proposed treatments unsuitable for you, or has reason to doubt the reliability of the treatment or practitioner, that may be information you need to know. If, however, your doctor displays pure prejudice, then you have to consider whether this particular doctor is going to be the best person for you to work with.

The words 'working with' are key here. If you feel you are unlikely to develop a partnership with your doctor without feeling compromised, then you might want to think about changing to a team that will better fit your needs. Though this may seem drastic and difficult to consider when feeling under pressure, bear in mind how important it is that, in the long term, you are involved in your own decision-making process, that your opinion is listened to and that you are 'choosing your treatment', not being 'given it'.

In summary, when diagnosed with cancer and evaluating treatment options:

- Get the facts about your illness
- Make a list of questions you want answered (see Chapter 3)
- Ask to see the consultant (rather than the juniors) responsible for your care
- Do not be afraid to ask anything, but let your team know how much you want to know
- Insist on being told the truth
- Make sure you know what alternative and complementary approaches are available
- Take a relative or close friend with you to make notes (or take a cassette recorder, although this might be intimidating for medical staff and often means that their answers will be far more guarded)
- Discuss any queries with your GP
- If you are not happy about any aspect of your care, tell your doctors or the cancer services manager of the unit where you are being treated
- Talk to nurses, radiographers and pharmacists, who are often useful sources of information and have more time to explain things that you may not have understood in the short time spent with the doctor
- If you are unsure about what to do, ask to see the consultant again or seek a second or third opinion
- Take steps to prepare and support yourself and your immune system throughout your treatment programme (see Chapter 7).

Current Medical Treatments

The main treatments used currently for cancer are:

- surgery
- radiotherapy
- chemotherapy
- hormone therapy.

Surgery

Often, the first step in cancer treatment is surgery. The aim of cancer surgery is to remove the whole tumour, leaving behind as much of the normal tissue as possible. The tumour must be removed in its entirety for the operation to be a success and the pathology department must find that there are clear margins of healthy tissue around the entire tumour. If not, then further surgery will usually be recommended.

You may have heard that operating on a tumour can encourage it to spread. That is a consideration your surgeon will take into account, and great care will be taken to minimize the risk of spread during surgery. If your surgeon thinks this might have occurred, he may well recommend that you have follow-up systemic treatment, such as chemotherapy, to take care of it.

Both orthodox and integrated cancer doctors agree that the risk of cancer spreading during surgery is far outweighed by the risk of leaving the tumour to continue to grow, metastasize and cause further problems. New evidence also shows that existing tumours secrete proteins that can facilitate secondary growth in other organs. So, the removal of all possible cancer from the body is vital.

Success with cancer surgery comes from knowing exactly how much tissue needs to be removed, so an accurate assessment of tumour size and shape is essential before deciding on the type of operation for your particular type of cancer.

Cancer Surgery: The Key Issues

- Find out what sort of operation is being proposed.
- Establish how experienced and skilled at this type of surgery your surgeon is.
- Find out if there are any new developments in surgery for that operation.
- Find out how long you will need to be in hospital and need to take off work afterwards.
- If you are having surgery done privately, make sure you know all the costs involved.
- If you have health insurance, make sure in advance that all the fees will be covered.
- Do not sign the consent form to surgery unless you fully understand what is being proposed and the potential long-term side-effects.
- Make sure you are prepared physically, psychologically and practically before you undergo the operation (see Chapter 7).

If you are told your tumour is inoperable, you should certainly consider getting a second or even a third opinion. There may be a great variance in opinion, depending on the particular surgeon's skill and experience, and certain hospitals specialize in certain types of cancer. You may find a surgeon who is specialized in your particular type of cancer and is highly skilled in removing difficult tumours. For example, some neurologists will operate to remove bony secondary tumours from the spine and reconstruct the vertebra using a titanium prosthesis whereas, in other places, only radiotherapy is on offer. Your scans and X-rays can also be sent to specialists in other countries for their opinion of the possible surgical help for more complex tumours.

Following Surgery

If your tumour has been completely removed and no spreading to other tissues is detected, you may not need follow-up treatment. However, you will usually be offered either or both radiotherapy and chemotherapy, as well as hormone therapy if your tumour is hormone-dependent.

Radiotherapy

Radiotherapy uses ionizing radiation in the form of X-rays to treat cancer. Wilhem Roentgen discovered X-rays in 1895. Within a year, they were being used in the treatment of cancer. We have come a long way since then, and radiotherapy for cancer treatment is now incredibly sophisticated. Often, radiotherapy is given to effect a complete cure – called radical radiotherapy. Alternatively, it can be used after surgery to 'mop up' any stray cancer cells persisting around the operation site. Another important use of radiotherapy is for symptom control in palliative care.

Types of Radiotherapy

The most common type of radiotherapy is the use of an external radiation source produced by a linear accelerator, a large machine that delivers a precise dose of radiation to a particular site of the body. An alternative form uses internal radiation, where a radioactive source – such as radioactive needles or 'seeds' – is temporarily placed in the part of the body affected by tumour, such as the womb or prostate gland.

Different types of X-rays are used as each has a different level of penetration. Laboratory evidence tells us that radiotherapy works by damaging DNA in the nucleus of rapidly dividing cells. The DNA molecule has a particular sequence, creating a vital code for proteins that have important functions both inside and outside the cell. Radiation breaks the 'backbone' of the DNA molecule so that, when the strands join back together, the coding sequence is altered, resulting in the cell's death. It only affects cells that are reproducing, which is why radiotherapy is given in multiple doses – to catch the cells at different phases of their growth cycle.

Radiotherapy damages cancer cells whereas normal tissue is usually able to repair itself. We have learned how to exploit this difference, and establish a balance between destroying cancer cells while causing minimal damage to normal tissues. Also, the delivery systems for radiation are now so precise that it is almost possible to irradiate only the tumour. However, if the individual survives for some time after radiotherapy, it is possible for a new, different second cancer to arise as a result of the radiotherapy treatment.

The Radiotherapy Process

A consultant radiotherapist will be in charge of your radiotherapy treatment and will help with decision-making. So, discuss any problems or questions you have with him. When receiving radiotherapy, the radiographers who deliver the treatment will see you on a daily basis. They are an excellent source of information and can often be far more helpful than the consultant. Despite a lot of adverse publicity, radiotherapy is a remarkably safe form of treatment. There are clear guidelines for the calibration of the machines, and it is a legal requirement that the machines be frequently checked.

Having decided on radiotherapy, the next part of the process is the planning. This is usually done on a machine called a 'simulator', which simulates your treatment on the X-ray therapy machine to set up the exact position of the intended treatment. The area to be treated is marked on your skin with an indelible pen so that the markings last throughout the treatment period. However, if the areas are complicated or where marks are unsightly or less likely to stay put, a perspex shell can be contoured to fit your body precisely and act as a marker. This shell can also prevent even the slightest movement during treatment so that the X-ray beam only strikes those tissues it is supposed to hit. If intended for the head, holes are cut out of the shell to leave your eyes, nose and mouth uncovered.

As no two individuals are the same, do not be alarmed if you compare notes with others and find that your radiotherapy is different from theirs. There are all sorts of reasons for this. If you are at all worried, question the radiographers during one of your visits or ask to see the consultant oncologist who has planned your treatment.

Different centres may use different machines, with larger centres having a wider choice for more specialized treatments. But it may be appropriate to be treated at a small centre nearer home to cut down on the hours spent travelling to and from the hospital each day. Once again, a relative-benefit evaluation needs to be done, involving both you and your doctor.

If the most important aspect of treatment is the cosmetic result, then this may necessitate a lengthier treatment using a relatively lower dose to avoid long-term skin damage from the radiation. However, if the final appearance is not of concern and the area being treated is very small, it may be possible to have a shorter course of radiotherapy using a higher dose. Radiotherapy treatment is flexible, and it is important that the patient makes his needs apparent at the outset so that the consultant can tailor the treatment appropriately.

New research by Professor Kedar N. Prasad in the US has shown that, far from potentially diminishing the effectiveness of chemo- and radiotherapy, high-dose vitamin and mineral therapy can potentiate both forms of treatment. This is because the abnormal tumour cells become more vulnerable after having taken up high levels of antioxidants (see Chapter 5).

Side-effects of Radiotherapy

A full description of remedies to reduce the side-effects of radiotherapy are found in Chapter 7.

Fatigue and Nausea

One side-effect that many people experience during their radiotherapy treatment is general fatigue and nausea. This is thought to be due to:

- your body having to work harder as cells are destroyed
- the toxicity of the radiation
- the disruption to your body's natural energy fields.

So, you should not be at all surprised if you need an extra two or three hours of sleep every day, and spiritual healing to lift your energy and spirits. See Chapter 7 for ways to help your body cope with this treatment with the help of homoeopathic remedies and acupuncture, which releases the stored heat and energy radiotherapy causes.

Nausea may be experienced at the beginning of treatment, but this should gradually improve with time. This may occur especially when a large part of the body is being treated, and is particularly common during radiotherapy to the abdomen, although it may also arise when having treatment to nearby areas.

Skin Burns

With skin cancer, the area being treated is likely to be affected by the radiation, leaving your skin red and sore, rather like sunburn, towards the end of treatment. (Again, for information on helpful radiation cream, see Chapter 7.) Individuals vary in their sensitivity to radiation.

The same dose may produce a severe skin reaction in one person and only a mild reaction in another. As a rule, symptoms are worse towards the end of treatment, often reaching a peak after four or five weeks.

Difficulties with Eating and Drinking

If treatment affects your oesophagus or throat, you may find it becomes rather inflamed and sore. This is because radiotherapy initially causes an inflammatory reaction. You may have difficulty swallowing, and find eating and drinking painful. Discuss this with your doctor to try and prevent this as much as possible, as this problem is unpleasant and can make you feel miserable. A nutritional advisor would be helpful at this time for advice on suitable food, drinks and remedies, and also to support you if the going gets tough. Again, see Chapter 7 for any complementary therapies that may help. You may also experience diarrhoea if the bowel is irradiated.

Possible Flare-up of Symptoms

Because the effect of radiotherapy builds up over weeks and because the tissues being irradiated become inflamed, your initial symptoms may temporarily get worse before they get better. For example, if the problem is a bony secondary tumour pressing on a nerve, then, for up to six weeks post-treatment, the pain or nerve impairment may get worse. But as the inflammation subsides, relief will be experienced.

Infertility

Radiotherapy to the reproductive organs may affect your ability to have children. Some effects are transient and return to normal after a while, whereas others are permanent. If you are considering having children in the future, check with your doctor about the possible risks, and find out what steps can be taken to aid fertility in the future. For example, men may wish to have sperm frozen for use later or, for women, egg collection and later IVF (*in vitro* fertilization) may be considered.

Limitations of Radiotherapy

Tumours are given a dose of radiotherapy that is close to the maximum tolerated by the normal tissues in the area being treated. The risk of damage to normal tissue is the major factor limiting the dose of radiotherapy given. There is also an overall limit to how much radiation can be given to one area or the whole body.

Should the tumour recur, further radiotherapy to the previously treated area may then exceed the normal tissue tolerance, so it is unusual to be able to repeat a course of treatment if there is a recurrence in the same place. Especially sensitive structures include the brain, spinal cord, lungs, liver and bone marrow, and great care is taken not to cause radiation damage in such areas.

It can be very frustrating for someone who responded well to radiotherapy the first time not to be able to have further radiotherapy for a tumour recurrence at the same site.

Radiotherapy, like surgery, is a form of local treatment. So if the tumour has spread beyond the confines of its primary site, radiotherapy cannot be considered a curative treatment.

Palliative Radiotherapy for Symptom Control

Radiotherapy is often used to control symptoms in a palliative setting. In general, palliative care is aimed at improving your comfort and quality of life. Palliative radiotherapy is given in short bursts or sometimes as only a single treatment.

Radiotherapy can be very effective for pain relief, especially of that caused by bone metastases. Studies have shown that single treatments for pain can be as effective for many symptoms as a long drawn-out course requiring many hospital visits. If you are in any doubt as to the usefulness of radiotherapy for your symptoms, ask the oncologist, the radiographers or a palliative care consultant.

Here is a checklist of questions for the radiotherapist:

- What is the treatment being offered?
- When will the treatment be planned?
- How long will this take?
- When will the treatment start?
- How many treatments will I have and how long will each one last?
- Can I drive myself to treatments and, if so, where can I park my car?
- Can I stay in hospital or in a hostel nearby during my treatment period?
- Can I choose the time I will be treated each day?
- Are there any days that I will not be treated?
- What are the immediate side-effects and what should I do about them?
- Will it affect my fertility?
- Is there anything I should avoid, such as sunbathing, swimming or washing?
- When will I next see a doctor?
- What happens when I finish the course of treatment?
- Is there any support available if I am frightened or upset during treatment?

Leading-edge Developments in Radiotherapy Treatments

There are ever-changing and more sophisticated methods of tackling cancer cells with radiotherapy. However, some of the treatments described here have not yet reached the UK.

Intensity Modulated Radiation Therapy

This is precision radiotherapy that targets the tumour with a high dose over less time. Because it is so precise, it reduces radiation exposure to healthy tissues.

In addition to boosting effectiveness, the combination of accuracy and increased dose also cuts treatment time by 90 per cent compared with conventional radiotherapy. This significantly reduces side-effects and improves tolerance of treatment.

Treatment outcomes are expected to be the same as with standard radiotherapy. So far, this has been used on a wide range of tumours, with much better cosmetic effects when used on breast cancer. It is likely to become a standard method in the future.

Its main disadvantage – as with any precise treatment at this time – is that your doctor has to be absolutely certain that he is able to target the entire tumour within the exact treatment field. If this is not possible, your doctor may choose to use a more conventional form of radiotherapy.

Intraoperative Radiotherapy

Intraoperative treatments involve a miniature X-ray source inserted into the body during surgery to administer the radiotherapeutic dose.

This may be used to apply radiotherapy to where the surgeon has just removed a tumour or to a space where a tumour has been removed previously. While this treatment has been around for a while, new developments mean that more precise technology can deliver the radiotherapy to the appropriate tissue without damaging the surrounding areas.

Radiofrequency Ablation

This uses electrical energy to create heat at a specific location up to a specific temperature and for a specific period of time and, ultimately, results in the death of unwanted tissue.

The ablation probe is placed directly into the tumour tissue. The radiofrequency energy flows through electrodes, causing ionic agitation and, therefore, friction in the nearby tissue. This friction creates heat and, once sufficient temperatures have been reached, the heat will kill the target tissue within a matter of minutes.

This procedure can be used for liver tumours:

- by putting an electrode through the skin and using an ultrasound, CT or MRI scanner to guide the needle to the tumour
- during open abdominal surgery, when the specialist has direct access to the liver
- during a laparoscopic or 'keyhole' surgical technique.

Heat is a very effective means of killing cancer tissue. As tissue temperatures rise above 113°F (50°C), protein is permanently damaged and cell membranes fuse. The process is rapid, typically requiring less than 10–15 minutes of exposure for a 3-cm tumour. This can be done without causing too much damage to surrounding tissues. There are some specialists in the UK who use this procedure, but it is only useful for tumours that are 5 cm or less in size.

Effects are similar to that of a microwave, where heat is generated from the inside out. Destroyed cells are reabsorbed by the body over time.

Therasphere

This is a system whereby millions of microscopic glass beads embedded with a radioactive element are delivered directly into the blood vessels feeding a tumour.

It is currently used for tumours in the liver – both primary and secondary. The tiny beads (one-third the diameter of a human hair) are passed through a catheter placed in the femoral artery (in the thigh). They are then guided via the hepatic artery (the main blood vessel in the liver) to the blood vessel supplying the tumour. The beads remain in the body and lose their radiation within two weeks.

Patients can return home the same day, and there is no risk to family members. Possible side-effects include vomiting, mild fever, abdominal pain and gastric ulcers but, so far, the main complaints have been fatigue and nausea.

Clinical trials in many different countries so far show that patients are living twice as long with this treatment – and with good quality of life. It has also been successfully combined with chemotherapy. There have even been one or two recorded incidences where a liver cancer had shrunk sufficiently to become operable, or potentially curable. Its limitations, as with all forms of treatments involving radiation, are related to the size and volume of the tumour, as too large a tumour would require an unsafe dose of radiation.

Fractionated Stereotactic Radiosurgery

This is a non-invasive therapy for brain tumours that, in the past, have been very difficult to treat. It directs precisely guided beams of radiation from many hundreds of different angles to converge on the tumour. It is called radiosurgery because the surgeon uses the radiation beams like a knife to cut out the tumour. By focusing these beams from so many different positions, the effects on the normal healthy brain and tissue are minimized while striking only the target with the prescribed treatment.

The main difference between standard radiation and fractionated stereotactic radiosurgery is that standard radiation will also irradiate large amounts of normal healthy brain compared with radiosurgery, which is focused almost exclusively on the tumour.

This approach is also proving effective for treating tumours of the head and neck, where there are many important nerves and structures very close together in one area.

Traditional surgery may result in a degree of facial paralysis and functional loss, so this form of treatment, if available, is highly desirable.

Brachytherapy

This is being used for prostate cancer that has been detected early and not spread beyond the gland. In this case, tiny radioactive 'seeds' or pellets, containing radioactive iodine, are implanted directly into the middle of the cancer via thin needles, where they will keep on giving off radiation for up to a year. Up to a hundred pellets are implanted through the skin, under either a spinal or general anaesthetic.

The radioactivity of the pellets slowly decays during the months after the operation; few long-term risks have been reported with this treatment.

Chemotherapy

We have seen how surgery and radiotherapy are used to deal with disease that is localized in a particular area. But if the disease has spread, or metastasized, then the treatment has to reach all parts of the body to eliminate cancer cells wherever they have lodged. Such treatments are called 'systemic', as they go right round the system. Since the 1940s, around 150 drugs with anti-cancer effects have been developed. They act in various ways to destroy or slow down the growth of rapidly dividing cancer cells.

There are several ways in which different types of anti-cancer drugs work:

- by preventing the DNA in the cancer cell nucleus from being copied, a vital process for cell division and growth of the tumour
- by depleting the cancer cell of the building blocks for DNA so that fewer raw materials are available for DNA to replicate itself
- by preventing the binding of enzymes that enable the production of key protein molecules in the cancer cells

- by blocking protein synthesis, especially those that maintain healthy cell activity as well as cell division.

The Discovery of Anti-cancer Drugs

The majority of anti-cancer drugs were discovered by accident. Initially, a few were designed specifically to inhibit tumour cell growth, but this is now changing.

Many successful cancer drugs come from natural sources – adriamycin comes from a fungus found on buildings on the Adriatic coast; vincristine originated from the pretty blue *Vinca* (periwinkle) plant, often seen in English gardens; taxol and taxotere, collectively called taxanes, were derived from the Pacific yew tree – and were also found by accident. There are now several other derivatives synthesized in the laboratory.

Chemotherapy Regimes

Chemotherapy is often given as a mixture of two or three drugs in a fixed pattern, known as a 'chemotherapy regime'. There are many regimes, which are constantly changing, as research is ongoing to define the optimal combinations for the best effects. Specific regimes are not covered here as they would quickly become out of date. Once you know what chemotherapy drugs your oncologist is offering, further information about them can be obtained from:

- CancerBACUP. This organization has excellent leaflets about the various anti-cancer drugs, and a website with a comprehensive section on chemotherapy (www.cancerbacup.org.uk)
- Pharmacologists in the information departments of major hospitals
- Part 2 of the Resources Directory. This lists other useful websites and resources for more information about your treatment
- The UK Cancer Options team, which offers in-depth information, including the results of clinical trials using the drugs, the rates of responses, and how frequent and severe the side-effects were. It will also research the clinical evidence for you and let you have the facts.

Administration of Chemotherapy

There are several ways drugs can be given for cancer. Some can be taken as pills or capsules, but the majority are given through an intravenous drip. They may sometimes be delivered straight into a body cavity such as the bladder or abdomen. Most can now be given via an outpatients clinic.

Chemotherapy suites with comfortable reclining chairs and a bright, supportive atmosphere have sprung up throughout cancer-treatment centres. These are usually run by nurses, who are expert at dealing with the administration of chemotherapy. They are huge founts of knowledge about the side-effects, any likely problems that may be encountered and how to deal with them creatively.

The Side-effects of Chemotherapy
Effects on Fast-growing Tissues
Because tumour cells are so close in structure and function to normal cells, it is not surprising that any drug that reduces cancer growth also affects normal cells. This means that many cancer drugs have very potent side-effects, and are only prescribed by specialists in the field. Anti-cancer drugs inhibit cell turnover in general and so affect most severely the most rapidly dividing cells in the body. These include those in the bone marrow that form blood cells, and those in the lining of the intestines, skin and hair follicles. A depressed immune system is common with many anti-cancer agents because of their effect on bone marrow. Therefore, when considering your treatment plan and assessing your tolerance levels, you may wish to consider how to offset this effect on immune function by immune stimulation (see Chapters 5 and 7).

Nausea, Vomiting and Diarrhoea
The side-effects of chemotherapy are nausea, vomiting, diarrhoea and fatigue, from both the immediate shock to the tissues and bodily systems, and your body's ongoing natural reaction to expel toxic substances from the body. This is the same mechanism that comes into play when you inadvertently eat something that gives you food poisoning, and is a normal defence mechanism.

Infertility
As with radiotherapy, there are potential effects to your fertility that can be permanent. If infertility is unacceptable to you, make sure you check this before starting the chemo, and look into the other options available.

Depression
Often not mentioned, this can be a direct result of the depressant effects of chemo. It is therefore vital to set up a good emotional support network while going through chemotherapy.

Tiredness

Receiving chemotherapy can be very tiring, and it is helpful to boost your energy with healing. Be prepared to limit your social and work output.

Dealing with Side-effects

How you handle the side-effects of chemotherapy comes down to your personal levels of endurance and your personal philosophy of treatment. The drugs given to deal with these side-effects are usually a combination of anti-sickness tablets and steroids, taken for only a few days.

These are given with two main objectives:

1. To make you feel more comfortable
2. To help the body retain the drug long enough to kill the cancer cells.

Your oncologist will be giving you a measured dose of chemotherapy according to your body mass. The aim is to give you as large a dose as you can tolerate while deriving the most benefit.

This is where generalizations should end and your role begins.

When you first begin chemotherapy, there will be a period of adjustment, at which time you report your symptoms while the side-effect medication is altered to find what works best. Some of the undermining effects of chemotherapy, such as fatigue, nausea and depression, can worsen as the treatment continues. You will also then notice effects on your body, mind and spirit, and your ability to cope with these problems may also change. Sometimes you will cope very well, and feel determined and strong; at other times, you may find it more of a struggle, and need to call on your support team and self-help plans to get you through it.

It is important to ensure that your levels of tolerance are communicated to your doctor, as he will want to give you as much chemo as you can tolerate. But the only guide he has is the feedback from you. Tolerance varies from person to person, and you may require a dose alteration to be able to carry on with your treatment. You must make sure that you tell your doctor if you feel the toxicity is too much for you. Frequently, people suffer at home between courses and then play down how bad it was for them. While stoicism may be an attribute and your desire to receive an effective treatment natural, you should be aware of the need to look after yourself in a measured way. Taken to an extreme, ignoring or 'toughing out' bad reactions to chemo may even be fatal!

New Developments in Chemotherapy

Preoperative Chemotherapy

A development that is proving successful is to give a course of chemotherapy prior to surgery. This can shrink the tumour, making it easier to operate within good safety margins. It has proved useful for cancers of the oesophagus and bowel, and its potential is being considered for other types of cancer. It is likely that tumours removed post-chemotherapy are also safer as they are less likely to cause recurrence by shedding active cancer cells.

Under review is a system called 'chronomodulated therapy' whereby a regime of four different chemotherapy drugs are given according to a strict dosing schedule. Results have been very good, but it is not yet clear whether this will become a standard treatment.

Preoperative chemotherapy is not suitable for everyone as it can be quite taxing on the body, but it is likely to become more widely used.

Rotating Regimes

As already mentioned, cancer cells can build up resistance to chemotherapy. In the past, this has meant moving on to another batch of drugs until the availability of suitable treatments is exhausted.

Many oncologists are now having success by rotating the drugs you receive. They have found that, by going back to a drug after stopping it for a period of time, cancer-cell resistance has decreased.

Hepatic Artery Infusion

For cancer of the liver, infusing the chemotherapy directly into the hepatic artery may be an option. The hepatic is the main artery feeding into the liver and carries a large blood supply. The chemo is delivered directly into a small catheter placed into this artery. This has the potential advantage of delivering higher doses of anti-cancer drugs straight to the cancer cells while avoiding the side-effects of chemotherapy delivered systemically (throughout the body).

Following the chemotherapy infusion, embolization is performed, which involves placing a small gelatin sponge into the relevant hepatic artery to block further blood flow to the cancer. This reduces the volume of blood going to the cancer, allowing the chemo to spread throughout the tumour and remain there in sufficient concentrations without being washed away too quickly.

These liver-directed treatment approaches are highly specialized procedures and, when performed by experienced professionals, have produced encouraging results.

Chemotherapy Gel

An injectable gel containing the chemo has proved effective for cancer in the region of the head and neck, traditionally considered an area where cancer is difficult to treat.

When the drug cisplatin is given intravenously, it is known to have severe side-effects, but when the gel is injected directly into the tumour, these side-effects are greatly reduced.

Hormone therapy

Hormone blockade can be used to inhibit the growth of hormone-dependent cancers. Hormones are chemical messengers produced by the endocrine glands, including the pituitary at the base of the brain, the thyroid in the neck, the adrenals above the kidneys, the ovaries in women and the testes in men. Many hormones control the normal growth of specific tissues. For example, the female sex hormone oestrogen is produced by the ovaries, and stimulates the growth of cells in the breast and lining of the womb.

In 1896, George Beatson, a Scottish surgeon, removed the ovaries of two young women with advanced breast cancer. In both cases, the disease stopped growing and disappeared. Although the tumours later returned, this was the first demonstration that changing the circulating levels of hormones could be effective against cancer. Since then, anti-hormonal therapy has been widely used for cancers in tissue susceptible to hormonal influences such as the breast, prostate and uterus.

There are five ways to influence hormonal activity:

1. Destroy the gland that produces the hormone by surgery, radiotherapy or drugs
2. Stop production of the hormone chemically, using drugs such as Arimidex and Zoladex, as in the case of breast cancer
3. Change the hormonal balance of the body – for example, female hormones are used for prostate cancer to reduce the growth of male hormone-driven tissues, and many women treat oestrogen-sensitive tumours with progesterone (but only if the tumour is NOT progesterone-positive). Removing oestrogen-sensitive tumours during the second half of the menstrual cycle, when there are high levels of progesterone, also lowers the risk of future metastases. This is presumably because there is a less receptive climate in the body for the seeding of new growths.
4. Use drugs that block the effects of hormones. For hormones to work, they have to interact with receptors in the target tissue working rather like a lock and key do. If another agent fits the same lock, but does not activate it, the effect of the hormone is effectively blocked. Such agents are called 'anti-hormones'. The best example is tamoxifen, which blocks the action of

oestrogen, and is often used to treat breast cancer. Another is bicalutamide, which blocks the action of the male hormone androgen to encourage prostate cancer cell growth.

5. Change the balance of hormone production. This can be done naturally with indole-3-carbinol, derived from plants such as cabbage and broccoli. It changes oestrogen metabolism to favour the production of milder forms of oestrogen (oestriol and oestrone) rather than the more stimulatory form (oestradiol).

Not all tumours respond to hormone treatment, not even those arising in hormonal tissue. Hormone treatment has fewer side-effects than chemotherapy, as there is no bone marrow depression or hair loss. For this reason, hormones are often used as the main form of therapy for those tumours likely to respond. However, tamoxifen itself carries a 5–10 per cent risk of causing cancer of the womb lining (endometrium), so the womb needs to be monitored regularly by ultrasound throughout this form of treatment.

The problem with most chemotherapy and hormone treatment for common tumours is that they tend to stop the disease for only a limited period of time. Resistance can develop, allowing the disease to recur after a time.

Newer Treatment Approaches

The recent developments in cancer therapy are moving us away from radiotherapy and chemotherapy, which have been the mainstays of treatment for some time. Scientists are rapidly increasing their knowledge about the complex life and workings of the cancer cell. As their understanding grows, specific treatments are emerging that will eventually enable cancer to be treated much more effectively and with much less damage to the body.

Laser therapy

Lasers generate light energy to destroy tumours. A fibreoptic cable is placed within a tumour, and light from the laser is passed through the cable, resulting in heat that can destroy a spherical mass of tissue surrounding the laser tip. The amount of laser energy needed to destroy the entire tumour can be calculated according to the size of the tumour (including a margin of healthy tissue). The procedure has been performed safely with minimal pain, and is a form of hyperthermia.

Laser-induced Interstitial Thermotherapy

One of the most recent developments in laser therapy, it uses the same idea as hyperthermia (heat treatment) – using heat to help shrink tumours by damaging the cells or depriving them of substances they need to live. In this treatment, lasers are directed to interstitial areas (between organs) in the body. The laser light then raises the temperature of the tumour, which damages or destroys the cancer cells.

Cancers currently being treated with lasers include cancers of the:

- vocal cords
- cervix
- skin
- lungs
- vagina
- vulva
- penis.

Laser Surgery for Head, Neck and Throat Cancers

Laser surgery to treat some throat cancers is less risky than conventional surgery, and offers a better quality of life afterwards as it avoids the invasive treatment and potential disfigurement that previous surgery entailed.

Many types of head and neck cancers can be treated by laser. Whereas early on only small early tumours were treated with this technology, further developments have meant that more advanced tumours can now be excised with lasers.

With the new technique, the surgeon uses a natural passageway such as the mouth rather than an incision to reach the tumour. Special fibreoptic videoscopes and a 'micromanipulator' tool allow the surgeon to guide the laser beam around the edges of the tumour with pinpoint accuracy.

Radiotherapy and chemotherapy are often used in combination with laser surgery to treat mouth and throat cancers.

Laser Treatment for Breast Cancer and Palliative Care

We will see lasers playing an increasingly major role in surgical techniques over the next few years. Laser therapy for small breast tumours, rather than a lumpectomy, is already an option in some parts of the US.

In addition to its use to destroy the cancer, laser surgery can also relieve symptoms caused by cancer (palliative care). For example, lasers can shrink a tumour blocking the windpipe, making it easier to breathe. It may also ease colorectal and anal cancers. We are likely to see more use of laser treatments as more doctors become trained in its use.

Cryotherapy/cryosurgery

Occasionally performed with a laparoscope, cryosurgery is usually done during open surgery. It destroys tumours (including a margin of healthy tissue) by freezing them.

Probes are placed directly into the tumour and supercooled liquid nitrogen or argon gas is pumped through the probes to freeze the target area. The cancer cells crystallize, which damages their cell membranes, and thawing causes further damage. Usually, two 'freeze–thaw' cycles are carried out in each area, as this has proved better for destroying cancer cells than just doing it once.

These procedures are used for liver, prostate and breast tumours at the moment, and are most effective when there are only one or two tumours to treat. The technique is constantly being improved and refined to treat tumours that are more difficult to reach.

Ultrasound and microwave thermotherapy

Some of the techniques mentioned require the placement of a probe within the tumour to achieve their results. But newer technologies are being investigated to treat cancers that are more remote. This means that the tumours are heated from outside the body.

One such method is called 'high-intensity focused ultrasound' (FUS). When used for imaging scans, ultrasound uses a wide range of high-frequency sound waves to bounce off tissues in the body. But when these ultrasonic beams are focused intensely onto one spot, they can heat the tissues and destroy the cancer cells. Early trials of early-stage breast cancer have produced impressive results. So far, however, this technique is only used in the US and in research projects in the UK.

Focused Microwave Thermotherapy

This technology uses a different technique for heating cells in the tumour. It takes advantage of the difference in water content between healthy and cancerous cells, and can heat tumours without burning the skin. However, both focused ultrasound and microwave thermotherapy need much more research to determine if they can effectively treat breast and other cancers. Nevertheless, results so far are promising and ongoing research is being done in the US.

These treatments, known as 'ablation techniques', hold great potential for the future. Early signs are that they can be performed safely, with little discomfort to the patient and without the need to stay in hospital. Their only drawback is the difficulty in establishing whether the whole tumour has been removed. When a way to confirm that is perfected, we should be seeing these techniques in far wider use than they are at the moment.

Percutaneous ethanol injection

This is used to treat inoperable primary cancers of the liver, but is not effective for metastatic liver cancers. It can treat single lesions less than 5 cm (about 2 inches) in diameter, or two to three tumours if each one less than 4 cm in diameter.

Ethanol injections are performed as an outpatients procedure, and require two or three treatments each week, for a total of six to eight treatments per cancerous lesion. Ultrasound is used to locate the tumour, and absolute ethanol is injected into it, causing cell death of the tumour mass.

Recovery time is short due to the lack of complications.

Photodynamic therapy

At present, this is being used for oesophageal cancer and early-stage lung cancer. It can also serve as an investigational technique for obstructive lung cancer, Barrett's oesophagus, and cancers of the head and neck, bladder and skin.

This is a two-step procedure done on an outpatients basis. The patient is first injected with a light-activated drug – Photofrin – which targets or 'sticks to' cancerous cells. (In the case of a skin cancer, cream is applied and treatment commences 2–4 hours later.) Approximately 24–48 hours later, a laser light is directed through a scope onto the tumour, exposing the cancerous tissue to a specific spectrum of light that 'switches on' the drug and then destroys the cancerous cells, without damaging the surrounding healthy tissues.

Light and heat therapies are also being developed by alternative medicine doctors (see Chapter 5).

This is a relatively pain-free procedure requiring minimal sedation and proven to be relatively safe. However, there are side-effects:

- local swelling and inflammation, which may occur in and around the tumour, causing discomfort or a temporary worsening of obstruction if situated in the oesophagus or lungs
- photosensitivity for approximately 30 days due to the continued presence of the drug in the body. Particularly affected are the skin and eyes, which will be sensitive to bright light. Exposure to bright light or direct sunlight should be avoided to prevent sunburn, redness and swelling.

A disadvantage of the treatment is that argon laser light cannot pass through more than 3 cm of tissue. For this reason, it is mainly used for tumours on or just under the skin, or just beneath the lining of internal organs. It can be directed through a bronchoscope into the lungs, through an endoscope into the oesophagus and gastrointestinal tract, or through a cystoscope into the bladder.

Cancer Treatments in Development

Cytoreductive surgery and hyperthermic intraoperative intraperitoneal chemotherapy are two new treatments that are used together when there is extensive spread of tumour throughout the abdominal cavity.

Cytoreductive surgery

This involves the aggressive removal or destruction of all visible tumours present throughout the peritoneal surfaces. The peritoneum is a membrane that covers the abdominal organs and cavity. Sometimes, an abdominal tumour is found to have spread deposits throughout the peritoneum. With cytoreductive surgery, its removal or destruction is attempted using a combination of surgical techniques, including electroevaporation, lasers, ultrasonic dissection and an argon beam coagulator.

The long-term results depend on the ability of the surgeon to remove all visible tumours. The long-term benefits are directly related to the size of the cancer deposits that may be left behind. The smaller they are, the greater the chances that they will respond to the intraperitoneal chemotherapy that follows.

Cytoreductive surgery is an extensive, lengthy procedure that lasts, on average, more than 10 hours. Frequently, it is necessary to remove segments of the small and large bowel, spleen, stomach and pancreas to achieve adequate cytoreduction. The extent of cutting will depend on the location and size of the tumour. The operation is combined with the following treatment.

Hyperthermic intraoperative intraperitoneal chemotherapy

This is the intraoperative (during surgery) administration of heated chemotherapy into the peritoneal cavity, once the extensive removal of tumour (cytoreductive surgery) has been completed. The technique permits the delivery of high concentrations of selected drugs into the abdominal and pelvic areas. The drugs make contact with all of the peritoneal surfaces, including the tumour-resected areas.

Previously, the spread of tumour throughout the peritoneum has been regarded as a terminal condition, with most oncologists considering it a condition for palliative treatment only.

Aggressive cytoreductive surgery with or without intraperitoneal chemotherapy has proven beneficial in several studies. First reported in the 1980s, intraperitoneal chemotherapy has been described as a safe treatment, and is currently under evaluation at several centres around the world. The administration of hyperthermic intraperitoneal chemotherapy at the time of surgery has achieved long-term disease-free survival.

Cancer vaccines

These cover a wide range of products, and are a crossover area between mainstream and alternative cancer medicine. A form of immunotherapy, they all have the potential to stimulate or reactivate the immune system to kill cancer cells and protect against tumour recurrence. There has been some success with general vaccines – called 'non-specific' because they are not derived from cancer cells in particular. For example, the BCG or tuberculosis vaccine has been used for some time with notable success. In bladder cancer, it is given directly into the bladder, where it acts as an antigen to stimulate a general immune response against the cancer cells.

Perhaps the most exciting products are the therapeutic vaccines, which can induce cancer cell-killing by specifically reactivating immune mechanisms that have ceased to recognize and attack cancer cells. We know that tumours evoke an immune response in both animals and people – but the response is usually very weak. If we could develop ways to enhance this response, then we might have an effective anti-cancer weapon. Enhancing the immune response is the basis of many of the alternative treatments covered in Chapter 5.

Dendritic cell therapy

This area of active research into cancer immunotherapy involves a unique immune-system cell known as 'dendritic cells'. They trigger an immune response by taking up cancer antigens and processing them into a form that other immune cells can then respond to. Dendritic cells can be removed from the bloodstream, grown in the laboratory and exposed to tumour antigen in culture dishes. When these dendritic cells are then injected back into a person with cancer, an immune response is generated, causing the tumour to shrink. There are several clinical trials taking place in the UK with dendritic cell vaccines, most notably under immuno-oncologist Professor Gus Dalgleish, of St George's Hospital in London. This therapy is also available from alternative cancer practitioner Dr Julian Kenyon in Winchester and immuno-oncologist Dr Thomas Nesselhutin in Germany (see Resources Directory, page 331).

Over the last 10 years we have understood a lot more at the molecular level about how antigens are presented and immune cells activated. We also have more clinical information from studies of cancer vaccines. However, it takes a very long time for a cancer vaccine to be shown to work for slower-growing cancers. In early breast cancer, for example, it may take 10 years of studying patients that have or have not received a vaccine to determine any benefit. For this reason, most studies have involved patients with a poor prognosis, such as melanoma skin cancer or kidney cancer that has already spread.

It is hoped that future developments will bring us specific, targeted cancer vaccines that can latch onto cancer cells and enable the body's own immune mechanisms to destroy the cells effectively.

Gene therapy

This involves the use of specific DNA sequences to treat a disease by correcting faulty DNA or replacing lost DNA. The main problem is how to get the new genes into every cancerous cell. If this cannot be achieved, then any cells that remain unaffected will emerge as a resistant group. Transferring DNA uses carriers called 'vectors', such as viruses, which can often be adapted to carry therapy genes. But, as yet, no ideal vectors exist. Nevertheless, using a variety of ingenious systems, more than 400 studies of gene therapy have now been carried out involving over 5,000 cancer patients worldwide – but mostly based in the US.

Several strategies are under investigation, including:

- tagging cancer cells with a foreign gene to stimulate the immune system
- targeting immune-stimulating factors to tumour cells
- inserting genes that activate anti-cancer drugs
- suppressing or replacing defective cancer-causing genes in patients.

Experimental gene therapy is currently being used to treat brain, colorectal, prostate and breast cancers.

The accurate delivery of the foreign gene to the tumour cell is key so, until better delivery systems become available, it is difficult to see how gene therapy will have a major impact on cancer treatment. However, it is likely that, by the end of this decade, extremely sophisticated systems will have solved the delivery problem – so watch this space!

One example of progress in gene therapy, developed by scientists in England, could potentially block breast cancer-cell spread throughout the body by targeting cancer cells with a fragment of DNA called a 'mini-gene', housed inside of a specially modified virus. Cancer cells contain a molecule that instructs them to move; this gene therapy is targeted at this molecule to prevent the cancer from spreading round the body. In future, treating people with the modified virus before surgery could hold cancer cells in place within the tumour, thus improving the chances of a successful operation to remove it.

Viruses

Research scientists in London believe that genetically engineered viruses will prove to be more effective than conventional chemo- and radiotherapy in the future. A team from The Hammersmith Hospital is launching a series of pioneering clinical trials to discover whether the technique can produce tangible results. They hope that such an approach could increase patients' survival rates. While effective in the laboratory, success has now to be proven in humans.

These viral approaches are not only potentially more potent, but they also do not rely exclusively on triggering generalized cell death, the underlying method of many of the treatments used today, and the cause of so many of their unpleasant side-effects. In contrast, these viruses can target and infect only the cancer cells, which will multiply and eventually die, releasing more viral particles to infect other targeted cancer cells. It is also thought that the viral approach may lead to fewer side-effects than do some of the current therapies.

Virus-directed Enzyme Therapy

This treatment is becoming more commonplace, although still only within clinical trials. A modified (harmless) virus carries an enzyme into the cancer cells. Once there, an inactive form of a chemotherapy drug – called a 'prodrug' – is given to the patient. When the inactive prodrug reaches the cancer cells, the enzyme within converts the prodrug into an active chemotherapy drug to kill the cancer cell.

Again, this type of treatment is targeted only to cancer cells. As normal body cells should not be affected, there should be fewer side-effects with this treatment. How effective the treatment is and its side-effects are being tested in clinical trials now in progress in the UK as well as internationally.

Other developments

Smart Scalpel

A 'smart scalpel' has been developed in the US that can detect the presence of cancer cells as a surgeon cuts away a tumour. The device, called a 'biological microcavity laser', should help surgeons be more accurate when cutting away malignant growths, thereby minimizing the amount of healthy tissue removed. In effect, the device tells the surgeon when to stop cutting.

Cells are pushed through a micropump, and any abnormal cell proteins (present in cancer cells) are identified. The resulting analysis is shown on graphics, so the surgeon can see when he is cutting into normal tissues.

Adoptive Transfer

This approach replaces a patient's immune cells with cancer-fighting ones.

Using a small piece of the patient's tumour, immune cells known as 'T cells' are activated in the laboratory against the tumour. Once the T cells have multiplied to a sufficient number for treatment, they are administered to the patient. The T cells remain active against the tumour for up to four months.

Patients are also given a high dose of a protein called interleukin-2, which stimulates continued T-cell growth in the body. Prior to the immunotherapy, chemotherapy is used to deplete the patient's own immune cells as they have proved ineffective at fighting the cancer.

The results have so far been impressive, with promising results for metastatic melanoma that has not responded to standard treatments. With further research, scientists hope to apply this approach to many types of cancer as well as infectious diseases such as AIDS, where immunity is also compromised.

Tests show that, in many of those who respond favorably to the treatment, the administered immune cells are thriving, multiplying rapidly and attacking tumour tissue.

Thalidomide

Many people have heard of the drug thalidomide, which caused severe birth defects in a large number of children in the 1960s, when the drug was being used as an anti-sickness drug for nausea in early pregnancy.

The birth defects arose because thalidomide interferes with the body's ability to form new blood vessels. This mechanism is now being used against cancer, limiting the tumour's ability to develop a blood supply.

It may also ease some of the symptoms associated with serious cancers, such as sweating and severe weight loss.

A number of clinical trials are ongoing with thalidomide being tried against a wide range of cancers. So far, the drug has been proved useful against malignant myeloma, a form of cancer that is particularly difficult to treat.

Tumour-targeted Super-antigens

The term 'super-antigen' is a collective term, referring to a number of substances that stimulate the human immune system. They mainly stimulate T cells, which identify and eradicate abnormal cells in the body.

The super-antigens are designed to make cancer cells easy to recognize and to stimulate the body's own immune system to rid itself of them. Other methods aim to stimulate the immune system, but this one is a step forward as it identifies and targets cancer cells in a precise way. To seek out tumour cells, the super-antigens are linked to an antibody which, in turn, recognizes a marker found on most cancer cells. The technology can, in principle, be used to treat any type of tumour. Clinical trials are underway in the UK involving cancers of the lung, kidney and pancreas.

Clinical Trials

You may at some stage of your treatment either be offered, or decide that you wish, to take part in a clinical trial. Any such trial of a new drug or treatment approach must have first gone through extensive laboratory and animal testing. You need to know at which phase of testing the treatment is.

- Phase I trials are the first studies in people to evaluate how a new drug should be given (by mouth, or injected into the bloodstream or muscle), how often and at what dosage. Only a small number of patients are enrolled, sometimes as few as a dozen.
- Phase II trials continue to test the safety of the drug, and evaluate how well it works. These studies usually focus on a particular type of cancer.
- Phase III trials use a new drug, a new combination of drugs or a new surgical procedure and compare it with the current standard drug, combination or surgery. Study participants are usually randomly assigned to receive either the standard or the new drug (randomization). Large numbers are often enrolled, sometimes at many hospitals nationwide or even across many countries. If entered in this type of trial, you will not know which treatment you are receiving and neither will your doctors (double-blind). The randomized double-blind trial is considered the 'gold standard' in clinical research, and forms the basis of all serious scientific evaluation of medical treatments.

You may be able to find a relevant clinical trial through your doctor, or you yourself can check for any new treatments you feel may be of benefit to you. There are several websites that list the open clinical trials both in the UK and elsewhere. The UK Cancer Options team can also provide you with such a list.

However, you can only enrol into a clinical trial through your doctor. Trials are carried out at main cancer centres. Trial protocols explain:

- the reason for doing the study
- how many people will be in the study
- who is eligible to participate in the study
- what study drugs the participants will take
- what medical tests they will have and how often
- what information will be gathered.

The obvious benefit of taking part in a trial is that you may gain access to a new treatment that may be effective for you years before it becomes generally available.

The disadvantages are:

- You may receive a drug that does not work for you or is no better than other treatments you've been offered.
- The new drug may cause unexpected side-effects.
- If the trial is randomized, you may be allocated to an untreated (control) group, and you will not be aware of this during the trial. (However, not all trials are randomized, so you might be given the trial drug if your condition deteriorates while in the control group or when the trial ends.)
- If you decide to take part in a clinical trial abroad, be sure you know how much follow-up assessment and costs are involved, as the researchers will expect you to return for check-ups and evaluation.

Judging breakthroughs

A major problem facing both patients and doctors is the false hope raised by many so-called 'cancer breakthroughs'. These appear with great regularity, often as short newspaper articles triggered by a press release.

There is tremendous media interest in all cancer treatments – especially those that are new or sensational. Cancer research is funded by charities, which have to raise money in competition with an ever-growing list of other good causes. Such charities have had to become far more business-like in their approach to fund-raising and often have effective public-relations departments. Stories are usually released as honest reports but, just like a game of Chinese whispers, so cancer cure stories tend to become exaggerated. Hopes are raised, which can add greatly to the distress of relatives and friends of patients who later find out that the hopes were groundless.

To go searching for an experimental treatment without at least discussing it with your oncologist is unwise. One problem when investigating any new type of treatment is that only certain types of patient may be suitable for the clinical trial. Worse still, you may find that the breakthrough is still at the 'test-tube' or animal stage and nowhere near ready for trials in humans.

To help you in judging so-called breakthroughs:

- Carefully read the information you have found.
- Make sure it has been used in people and that it is not just another mouse experiment.
- If a research charity is mentioned, contact its public relations office for accurate information.
- If from a pharmaceutical or biotechnology company, contact its information department or look it up on its website. Recent press releases are usually available and may provide far more information than the article in the paper.
- If you think the treatment is for you, contact the investigator responsible for the study.
- If you cannot find out anything about a treatment, contact a cancer information charity such as CancerBACUP in the UK. If the treatment is from the US, contact the National Cancer Institute or see its website.
- The Internet is the easiest, quickest and most reliable way to find out about potential cancer breakthroughs. Most cancer organizations now maintain an excellent website (see the Resources Directory pages 257–63).
- Use the UK Cancer Options service to help you decide whether you should go for inclusion in any clinical study.

Using the Internet

The Internet is the best frontier-scouting tool available. If you cannot use it or have no access, then find a friend who can, or get help from your local library or cancer information centre. Young people are great as they know exactly how to get Internet results quickly. Two hours of browsing the World Wide Web will turn up a lot of information on any aspect of cancer care, but you need to know how reliable the information is. Some websites are clearly promotional; crooks with powerful vested interests run others. Chapter 3, the Resources Directory and the list below recommend sites with reliable information.

The box on page 49 can get you started at excellent sites with up-to-date high-quality information. Most are hyperlinked to other websites, and many have chat rooms so you can share your experiences with other people with the same type of cancer.

How much information you want is up to you. The upside is that information is the key to empowerment. If you wish to be involved in decisions about your care, you need to understand your options as well as their advantages and disadvantages. It can also help you to discover whether rationing is preventing you from getting what to others may be standard at a nearby hospital. Above all, it can enable you to make an informed choice.

But there's a downside, too. It can be depressing to plough through gloomy information and statistics. You may find it hard to understand because of all the medical terms. As the general public in the US are usually more aware of medical developments than in Europe, American websites can be difficult to follow. You might also misinterpret things, so use your medical team or Cancer Options (see page 259) to make this part of learning about cancer easier for you.

Beating the UK's national health system

Britain's NHS is a remarkable institution – and, for some reason, we all love it! We know that it is possible to obtain the best possible cancer care in the world in Britain and, yet, many are still getting substandard care. How can you beat the system to make sure you are getting the best? My advice is to take control of your situation, however difficult that may seem. Dr Daniel's Health Creation Programme will help you psychologically, spiritually and physically, but you can help yourself obtain the best possible treatment. Arming yourself with such information will empower you to work effectively with the professionals looking after you.

A word of warning, though – professional attitudes vary enormously. The best advice is not to get into confrontational situations that are highly emotionally charged with your doctors. Starting off on the basis that they are giving you the wrong treatment is not a good way forward. Constructive discussion over the various options available, and how applicable is the background material you may have found during your frontier scouting, is a far more useful approach. If you don't take the responsibility for getting the right treatment, why should anyone else? You are entitled to know exactly what plans the doctors have for your treatment in hospital, and this Directory will help you understand the issues. Discuss the situation with your own GP as well as the consultant. Further information can be obtained from the entire cancer healthcare profession, which is increasingly becoming specialized, and fully aware of the implications of surgery, radiotherapy and chemotherapy.

People often don't ask questions because they are afraid to appear stupid, ignorant or difficult. Don't be. Always question until you feel satisfied that you have enough information or, if necessary, know where to get even more. Be assertive, but not aggressive. Show that you want all the information available and that you want to be empowered to make your own decisions.

The most powerful route to use when you feel your questions are not being answered is via a second opinion. This can be done on the NHS, or through your GP or an integrated medicine cancer doctor. Cancer Options can advise you on how to go about this, and help you make the necessary arrangements with your own and the new doctor.

Rationing abounds in the NHS despite denial by both politicians and administrators. 'Postcode prescribing' still exists, although the National Cancer Plan is trying to eliminate it. The best way to make sure that you are not missing out on something that is available to some, but not others, in the NHS is to arm yourself with information. You have to be sure that the treatment really is indicated for you. If you are denied it, establish with your own consultant the reasons why you cannot have the treatment. It may be due to a problem in your liver or kidneys rather than financial constraints in the hospital. If, however, it is the cost, then ask for a second opinion in a different area where you know the drug you want is being used.

Alternatively, get the drug privately. Private medicine confers certain advantages – mainly, more time with a consultant and avoiding having to see a series of doctors who may not be familiar with your case. You may not be able to cover the costs but, if you ask your friends, family, colleagues or local community fundraisers, they may be able to raise the money you need. You must not feel too embarrassed to ask for help directly or via a supporter, as help like this could save your life. If you have health insurance, make sure it will cover the cost of chemotherapy before you begin it. This is normally included in insurance cover but, for your own peace of mind, you should make sure you will not be given a top-up bill to pay.

Don't be worried about seeming to be overly persistent. As already mentioned, research has shown that 'difficult patients do better'. Persistence, empowerment and information are the keys to making sure you get the right treatment for you.

A Note about the Authors of this Chapter:

Professor Karol Sikora, who wrote this chapter, is an ideal UK consultant for a second opinion. He is London-based and has a clear perspective of the national and international cancer picture. He can be found at the Harley Street Cancer Centre, 81 Harley Street, London, tel. 020 7935 7700.

Patricia Peat, co-author of this chapter, runs the UK consultancy Cancer Options to help you find state-of-the-art cancer treatment both nationally and internationally. The number to call is 0845 009 2041.

CHAPTER 5

Alternative cancer medicines: the best of today

Written with help from research chemist Andrew Panton

This chapter presents the latest developments in alternative cancer medicine in the fields of:

- Anti-cancer nutrients
- Herbal medicine
- Hormone therapy
- Metabolic therapy
- Immunotherapy
- Neuroendocrine therapy
- Physical therapies
- Nutritional therapies
- Mind–body medicine.

A full description of how to use and find each of the following best-known alternative cancer medicines can be found in the Resources Directory.

While the number of options available may perhaps make it difficult to choose what is right for you, it will give you a good basis for discussion if you choose to visit any integrated or alternative cancer doctors or clinics.

Understanding Alternative Cancer Treatments

Alternative cancer medicines are defined as those that may be used as an alternative to orthodox cancer treatment.

This is the most controversial area of integrated medicine as most oncologists believe there are no genuine alternatives to orthodox cancer treatment. This is mainly because of the lack of hard evidence of the randomized controlled trial variety used in orthodox medicine to judge treatment efficacy. However, this is changing as money and high-level research skills are being diverted to alternative areas of research by public demand. This trend was led by the US in the mid-1990s, when an Office of Alternative Medicine was established within the National Institutes of Health. Within this office, there is a specialized cancer section, and research results are beginning to come forward from their early trials with commonly used anti-cancer alternatives. This lead is now being followed in 2004 by the UK National Cancer Research Institute, which has set up a specialist research group in this field, although it is likely to focus on qualitative research of complementary supportive care rather than evaluation of alternative cancer medicines.

Your doctor's main concern will be whether the approach you are considering could harm you or interfere with your medical treatment and whether you are being exploited financially. These are legitimate concerns for your protection. So, decide first whether you think your doctor is open-minded enough to give you an unbiased opinion.

Another reason why many alternative cancer treatments have not yet become mainstream, despite the evidence of benefit in many patients who have used them, may have much to do with the 'political' control over the cancer-medicine 'market'. The politics of cancer are believed by many to have an overriding influence on the direction of cancer science – what we are led to think and believe about cancer, and what you can expect to be offered as treatment options.

The issues behind this controversy are beyond the scope of this book, but if you wish to make up your own mind on this matter, there are numerous agencies to refer to such as What Doctors Don't Tell You and Philip Day's Campaign for Truth in Medicine. Two of the liveliest and most controversial sources of information and opinion on this subject come from Dr Samuel Epstein in his book *The Politics of Cancer* and Dr Ralph Moss in his book *The Cancer Industry: Unravelling the Politics*. In effect, herbal remedies, nutritional substances and mind–body approaches are not patentable, so there is little motivation for research trials to be carried out as no one will seriously profit (and the cost of research trials and product licensing is huge). But worse than that, the cancer-drug industry is worth billions so, again, there is little incentive to prevent cancer or find the answers within natural medicine.

Evaluating alternative cancer medicines

In the Resources Directory (pages 269–318) you will find more specific information about each alternative cancer medicine described in this chapter, classified under the following headings:

- Uses and dosage: the primary uses of the agent and typical dose ranges
- Drug interactions and special precautions: known cautions and information to be aware of when using the treatment
- How to use: whether the treatment can be purchased and self-administered, or whether it must be prescribed and administered by doctors or nurses in a medical setting; also, whether it is safe to use with conventional treatments
- Mechanism of action (MOA): if known, this is described or, alternatively, the theory upon which its use as treatment is based
- Level of evidence: the evidence supporting its use as treatment is classified as:
  - Randomized controlled trial (RCT), the 'gold standard' of high-quality scientific research, in which study subjects have been matched with controls, who do not receive the study treatment, and neither the patients nor the doctors know who is being actively treated. This methodology eliminates bias and placebo effects, enabling the effectiveness of the treatment to be assessed objectively.
  - Pure science, where a treatment has been tested in the laboratory (in vitro) to establish the active constituent and probable mechanism of action
  - Case study, where a series of patients who have taken a treatment have been studied by doctors, and a clinical impression has been gathered over time as to the value of the treatment
  - Anecdotal evidence, where the benefits of a treatment are described and passed on from patient to patient on the basis of personal experience
  - Traditional treatment, where a treatment is part of an ancient system of medicine that has been passed down by practitioners from generation to generation
  - Epidemiological, where the disease patterns in a population are studied.
- Source and price: where the treatment can be obtained and the approximate cost at the time of publication
- References: to find the research study material cited.

Alternative approaches to cancer are based on the need to:

Destroy cancerous tissue with naturally occurring cytotoxic substances, and physical agents such as heat (hyperthermia) and light (cytoluminescence)

Detoxify the body by complete detoxification of the system, ridding the body of its load of organic and inorganic chemicals that have accumulated due to poor nutrition, environmental pollution, infections and medical procedures, which may impede resistance and healing mechanisms

Nourish the body with supernutrition and anti-cancer foods

Repair damage to the genes and tissue-healing mechanisms

Defend the body with immune stimulation

Energize the body with bioenergy medicine.

Some advocates of alternative cancer medicine are adamant that their treatments cannot be taken with conventional medicine at all because the emphasis placed on complete detoxification, immune stimulation and cellular regeneration is directly in conflict with the toxic nature of chemo- and radiotherapy. It is this extreme position that has frightened conventional cancer doctors as there is then a genuine risk that you may not be receiving treatment that could be lifesaving or greatly reduce your suffering. So, if you are contemplating alternative medicines, the main decision to make is where you stand in relation to this thinking.

There are a number of possibilities to look at:

- You may wish to take a window of time out to try alternative cancer medicines before you embark on an orthodox medical treatment (but only if your cancer is not too serious or not fast-growing).
- You might try both approaches at the same time to minimize the damage being done to the system by the harsher orthodox medicines, and aim to get the best of both worlds.
- You may choose to wait until you have had conventional treatment before embarking on alternative treatments, seeing them as a way of repairing the tissue damage done by conventional medicine and as a long-term insurance policy.
- You may choose to keep cancer alternatives as a 'last-hope' option, for when you are told that conventional medicine is no longer working.

It may be helpful to consult an integrated medicine doctor (see the Resources Directory) to help you decide what is right for you. Remember, you are not being actively advised by this doctor, but only enabled to reach your own conclusions. You may also want to consult the advocates of alternative cancer medicine directly to help you make a decision. Contact points for the main alternative cancer clinics worldwide are listed in the Resources Directory, and there are many websites that can help you to find and explore alternative options.

As already mentioned, your conventional doctors may well be the first to admit that they have not studied either the theory or practice of alternative cancer medicines, so their opinions may well be based on personal feelings rather than specific knowledge. This is the same for many alternative cancer specialists, who may not have studied conventional cancer medicine. This is why a more neutral integrated medicine doctor with a 'foot in both camps' may be in a better position to help you reach a balanced conclusion.

The main point is to try not to be too rigid. There is a time and place for everything – the skill lies in judging when it might be necessary to shift your position and change the type of help you are seeking.

The need for regular medical monitoring

If you wish to go entirely natural in your approach to fighting cancer, it is advisable to do so with the back up of regular monitoring by your medical team, and regular guidance from a good integrated medicine doctor, or your GP if he or she is open-minded. Ideally, you need to know whether your efforts are holding your cancer stable, causing it to regress, or if it is still growing despite your best efforts.

With this information, you will be able to decide whether you need to change your course of action and consider a more conventional approach, or move to a 'best of both worlds' approach.

Alternatives on the Internet

You can find more information in alternative cancer medicine books and via the Internet. However, be aware that the 'Net may present you with an overwhelming number of alternative cancer medicines, the scientific evidence for the effectiveness and safety of which may not be available or known. Please be advised by a qualified doctor before buying or trying anything, especially if it is new or very expensive. This chapter will give you a good starting place to look for alternatives for which research has already begun.

The Resources Directory

In Part 2, you will find a list of the best known:

- alternative cancer medicines (Section 3.3).
- alternative cancer doctors (Section 4)
- alternative cancer clinics (Section 5)

It is not an exhaustive list, but represents the alternative resources that are the most widely used by people with cancer, which have stood the test of time and for which there is the most evidence. All the information given is based on the available knowledge at the point of writing and is given in good faith to help lighten the task of those with cancer who urgently need to find helpful information in order to explore their treatment options. However, mention of resources in the Directory does not constitute a recommendation. So please exercise your own discrimination when looking into the possibilities available and get the advice of your integrated medicine doctor to individualize your programme.

Using alternative treatments

Alternative cancer treatments are used singly in some cases and in combination in others. They ideally form part of an integrated treatment approach that includes nutrition, vitamin and mineral supplementation as well as self-help, support and energy treatments.

The exact combination of therapies and treatments depends entirely on the individual and your circumstances, needs and preferences. While it is perfectly safe for people themselves to begin using many of these treatments, the more complex regimes should be supervised by an alternative medicine doctor or alternative cancer clinic. It is also wise to take medical advice prior to starting these treatments, particularly while having other medical treatments or if pregnant. Any side-effects of treatment should be discussed immediately with your doctor.

Full details on the contents of Sections 1–9 are found in the Resources Directory (Section 3.3, pages 268–330).

1. Anti-cancer Nutrients

Diet and nutrition have been shown in over 10,000 scientific studies to play a key role in the prevention and treatment of cancer. A healthy diet with vitamin/mineral supplementation is an essential part of any anti-cancer regime. Nutritional supplements are known to be useful in helping maintain optimal nutrition, immune function and tissue-healing. Increasingly, products are being developed which contain the full range of antioxidant vitamins, herbs and minerals to make it easier for those with cancer to take. Examples include Transfer Factor, Wholly Immune and Immune Formula.

1a. Antioxidants

In recent years, antioxidant vitamins, minerals and plant extracts have been increasingly highlighted as playing an important role in protecting the cell's genetic material and membranes from free-radical damage, thus preserving normal cell reproduction and all-round functioning. They are now considered to be a vital element in all holistic cancer treatment and prevention plans. They are also important in boosting immune function and resistance to infection, and so form the cornerstone of any anti-cancer regime. The most commonly used antioxidants are vitamins C, E and beta-carotene (the safe form of vitamin A), and the minerals selenium and zinc, which are vital for the formation of enzymes needed in the antioxidative process.

Another way to take naturally-occurring antioxidants is through an excellent product called Juice Plus. This contains the nutritional essence of 17 different fruits and vegetables, dried under carefully controlled temperatures to eliminate most of the salt, sugar and calories, in a capsule format. The fruits and vegetables are vine-ripened, non-irradiated and treated to be sure they are herbicide- and pesticide-free. This is a very helpful solution for those who want the benefit of getting a high level of plant enzymes, co-factors and antioxidants without having to take in so much of the bulk and fibre associated with a wholefood diet. Juice Plus is backed by good-quality scientific research which can be found at www.childrensresearch.org and www.scienceandhealthnews.com. For more information on Juice Plus, go to www.juice-fit.com or ring +353 876 59 52 58.

1b. Herbal antioxidants

Many plants contain powerful antioxidants, and some people with cancer prefer to take their antioxidants in this form. Some good examples are pine bark extract (or Pycnogenol) or mixtures of plants antioxidants such as Cascading Revenol by Neways.

1c. Multi-mineral formulations

Numerous studies have shown the importance of minerals for regulating many physiological processes and in protecting the body against cancer. In particular, selenium, zinc, copper, chromium and manganese are important in cancer prevention because of their antioxidant properties, their role in maintaining the correct functioning of the immune system and for enhanced tissue healing.

1d. Essential fatty acids and essential sugars

Flaxseed (linseed) oil is a very rich source of alpha-linolenic acid (ALA), an important omega-3 essential fatty acid that is highly protective against cancer. It may be taken alone or as part of a mixture of essential fatty acids such as Udo's Oil. Mannatech provide essential sugars in their preparation Ambratrose.

1e. Co-enzyme Q10

Co-enzyme Q10 (ubiquinone) is a benzoquinone compound naturally synthesized by the human body. The Q and 10 in the name refer to the quinone chemical group and the 10 isoprenyl chemical subunits, respectively. Co-enzyme Q10 is present in most tissues as it is an essential component of our energy-producing system. The highest concentrations are found in the heart, liver, kidneys and pancreas where high levels of metabolic activity are maintained continuously. Tissue levels of this compound decrease with age, highly stressed lifestyles, increased requirements or insufficient intake of the chemical precursors needed for its synthesis. The ensuing deficiency contributes to ageing and disease processes.

1f. Immune stimulants

Inosito/IP6
This natural substance is a constituent of vitamin B and has very powerful immune-stimulating activity. It raises not only the number of circulating white cells, but also their activity. It is useful for preventing and treating infection, raising the white cell count during chemotherapy and as part of an ongoing cancer-treatment programme.

Biobran
This is another supplement which has been shown to have very strong immune stimulant properties.

2. Herbal Medicine

2a. Aloe vera
Aloe vera is a member of the lily family and has spiny, fleshy, white-speckled leaves. The plant is indigenous to Sudan and the Arabian peninsula, but is often grown as a houseplant worldwide.

Aloe vera has long been used medicinally for healing cuts, burns and various skin problems. For the cancer patient, this makes it ideal for preventing skin damage due to radiotherapy.

Aloe vera also soothes and heals the internal mucous membranes, and can help during and after chemotherapy to heal damage to the lining of the digestive tract.

Aloe is also believed to be able to treat cancer directly if taken in large-enough doses (e.g. 200 ml per day).

2b. Amygdalin or laetrile (vitamin B$_{17}$)
Among alternative cancer physicians, amygdalin is one of the most widely used supplements, with numerous positive reports of its therapeutic effectiveness against cancer.

Amygdalin is a nitriloside, cyanide-containing substance found in numerous foods, including the seeds of apricots, apples, cherries, plums and peaches.

When natural amygdalin is purified and concentrated for use in anti-cancer therapy, it is called 'laetrile'. It is claimed that laetrile targets only the cancer cells and destroys them through an enzymatic process involving cyanide. The use of laetrile in the UK was dampened down by legislation in the 1980s, but renewed interest has been sparked by Philip Day's book *Cancer: Why We Are Still Dying to Know the Truth*.

2c. Astragalus

This is the root of the *Astragalus membranaceus* plant, a member of the pea family. Native to northeast China, it has long been used as a traditional Chinese medicine to treat viral infections. Since 1975, *Astragalus* has been used in China for cancer patients undergoing radiation treatment and chemotherapy, in whom the plant seems particularly useful. Not only does it appear to help reduce the side-effects of treatment, it can also support damaged immune function and increase survival time.

2d. Carctol

This is a herbal formulation developed by Dr Nandlal Tiwari, based in Jaipur, Rajasthan, in India. Each capsule contains the herbs *Hemidesmus indicus*, *Tribulus terrestris*, *Piper cubeba* Linn, *Ammani vesicatoria*, *Lepidium sativum* Linn, *Blepharis edulis*, *Smilax China* Linn and *Rheum emodi* Wall. Dr Tiwari has been treating cancer with Carctol for over 20 years with notable success. Since prescribing Carctol in 2000, Dr Rosy Daniel has also seen remission of serious pancreatic, ovarian, kidney and brain cancer, and melanoma, with new success stories coming in every week. Help has now been offered by senior UK oncologists to independently validate these results and, if positive, formal research trials will follow.

2e. Cat's Claw (Uncaria Tomentosa)

This vine grows high in the canopy roof of the Amazon rainforest, and gets its name from the claw-like thorns that protrude from its woody stems. The plant has been used by many tribes in Peru for the treatment of inflammatory conditions, intestinal ailments, wounds and cancer.

2f. Echinacea

Also known as purple coneflower, this member of the daisy family is native to the US. Native Americans traditionally used the root on cuts, burns and other injuries to prevent infection, hence its native name 'snake root'.

Echinacea is an immune stimulant that can increase resistance to infections. It is also used to decrease inflammation and allergic reactions. The primary role of *Echinacea* for the cancer patient is to help provide protection against infection, a common and sometimes fatal complication in advanced-stage cancers or when the immune system is compromised after chemotherapy. It is used for approximately six weeks as a potent immune booster and should be started immediately at the onset of a cold or other infection.

2g. Essiac or Rene Caisse herbs

In the 1920s, Canadian nurse Rene Caisse discovered a non-toxic herbal tea for treating cancer based on a recipe from the Ojibway, a Native American tribe based in Ontario. She noticed that her Native American patients fared much better than her other patients and put their success down to the tea. She went on to publicize the tea widely, and it is now available as Essiac (Caisse spelt backwards), Rene Caisse herbs or Floressence.

The primary role of Essiac for cancer patients is to protect against infection, facilitate detoxification, particularly when undergoing chemotherapy, and boost the body's ability to fight cancer.

2h. Garlic

Garlic has long been recognized to benefit the immune system, improve general health, ward off colds and treat infections of all sorts. For the cancer patient, garlic can help to strengthen the immune system, facilitate liver detox and reduce free-radical damage due to its high levels of sulphur-containing amino acids. It may also have a direct anti-cancer effect.

2i. Green tea (catechins)

Green and black teas are derived from the same plant, *Camellia sinensis*. However, only green tea is rich in the polyphenols known as 'catechins'. The fermentation process to make black tea destroys the biologically active polyphenols of the fresh leaf. The catechins as a chemical group have significant free-radical scavenging properties and are potent antioxidants. Green tea and catechin tablets can be used for the prevention and treatment of cancer.

2j. Iscador (mistletoe)

Iscador is the trade name for a mistletoe preparation used by European physicians since 1920 for the treatment of cancer. It consists of fermented extracts of European mistletoe and was originally developed by Austrian scientist Rudolf Steiner, who pioneered the speciality referred to as 'Anthroposophical Medicine'. There are several different types of Iscador, depending on the type of tree the mistletoe grows on. In cancer patients, Iscador can stimulate the immune system and inhibit tumour formation.

2k. Mushrooms and their extracts

Many mushrooms have anti-cancer properties. The ones most commonly used in alternative cancer treatments are *maitake, shiitake, Coriolus versicolor* and *reishi*. The primary role of these mushrooms for the cancer patient is to boost the immune system.

2l. Noni juice

Noni (*Morinda citrifolia*) is a tropical plant indigenous to Australia, Malaysia and Polynesia, and has a long history of medicinal use for a variety of ailments throughout these areas. This small, blossoming shrub has rounded branches and dark-green glossy leaves that measure approximately a foot in length. Clusters of small white flowers sprout at different times and eventually evolve into bumpy egg-shaped fruit a few inches long. Noni juice is made from this fruit.

The primary role of noni juice for the cancer patient is to strengthen the immune system and protect against infection.

2m. Pau d'arco

This is a herbal extract of the inner bark of the *Tabebuia impetiginosa* tree, found in South American rainforests. Pau d'arco is used to treat and prevent cancer by boosting health and immune function.

2n. PC-SPES

This is a combination of eight medicinal herbs: *Scutellaria baicalensis, Glycyrrhiza glabra, Ganoderma lucidum, Isatis indigotica, Panax pseudo-ginseng, Serenoa repens, Dendranthema morifolium* and *Rabdosia rubescens*. Except for *Serenoa* (African dwarf palm or saw palmetto), these are all Chinese herbs. At the time of writing, it is difficult to obtain PC-SPES due to the controversial finding of contaminants in commercially available PC-SPES.

This has been used extensively, and successfully, by men with prostate cancer to halt progression of the disease. It may also be effective for lymphoma, leukaemia, breast cancer and melanoma.

2o. Turmeric (curcumin)

This is a member of the ginger family, and is native to India and China. It is a major herb in Indian cooking, and appears to exert antioxidant effects powerful enough to limit the development of cancer.

The plant's active constituent is curcumin, which protects against free-radical damage as it is a potent antioxidant. The primary role of curcumin for the cancer patient is to reduce free radicals in the body. It can therefore both prevent cancer, and protect the body from the side-effects of chemo- and radiotherapy.

2p. Other important herbal and food extracts

Graviola (Annona muricata)

Since 1976, there have been several promising cancer studies of graviola, an evergreen tree growing in the Amazon rainforest. However, the graviola extracts have yet to be tested on cancer patients. No double-blind clinical trials have been done, and such trials are the benchmark by which mainstream doctors and journals judge a treatment's value.

Nevertheless, graviola has killed cancer cells in at least 20 laboratory tests. The most recent study, conducted at the Catholic University of South Korea in 2002, revealed that two chemicals extracted from graviola seeds showed 'selective cytotoxicity comparable with Adriamycin' against breast and colon cancer cells in the test-tube. Another study, published in the *Journal of Natural Products*, showed that graviola is not only comparable to the conventional chemo drug Adriamycin, but dramatically outperforms it in laboratory tests. Results showed that one chemical in graviola selectively killed colon cancer cells with 10,000 times greater potency than Adriamycin.

Lycopene

This is found in tomatoes. In one study, men with prostate cancer who took a daily equivalent of 30 mg of lycopene underwent a 17.5 per cent drop in their PSA (prostate-specific antigen, a tumour marker). Oxidative DNA damage was also reduced by 28.3 per cent.

Plant Sterols and Sterolins

Plant sterols such as beta-sitosterols are known to reduce prostate symptoms, and gamma-tocopherol can reduce prostate cancer risk by five times (compared with alpha-tocopherol, which is more widely used in vitamin E supplements).

Saw Palmetto (Pygeum Africanum), Stinging Nettle and Lycopene

All of these have demonstrated efficacy in the treatment and prevention of prostatic hypertrophy. They are found in combination in the product ProstaCol. Another product – Gold Specifics Prostate Support Vegicaps, by Solgar – combines these agents with zinc, selenium and soy isoflavone seed concentrate.

Mangosteen (Garcinia mangostana)

This is a tropical fruit found predominantly in south-east Asia, and Xango is a dietary juice supplement made from the purée of the whole fruit (pulp, seeds and rind). The mangosteen plant has strong medicinal properties and has long been used in folklore medicine for a wide range of conditions. The fruit contains over 30 different xanthones (biologically active plant phenols found in only a few tropical plants), with powerful antioxidant activity, thus able to disarm free radicals while enhancing and supporting the immune system. The medicinal properties of the fruit have been studied: xanthones have been shown to be anti-inflammatory, antioxidant, antibacterial, antimicrobial, anti-cancer, antiviral and antiallergic. In laboratory tests with breast cancer cells and with leukaemia cells, xanthones also had strong anti-proliferative and apoptotic (cell-killing) properties, giving good cause to believe that this fruit may have a significant role in cancer prevention or treatment.

Wormwood (Artemisia Annua)

Wormwood is an ancient Chinese folk medicine shown to have anti-cancer properties. Researchers Professor Henry Lai and Professor Narendra Singh of the University of Washington have exploited the chemical properties of the wormwood derivative artemisinin to target breast cancer cells with surprisingly effective results. Their study, published in the journal *Life Sciences* (2001; 70: 49-56) describes a laboratory test in which the derivative killed virtually all human breast cancer cells exposed to it within 16 hours (the cancer cells were pre-loaded with high doses of iron).

The use of the bitter herb wormwood is nothing new; it has been used for centuries to rid the body of worms and malaria. One form of wormwood is also an ingredient in the alcoholic beverage absinthe, now banned in most countries. But it is likely that the medicinally active type, also known as 'Sweet Annie', contains the active ingredient thujone, found in high concentrations in wormwood oil.

Studies of artemisinin have also shown it to be effective against a wide variety of cancers, in particular, leukaemia and colon cancer. It was moderately effective against melanoma, and breast, ovarian, prostate, brain and kidney cancers. As treatment, it is given in combination with green tea, co-enzyme Q10 and pancreatic enzymes as well as a good anti-cancer diet.

In the UK, the medical herbalist Gerald Green is experienced with the use of wormwood. It may be administered orally and, as there is plenty of naturally occurring iron in the body, the prepriming with iron needed in the laboratory studies is not necessary.

The dose range is 200–1,000 mg/day (in divided doses), and it should always be taken with food. However, the dose does very much depend on the purity and potency of the herb. Care must also be taken as, at high doses, it can be neurotoxic, causing gait disturbances, loss of spinal and pain reflexes, breathing difficulties and even cardiopulmonary arrest.

Chinese Herbs

Many Chinese herbs are known to reduce tumour activity. Dr Robert Jacobs is among the few English alternative cancer doctors prescribing Chinese herbs. He particularly recommends *Da Quing Ye* (*Isatis*), which is similar to wode, and *Yi Yi Ren* (*Coix lachryma-jobi*) or Job's tears, in his anti-cancer therapeutic protocol.

Ukrain

This is made from the greater celandine (*Chelidonium majus*) plant, has a cytotoxic effect when given intravenously as part of metabolic therapy. This is a prescription-only product and, therefore, can only be obtained from an alternative medicine doctor (e.g. Dr Nicola Hembry).

3. Hormone Therapy in Cancer Treatment and the Menopause

Many cancers of the breast and prostate are hormone-sensitive, so progesterone cream and indole-3-carbinol can help to reduce the impact of oestrogen on the tumour.

3a. Natural progesterone

Human progesterone is produced naturally by the ovaries, adrenal glands and fat cells. Ovarian production stops after menopause, so synthetic progesterone is sometimes used to treat menopausal symptoms and cancer. The Mexican yam is rich in a natural precursor of progesterone – it turns into progesterone when absorbed into the body. This substance has come to be known as 'natural progesterone', in contrast to the synthesized progesterone given as a drug. The use of this natural progesterone from yam has been championed by Dr John Lee, the author of several books on the subject.

Progesterone vs Breast Cancer

Natural progesterone is taken by some women with breast cancer as an alternative, or in addition, to the oestrogen-blocking drug tamoxifen if they have an oestrogen-positive, progesterone-negative tumour. Building up levels of progesterone by using progesterone cream puts the body into a state of 'progesterone dominance'. In this state, it is much harder for tissues and tumours which thrive in an 'oestrogen-dominant' state to grow or be stimulated. This discovery was made when women with breast cancer operated on in the second half of their cycle were found to have lower cancer recurrence rates and better overall survival in the long term. So, when progesterone levels are high in the blood of those with oestrogen-dominant cancer, metastases are less likely to form. However, I do not advise the use of progesterone in those whose tumours are progesterone-positive, in case it stimulates the tumour. (This view is not shared by followers of Dr Lee who believes that, even with a progesterone-positive tumour, progesterone cream is beneficial.)

Progesterone vs the Menopause

Natural progesterone cream can also help to prevent hot flushes induced by tamoxifen – provided that the tumour is progesterone-negative. Building up progesterone also strengthens the bones, and nourishes the skin and mucous membranes, thus alleviating other menopausal symptoms such as dry skin and vaginal dryness.

3b. Indole-3-Carbinol (I3C)

This is a compound occurring naturally in cruciferous vegetables such as broccoli, cabbage and Brussels sprouts. Consumption of cruciferous vegetables has long been associated with a reduced risk of breast, colon and prostate cancers. I3C is being proposed as a possible natural alternative to tamoxifen, the oestrogen-blocking drug taken by many breast-cancer patients to prevent growth-stimulation of their cancer by oestrogen. I3C is also recommended for its direct anti-cancer effect.

4. Metabolic Therapy

This involves giving nutrients to the body in such high doses that they are being given as medicines and not food supplements. Usually given intravenously, the substances include:

> **4a.** High-dose vitamin C
> **4b.** High-dose vitamin B_{17} (laetrile or amygdalin)
> **4c.** Herbal extracts such as Ukrain.

(These are discussed above, pages 103, 105 and 111, and in the Resources Directory.) However, in the case of metabolic therapy, the high doses render them cytotoxic (cell-killing) rather than being used as immune stimulants or free-radical scavengers. They are, in effect, a form of natural chemotherapy. Evidence for their effectiveness as such comes from the fact that, following infusions of these substances, cancer antigens from disrupted cancer cells can be found in the urine. Also, large tumours can be seen to soften and shrink. These treatments need to be given daily for one to three weeks. Thereafter, there is a rest period, during which the state of the tumour is re-evaluated. Metabolic therapy can be used when conventional medicine has failed, or to reduce the size of the tumour prior to other types of therapy.

DMSO

This substance is sometimes included in metabolic therapy, and it also appears to increase the penetration of the B_{17} treatment.

4d. Shark and bovine cartilage

Cartilage is a tough, elastic type of connective tissue that does not develop a blood supply because it contains various 'antiangiogenic' substances to prevent the development of blood vessels.

The main use of shark and bovine cartilage in the cancer patient is to inhibit blood-vessel growth in a developing tumour, thereby cutting off its blood supply. This is the same mechanism of action as the drug thalidomide, sometimes used in conventional cancer treatment for the same purpose.

4e. Hydrazine sulphate

A synthetic chemical developed by Dr Joseph Gold in Syracuse, New York, its use is controversial, especially in the US. Hydrazine sulphate appears to inhibit the severe weight loss associated with major cancer. It is also believed to have indirect anti-tumour effects.

4f. Urea

A natural waste by-product of protein metabolism in the liver, the use of urea in cancer treatments was pioneered by Professor E.V. Danopoulos of the Medical School of Athens University.

It is used for treating liver cancer and preventing the development of liver metastases or secondary tumours as the liver is the only organ that shows high concentrations of urea after oral ingestion. As a therapy, it may not be effective against cancers other than those of the liver. The dose is individually determined.

4g. Enzyme therapy

In theory, enzyme therapy can help to break down cancerous tumours. The idea that 'oncolytic enzymes' could break down substances essential for tumour growth was first proposed by

John Beard in 1902. Early studies involved the enzymes trypsin, its precursor chymo-trypsin and pepsin, all delivered directly into the tumours. Another oncolytic enzyme is L-asparaginase, used to treat acute lymphocytic leukaemia. At present, there is an enzyme treatment called 'Wobe-Mugos' or 'Wobenzyme' that is widely used in Europe to control tumour growth. Another enzyme preparation is being tried currently under the name CV 247.

Enzyme therapy is often given with metabolic intravenous treatment as it is thought to increase the potency of such therapies. However, there is controversy as to whether enzymes taken orally can affect tumours in the body as it seems more likely that they would be deactivated in the gut or, if remaining active, cause havoc in other non-malignant tissues as well as the target tumour.

4h. Cesium

This metal is given by some metabolic clinics to alkalize the body to further potentiate the power of other metabolic therapies.

4i. The Rath vitamin C protocol

Matthias Rath, MD, a colleague of the late Linus Pauling, advocates the use of high-dose oral vitamin C along with the essential amino acids lysine and proline, and green tea extract. The daily regime includes:

- 14,000 mg of vitamin C
- 12,000 mg of lysine
- 2,000 mg of proline
- 1,000 mg of green tea extract.

4j. Amitriptyline

See Resources Directory, page 309.

4k. Aspirin

See Resources Directory, page 309.

5. Immunotherapy

The forefather of alternative immunotherapy was Dr Josef M. Issels, one of the 'gentle giants' to whom Penny Brohn, who started the Bristol Cancer Help Centre and who lived for 21 years with secondary breast cancer, went initially. It was while attending his centre that she had her inspiration for the Bristol Centre, which has pioneered such a radical change in cancer medicine in the 20th century.

Dr Issels became internationally known for his remarkable rate of complete long-term remissions of 'incurable cancers' such as advanced cancers of the breast, uterus, prostate, colon, liver, lung and brain as well as sarcomas, lymphomas and leukaemias. After completing the Issels treatment, these patients remained cancer-free for up to 45 years, leading normal healthy lives. The treatment also significantly reduced the recurrence of cancer after surgery, radiation and chemotherapy, thereby considerably improving cure rates.

In 1951, Dr Issels founded the first hospital in Europe for comprehensive immunotherapy of cancer of which he was the Medical Director and Director of Research. Of the patients treated at his hospital, 90 per cent had exhausted standard cancer treatment. In 1970, the hospital was enlarged from 80 to 120 patient beds. It had extensive research facilities, including immunological and microbiological laboratories. The hospital's programmes included research on tumour growth using *Mycoplasma* and bacterial vaccines to induce fever and hyperthermia.

During 1981–7, Dr Issels served as an expert member of and advisor to the Commission of the German Federal Government in the Fight Against Cancer. He also presented many papers to national and international medical congresses and within programmes of continuing education. He also published three monographs.

Dr Issels' concept of the development of cancer and its treatment

The Issels treatment is based on the idea that malignant tumours do not develop in a healthy body that has intact defence and repair mechanisms, but arise in a specific internal environment that promotes their growth. This environment develops over a period of time due to multiple causes and conditions that persist, and remain chronically active and risky even after removal of the tumour (whether by surgery, radiation and/or chemotherapy). The persisting immunocompromised biochemical milieu, he asserted, was responsible for allowing the formation of new tumours after local treatment in every patient with a secondary cancer.

Thus, the Issels treatment programme places equal importance on the removal of the tumour itself, and on the causes and conditions that led to the tendency to develop malignancies in the first place.

The Issels Theory and Treatment

Pre- and postnatal internal and external causal factors can lead to mutation-causing, toxic, sensitizing or neural effects in organs and organ systems which, in turn, lead to functional disturbances of the nervous, hormonal, excretory and defence systems. Secondary damage, especially an impaired detoxification system, will cause the body's internal environment to deteriorate, and can lead to the complex metabolic disturbances common to all chronic diseases and cancer.

When such a state persists, damage to the defence and repair mechanisms can occur. Depending on the inherited constitution and disposition, this can develop into a chronic degenerative disease and a 'tumour milieu', the ideal medium for cancer cells and the microorganisms found in cancer to grow. The body has then acquired the tendency to produce malignant tumours.

When a tumour appears, the disease has entered the recognizable phase. At this time, conventional cancer treatment uses weapons directed against the tumour and its symptoms only.

But treating the tumour alone is not treating the condition that produced it: the underlying cancer disease. Consequently, there is a high rate of relapse and recurrence.

According to the Issels concept, however, cancer is a systemic disease and the tumour is its late-stage symptom. Thus, the Issels treatment uses two lines of approach that are equally important and complementary:

1. A non-specific, basic therapy is aimed at eliminating causal factors, repairing damage, normalizing the internal milieu, and restoring the body's regulatory, repair and defence mechanisms
2. A specific therapy is directed against the malignant tumour itself and includes surgery, radiation, chemotherapy, hormone therapy, hyperthermia and cancer vaccines.

The non-specific therapy deals with the causes that led to the immune insufficiency and the development of cancer. This is modified to suit the individual patient's needs, and consists of:

- elimination of causal factors such as foci of infection, including those of the teeth, palate and tonsils, as well as malnutrition, abnormal intestinal flora, neurological disturbances, physical and chemical external factors, and internal and psychological factors
- desensitization of the body using autohaemolysates and colloids
- treatment of the secondary damage, metabolic disturbances, impaired detoxification and resulting defence weakness by general measures such as hyperpyrexia (fever therapy), and oxygen, enzyme, neural and organ therapies, with substitution or supplementation according to individual requirements.

This therapy is long term, but has no toxic side-effects, and aims to regenerate immune resistance. During such treatment, it was also frequently observed that eliminating infection in the head or the use of fever therapy rebalanced neurohormonal function.

Even in an advanced state of malignant disease, an immune reaction with complete tumour remission can be achieved. Many of the vaccine therapies seen today had their origins in the pioneering work of Dr Issels and, indeed, his hospital is still running today (see alternative clinics in Germany, the Resources Directory).

5. Vaccine therapy

The body's immune system plays a critical role in the fight against cancer. Specific vaccination immunotherapy techniques that support, enhance or restore optimal immune function may help to stabilize and reverse cancer without the adverse side-effects associated with conventional therapies.

5a. Coley's toxins

In the 1920s, Dr William Coley proposed that the rise in immune activity caused by certain infectious bacteria might stimulate a useful immune response against malignancies. The bacterial challenge was introduced into the body as a sterilized vaccine. Dr Coley found that his 'toxins' could give the body's defences a non-specific 'kick-start' against cancer cells by producing more white cells to attack cancer as well as bacteria.

5b. BCG (Bacille Calmette-Guerin) vaccine and melanoma vaccine

This vaccine stimulates a non-specific rise in immune function according to the same principles as Coley's toxins. A great deal of work has been done on melanoma vaccines for people with melanoma skin cancer. Pioneered at the John Wayne Clinic in California, this has been the specialist area of interest of Professor Gus Dalgleish at St George's Hospital in London. Melanoma vaccines are made from either the patient's own melanoma tissue or the tumour tissue collected from someone else with the disease. Professor Dalgleish has since extended his use of these vaccines to other types of cancer, and is pioneering dendritic cell therapy in the UK, as is alternative medicine practitioner Dr Julian Kenyon at the Dove Clinic.

5c. T/Tn antigen breast cancer vaccine

Cancer cells carry proteins, or antigens, on their surface that can be recognized by the immune system. The identification of certain cancer-related antigens forms the basis of this approach, developed by Dr Georg Springer. He showed that two antigens – T and Tn – play a vital role in the immune system's ability to respond to cancer. Since the early 1980s, Dr Springer has repeatedly shown, in both animal and human studies, that the immune response to the T and Tn antigens results in a much enhanced cancer cell-killing activity.

Using various biochemical tests, Dr Springer has detected the T and Tn antigens in over 90 per cent of all cancers. The less aggressive ones (those that are well differentiated) produce a higher proportion of T antigen whereas the Tn antigen predominates in the more aggressive (poorly differentiated) cancers.

Direct cancer vaccines are also being pioneered by Professor Dalgleish at St George's Hospital in London.

5d. VG-1000 cancer vaccine

Dr Valentin I. Govallo, MD, PhD, a Russian physician and immunologist, was the first scientist to reason that malignant cells survive and proliferate because they possess their own defence mechanisms that protect them from attack by the immune system of the host (the patient), a thesis now well established. After more than 20 years of work with cancer patients, he developed and refined the therapy now known as VG-1000, which works by undermining the cancer cells' defences, as described in his book *Immunology of Pregnancy and Cancer* (Nova Science Publishers, 1993).

VG-1000 is most beneficial against the sort of cancer known as 'carcinomas', the typical cancers from which most people suffer – breast, prostate, lung and colon cancer. VG-1000 is also helpful in melanomas, leukaemias and some sarcomas (cancers of muscle, bone and connective tissue). Patients who have recently had chemo or radiotherapy respond more slowly to VG-1000 as their immune systems are then depressed. However, patients who have had neither radiation nor chemotherapy can respond favourably. Thus, VG-1000 is clearly indicated as first-line treatment for those with recently diagnosed cancers as well as for preventing recurrence, or if the cancer is too advanced at the time of diagnosis for medical treatment to offer any real hope.

Since 1975, Dr Govallo has treated many patients, mostly those who had cancers that were considered incurable. It is claimed that more than 60 per cent of his earliest patients have survived for 10 years or longer.

5e. HANSI (homoeopathic natural activator of the immunology system)

HANSI treatment was developed as a treatment for cancer by Argentine botanist Juan Jose Hirschmann. This liquid compound, comprising the essences of plants and minerals found in the rainforests and deserts of Argentina, is available in various formulations for intramuscular injection, inhalation via a nebulizer or nasal spray, or sublingually (under the tongue).

HANSI is claimed to be effective against illnesses that alter the immune system such as cancer, AIDS, fibromyalgia, allergies, chronic fatigue, Crohn's disease, cystic fibrosis, lupus, Parkinson's disease and ALS (amyotrophic lateral sclerosis, or Lou Gehrig's disease). It is a powerful stimulant of the immune system, activating the NK (natural-killer) cells that attack cells which are 'foreign' to the body. According to the HANSI website, over 100,000 cancer patients have so far been treated, including those with cancers of the breast, pancreas, colon/rectum and prostate, as well as non-Hodgkin's lymphoma and malignant melanomas. In addition, when used with acupuncture, it helps to bring about relief of pain.

There are no contraindications, according to the manufacturer, so it is said to be safe for use while undergoing chemotherapy or radiation treatments. In fact, it appears to minimize the toxicity and side-effects of the drugs. The only listed warning is for those who have received a transplanted organ, as the rise in NK cells could conceivably trigger rejection of the transplanted organ.

5f. Dendritic cell therapy

This exciting new form of treatment involves priming the individual's dendritic cells with tumour antigen to reactivate the body's own immune response to the tumour. This is helpful because, in most people with cancer, the immune system fails to recognize – and therefore fight – cancer cells. Dendritic cell therapy greatly amplifies the effect of all other therapies aimed at immune stimulation as it makes the reactivated immune system much more tumour-specific. See also Chapter 3.

5g. Immuno-Augmentative Therapy

Immuno-Augmentative Therapy (IAT) was developed in the 1960s by Dr Lawrence Burton, a cancer researcher at the California Institute of Technology. Dr Burton isolated four blood-protein components in mice capable of crossing the species barrier and producing cancer remissions in humans. According to his theory, when the four components are balanced the body should be able to subdue cancer cells, but if any of the components are out of balance, the body cannot adequately defend itself. Thus, the aim of this therapy is to correct the balance of these protein factors to combat cancer.

According to Dr Burton's records, IAT has shown good results as a treatment for cancers of the bladder, prostate, pancreas and lymphomas.

5h. TVZ-7 Lymphocyte treatment

See Resources Directory, page 311.

6. Neuroendocrine Therapy

6a. Adrenaline therapy

German alternative-cancer-medicine pioneer Waltraut Fryda believes that cancer arises in the body due to adrenal exhaustion. This triggers a chain reaction causing the thyroid, in an attempt to compensate, to ultimately 'burn out'. The knock-on effects on the immune and endocrine systems then leave the door open for cancer to develop. The treatment involves correcting the disruption in neuroendocrine function and stimulating adrenal-gland regeneration.

6b. Insulin Potentiation Therapy (IPT)

This has been used to treat cancer for at least 18 years at his clinic in Tijuana, Baja California, by Dr Donato Perez Garcia, grandson of the discoverer of IPT, who also runs a training programme. Information about this little-known therapy is available at www.iptq.com (tel: + 52 (664) 686 5473).

7. Physical Therapies

The successful approach to reversing cancer and preventing it from returning is always multimodal – in other words, no single therapy, technique or substance can as yet prevail against the complexity of this disease. The exact combination of therapies and substances depends entirely on the individual patient, and the skill and knowledge of the physician. This section describes useful physical therapies that can potentially help the effect of other treatments.

7a. Heat therapy

In hyperthermia, pioneered by Professor Friedrich R. Douwes in Germany, the body temperature is raised to help destroy cancer tumours. Research shows that cancer cells are more sensitive to heat than normal tissues. Direct killing of cancer cells begins when the tissue reaches 104–105.8°F. Hyperthermia can greatly enhance the effectiveness of chemotherapy, radiotherapy and intravenous metabolic therapy.

7b. Light therapy

Also known as photodynamic or photoradiation therapy, phototherapy and photochemotherapy, this treatment combines a light source with a photosensitizing agent (a substance activated by light) to destroy cancer cells. The sensitizing agent collects in the cancer cells and, when activated by light, destroys the cells by releasing singlet oxygen, a potent free radical, which destroys the cancer cell from the inside out.

7c. Detoxification

An essential part of any cancer-reversal programme is detoxification of the body at the cellular level to promote excretion of toxins by the liver.

Clearing toxins and waste products from the body reduces immune system stress and tissue function in general. It is important to understand that cancer is caused not just by the presence of a carcinogen alone, but by a combination of this with the body's weakened ability to destroy cancer cells and tumours due to cellular toxicity.

There are a variety of detoxification therapies available for the intestines, liver, lymph, lungs and skin, all aimed at helping the body eliminate toxins. There are also specific herbal remedies to clear the toxic residues of both chemo and radiotherapy. Detoxification also includes eliminating unwanted viruses, bacteria and parasites from the body, which may also be weakening the body's ability to fight cancer, or be a direct cause of cancer.

Reducing Your Exposure to Environmental Pollutants

In addition to the above-mentioned internal detox, it is also desirable to reduce your exposure to the chemicals and toxins with which we commonly come into contact in our food and water, and our living environment, including the geopathic stress in our homes or offices. It is also helpful to eliminate foods and drinks to which we are allergic. Many of us have undiagnosed food intolerances, which can place a considerable burden on the body's defences.

Cancer usually arises where inflammation commonly occurs, which is what allergies cause, making the tissues of our gut and lungs vulnerable. Of course, the effect is worse when we regularly introduce strong toxins, such as tobacco smoke and strong alcohol, into the body. It is therefore advisable to stop smoking altogether if you have cancer and to keep the consumption of alcohol to an absolute minimum, saving it for special occasions only. It is helpful to have an allergy check for foods and drinks to which you may be allergic, so that you can eliminate these substances from the body to help reduce your immune system's load.

The elimination of electromagnetic radiation applies mostly to the extra-low-frequency radiation from electrical appliances. It is not healthy to live or work surrounded by electrical machinery, close to pylons or electrical junction stations. Protecting yourself from the geopathic stress created by electromagnetic forces generated by the intraction of different land masses is more controversial. However, there are studies that show that cancer is often clustered around areas of geopathic stress. If you suspect that your home or office may be part of your problem, it is wise to have this checked out.

7d. Oxygen therapies

Cancer grows best in anaerobic (low-oxygen) conditions in the body, and is thought to shrink in the presence of high levels of oxygen. Those with cancer can use hyperbaric oxygen chambers to saturate their blood with oxygen.

7e. Electromagnetic field therapies

An increasing number of electromagnetic devices are being used both to diagnose and to treat cancer. This is likely to be an important area of medicine in the future and may have numerous applications for the treatment of cancer symptoms, too.

8. Nutritional Therapies

Healthy eating is the foundation of all integrated cancer treatment programmes. It is currently estimated that at least 35 per cent of all cancers are caused by poor diet – mainly due to the relative lack of plant foods, and the excess amounts of animal fat and protein.

The lack of dietary vegetables starves the body of the vital phytonutrients needed to correct genetic damage in the cell nucleus. The body also misses out on the vital minerals and vitamins it needs to protect itself from free radical damage, and to maintain a healthy immune system. Excess animal fats and protein are associated with raised cancer levels because of obesity, the toxins and hormones stored within animal fat, and probably the infectious viral and bacterial material ingested, particularly where intensive farming has been practised and the animals are less than healthy.

Added to this are the problems created by diets that are high in sugar, salt, additives and refined foods from which protective nutrients have been stripped.

A further health problem arises due to the acidification of the body due to excess meat, coffee, acid wines, sour unripe fruits and soft drinks laced with citric acid. Many believe that the acidification of tissues provides an ideal environment for cancer cells to develop and thrive, and that getting the body alkaline again can be a major key in the prevention of cancer and its recurrence.

Nutritional therapies are focused on restoring a healthy diet that is based on:

- wholefood (replacing all 'white' foods with their 'brown' equivalents)
- non-acid fruits and vegetables with all meals
- vegetable juices
- dairy-free

- low-sugar and low-salt
- additive-free
- low in alcohol, coffee and tea.

If meat or fish are eaten occasionally, they must always be organic and (in the case of fish) wild. Individual circumstances will vary due to weight, type of illness, special needs created by illness, treatment being undertaken, cultural factors and individual preferences. It is therefore wise to seek the help of a nutritional therapist to establish a personal nutritional regime, and to have support in acquiring the necessary information and skills to make changes to your diet. Health Creation provides this type of help via our Nutritional Mentor Service, led by amazing chef and nutritional expert Jane Sen.

In her Cancer Lifeline recipes, Jane has devised recipes under three headings: Tough Times, for going through treatment or feeling unwell; Clean Machine, for detoxing after treatment or starting an integrated medicine approach; and Eat Right, to help you eat properly for the rest of your life.

The Resources Directory also lists organizations that will help you find a nutritional therapist (page 360). You may also need the help of a specialized hospital dietician if your illness has created special dietary needs, as these specialists are trained to assess your calorie and nutritional requirements in a scientific way.

Healthy eating should be adopted by all who have cancer or who wish to prevent it. But there are also some extreme forms of nutritional therapy where the accent is placed on food as a form of anti-cancer medicine in its own right.

Examples of this are the Gerson therapy, invented by Dr Max Gerson and now carried on by his daughter Charlotte Gerson and the Nutritional Therapy Trust, based on the work of nutritionist Lawrence Plaskett. These therapies are tough, involving around-the-clock juicing and daily coffee enemas, so are not compatible with having a job. Good support is required to keep these therapies going, and they must only be undertaken with medical supervision to ensure that any detox reactions are well managed and that there is no unwanted weight loss or metabolic upset.

One of the big issues with the more extreme forms of nutritional therapy is that it cannot be undertaken alongside the conventional treatments of chemo- or radiotherapy and that drug treatments of any sort are discouraged. So great is the emphasis on detoxification of the body that any medical intervention is seen as counterproductive. This can put patients in a difficult position and understandably worries conventional doctors. When undertaking these therapies, make sure you are also being monitored by a good integrated medicine or conventional doctor to make sure you are not missing out on potentially lifesaving medical treatment if your condition requires it or any helpful treatment that can reduce symptoms and improve your quality of life.

See the Resources Directory to find more about Jane Sen's services, and her books and videos, covering such topics as organizations offering nutritional therapies, nutritional-testing organizations and lists of foods which contain protective anti-cancer phytochemicals.

9. Mind–Body Medicine

Almost everyone with a diagnosis of cancer will initially need counselling or group support to help come to terms with the shock and disruption caused by the diagnosis. Further to this, there is also a need to examine whether your previous emotional experience or depression may have contributed to the lowered immunity and subsequent vulnerability to illness. We have already seen in Chapter 2 that recovery from serious illness requires an optimal frame of mind, and that many people will require therapeutic help to achieve this.

In essence, the goals are to:

- become free of depression
- become free of stress over which you feel you currently have no control
- express emotions freely
- offload old toxic emotions
- come out of isolation
- feel powerful in your own defence and believe in your own power to heal yourself
- believe in the power of others to heal you
- believe in the potential of a greater power to heal you
- develop strong affirmations, visualizations or hypnotic suggestions for yourself, and be able to see or feel yourself, healed and well, going on into the future
- develop inner peace
- become uplifted and happy
- become expressed creatively
- have a strong sense of purpose and meaning in life.

Help is at hand

There are a number of well-respected sources of mind–body medicine. In the UK, the world-famous Bristol Cancer Help Centre offers two- and five-day courses. In the US, the new Center for Mind–Body Medicine, which has established a cancer guidance training programme for cancer healthcare professionals, recommends the Cancer Treatment Centers of America and the Block Center for Integrated Cancer Care for those seeking mind–body approaches.

In California, there is the longer-established Commonweal Center, set up by Dr Michael Lerner. In Australia, there is the Yarra Valley Living Centre, run by Dr Ian Gawler, who survived, through his very strong meditation practice, a secondary sarcoma that had reached his lungs. In the north of England there is the Cancerbridge Trust in Hexham. The Breast Cancer Haven also offers mind–body courses both in London and Hereford.

The goal of the work of all these centres is to empower those with cancer and create healing at all levels – mind, body and spirit. The beauty of these approaches is that they can produce profound transformational healing as the crisis of illness is used as a wake-up call to get the life onto a happier and healthier footing than before. The emphasis on developing inner peace also means that people are greatly helped, if and when the time comes, to approach their death in a far more conscious and dignified way.

Not cancer-specific, but used by great numbers of people with cancer is the Journey process created by Brandon Bays, who healed herself of recurrent cancer through mind–body techniques. Brandon's inner work enables a profound emotional detox, freeing people of emotional burdens they have carried for years. This can be immensely liberating while also releasing a great deal of energy for healing and living life to the full. Another profound programme is the Order of Love, which can be used to heal old family conflicts.

My own contribution to this area is the Cancer Lifeline Kit and, within it, the Health Creation Programme. This is a six-month structured health and life review, which can be done independently or with the support of a Health Creation Mentor, who will coach you on assessing your state and needs each month, and on looking deeply at what currently inhibits or limits your life and how these self-sabotaging tendencies can be overcome. The programme's structure and self-assessment tools mean that you can see clearly each month where you are currently strong or vulnerable in all areas of your life. This allows you (and your Mentor) to clarify which areas you most need to work on. Over the six months of the programme, you will be able to observe your progress, and feel the benefits as you get your life and health onto a more sound and healthy basis at every level.

The types of therapies to improve your state of mind and, thus, your physical health include counselling, psychotherapy, hypnotherapy, emotional freedom therapy and neurolinguistic programming (NLP), group work, art, music, drama, journaling, story-telling, dream therapy, laughter and happiness training, drumming and voice workshops, and the self-help techniques of relaxation, meditation and visualization.

As for the body, there are therapies and training that can also profoundly improve your state of mind, such as hatha yoga (achieving peace of mind through physical postures that balance the mind and body), pranayama (breath training that stills the mind and energizes the body) and tantric yoga (the yoga of bliss through exploration of the sexual energies). Dance therapy can also liberate healing energy; one of the best is the Five Rhythms training created by dancer Gabrielle Roth. Often, those who feel emotionally stuck and trapped in destructive relationship patterns can achieve greater progress through more physical therapies. A form of psychotherapy which specifically bridges the mind–body divide is Gestalt, where therapists often work with the 'felt emotion' in the body rather than the mind.

Getting the Best of All Worlds

Dr Nicola Hembry is one of Britain's leading integrated medicine physicians who uses nutritional, allergy and environmental medicine as well as offering intravenous metabolic treatment. She is a truly holistic practitioner who cares for her patients at all levels of the mind, body and spirit. She is medically sound and scientifically based, while also having total respect for her patient's choices and a huge range of alternatives to offer them. The following is her view of the integrated approach to cancer, demonstrating the ideal stance you are looking for in a true integrated medicine physician:

> 'The therapeutic approach I currently offer cancer patients is what I describe as an integrated one, aiming to complement orthodox treatment with predominantly nutritional medicine and metabolic therapy. As much of the epidemiology relating to current increases in cancer incidence relates to dietary factors, and particularly to the erosion of defence mechanisms that occurs as a result, I strongly believe that the fundamental aim of treatment must be to restore the groundwork and foundation for health by restoring and optimizing one's physiology. This means restoring immune function, detoxification mechanisms, DNA repair mechanisms, processes for apoptosis [cancer-cell death] and redifferentiation of cancer cells, as well as anti-inflammatory mechanisms, to name but a few.
>
> 'Diet is an obvious part of this, but due to changes in agricultural practice such as monocropping and selective nutrient replenishment (NPK), as well as the use of chemicals which destroy the mycorrhiza in the soil and, by so doing, reduce mineral availability to plants, there is actually no evidence to support the much-quoted

premise that we should be able to get all the nutrients we need from a well-balanced diet. The evidence today is actually to the contrary, with many individuals having significant nutrient deficiencies – particularly in selenium, zinc, magnesium and vitamin D. Our diets have reduced in flavonoid content by 75 per cent over recent years, and these particular phytochemicals and nutrients play a major role in cancer prevention. They have a number of roles including promotion of apoptosis (cell death), redifferentiation (when "wild" cancer cells become normal again) and angiogenesis inhibition (stopping the formation of a blood supply to newly forming abnormal tissue).

'In my practice, the first thing I discuss with patients is diet – encouraging them to eat more fruit and vegetables (including fresh juices and smoothies), to cut out dairy products and all processed foods – placing the emphasis on whole, fresh, unadulterated foods. Depending on the individual situation, I also encourage deep-sea fish, organic free-range eggs and occasional meat (good-quality organic or wild meat). My view is that patients should thrive on their diet; therefore, finding a way for them to eat well, but also enjoy their food and have healthy treats, is really important. This is a major way that they are building up their resources and defences and will to fight, and it is important when healing not to feel hungry, weak and deprived.

'My treatment plan builds on the diet, with additional selenium, flavonoids, particular vitamins such as vitamins A and D, which both have redifferentiating functions as well as vitamin D's anti-inflammatory actions. I use immune modulators and substances with anti-inflammatory and anti-angiogenesis actions. I also use B17 as part of my basic regime. For some people, this is enough to keep them well and their disease under control, but for those with metastatic disease, I will use more specific cytotoxic agents, including intravenous treatments with Ukrain, B_{17} and high-dose vitamin C infusions, but also sometimes Carctol, fermented soy and Iscador.

'My aim is to help build the patient's own resources to keep the disease under control, and to produce remission if we are lucky. But sometimes additional non-toxic natural cytotoxic treatments or conventional chemotherapy and radiotherapy may be required to help achieve this (if they have not reached the end of their mainstream treatment options).

'I usually encourage surgery, where possible, to reduce the tumour load, and I have no issue with chemotherapy except when it is used rather indiscriminately because there is nothing else to offer the patient. Chemo is often suggested when there is only a very low chance of even a partial response, whilst causing significant damage to the

individual's immune function and general well-being and a negative impact on their quality of life.

'The ideal in my view is the integrated approach where mainstream treatments are used appropriately alongside supportive, non-toxic regimes which can help to support the immune system and organ function, and to mitigate side-effects, and which may in their own right help to keep the disease under control. In some cases, I certainly think there are non-toxic regimes that might be tried first, before resorting to chemotherapy, and there may be treatments which could be better for an individual than their mainstream options, for example, using intravenous Ukrain for pancreatic cancer.

'Although, so far, I have concentrated on largely physical approaches, I am very mindful of a more holistic perspective in relation to the individual and their circumstances. For example, while chemotherapy may be the "right" thing for one person with a particular disease, for another with the same disease, it may be an inappropriate choice for a number of different reasons. Working holistically takes these factors into account, as well as considering lifestyle factors generally and ways an individual may improve their well-being and optimize their outcome. This may involve other physical approaches, including exercise, stress reduction, relaxation techniques and pain management, as well as emotional, psychological and spiritual support.

'Although focusing largely on physical treatments in my own practice, I feel it should be emphasized that this is only one part of the process – and in a sense is like preparing the "ground" for their recovery. There may, however, be other ways in which a fuller process can be facilitated for the individual. I look out for this, and refer or make suggestions to guide the individual on to someone or something which can help to support this process.

'I think that although we understand that cancer is a very complex condition – with many different processes involved both in the development and spread of the disease – the fact that we continue on the whole to focus on chemical cytotoxic treatments is illogical and very unlikely to solve the problem.

'Cancer is complex – with many different processes involved in its prevention and cure, such as:

- *restoring normal control of apoptosis*
- *redifferentiation of abnormal cells*
- *controlling inflammation and angiogenesis*
- *repairing DNA*

• *correcting immune surveillance and detection of cancer cells*
• *restoring optimal nutrition*
• *stimulating mind–body interactions which can improve cellular function.*

'In my view, the only logical approach to cancer must be a multifaceted one which addresses the problem from all these different angles.

'Ultimately, to find the solution, we have to address the cause, and it is illogical to think therefore that one day we will find a magic bullet "cure for cancer" which will bypass all the factors which have given rise to the problem in the first place.

'Yes, it is exciting and groundbreaking when new treatments are discovered – particularly, in my view, if they are targeted and minimally toxic to the rest of the body. It is even better in the case of cancer vaccines, when the body can be encouraged into more effectively fighting the disease itself. But if the body is poorly nourished, selenium- and zinc-deficient, without the active defence mechanisms offered by a good dietary intake of flavonoids, with poor detoxification mechanisms and poor DNA repair mechanisms, with excess cortisol and stress hormones from chronic stress due to lifestyle factors – physical, social, and psychological … then these treatments may work for some, but they may not work for long, if at all.

'The most progressive approaches to cancer now are those which look at integrating a range of approaches built on the foundation of optimal nutrition and a happy lifestyle for the individual.'

Continuing to build the picture

If you have any other useful information or evidence relating to these alternative cancer treatments, I would be very interested to hear from you, as this is a living document which will be updated as new information becomes available. We would also like to know if you think we have omitted any important form of alternative cancer treatment. Please send your contributions to:

The Cancer Directory,
Health Creation,
77a Alma Road,
Clifton,
Bristol BS8 2DP

CHAPTER 6

Making your treatment decision

Once you have looked at all your treatment options, it will be time to make your decision as to whether you will undergo treatment and, if so, of what sort. It is important that you are happy with your choice and that you go back for more information if you are still unclear.

Getting a Second Opinion

If for any reason you are not 100 per cent satisfied with the information your consultant has given you, it is advisable to get a second opinion. You may wish to get this from:

- the same type of specialist as you are seeing in your local area
- a different type of specialist in your local area who will look at the problem from a different perspective. For example, the problem of nerve pain coming from a compressed nerve due to a bony tumour could be looked at by an oncologist, who might give chemotherapy or radiotherapy, a neurosurgeon, who might do an operation to decompress the nerve, an orthopaedic surgeon, who might operate to remove a bony tumour, or an anaesthetist/pain specialist, who might give you a permanent pain-blocking anaesthetic.
- a specialist of the same discipline as you are seeing, but at a national or international centre of excellence
- a holistic doctor
- an alternative cancer doctor.

It is your right to ask for a second opinion, both locally and nationally, if there is someone offering a more advanced service for your type of problem at another treatment centre.

The most important thing is not to feel embarrassed to ask for it. Nor should you feel that you are in some way being disloyal to your current consultant. It is generally better to take the advice on who to see for a second opinion from your GP, an integrated medicine doctor or another impartial cancer-information agency, rather than taking suggestions from your own consultant. This will avoid any embarrassment as well as the likelihood of being sent to someone who shares the same opinion as the consultant you are already seeing!

Giving Informed Consent for Treatment

When you undergo any medical procedure – be it surgery, investigations, radiotherapy, chemotherapy or other adjuvant (helper) medicines – you should do so only after having given your fully informed consent.

There is a huge difference between having been told about and signed up for a treatment or test and having fully understood it, agreed to it consciously and prepared yourself for it physically and mentally. It is estimated that we retain only one-eighth of the information given to us by doctors and nurses in medical situations because of the stress we are experiencing at the time.

Although this has already been said, it is worth stressing again: you should never embark upon any treatment or give consent until you have fully understood what the treatment is about, and you have genuinely understood the possible benefits and side-effects of the treatment. You should also take the proper amount of time to prepare yourself for the treatment before starting it.

Therefore, it is vital that you do not:

- let yourself be rushed or bullied into taking any decisions
- give your consent or embark upon treatment until you are ready for it.

Be assertive!

When you speak to your consultant:

- Feel free to ask about anything you need to know.
- Ask to be told the whole truth, if that is what you want.
- Take a relative or friend along for support. They can take notes while you are talking. Alternatively, take a tape-recorder so that you can listen later to what has been said when you are not stressed by the situation.
- Make sure you fully understand the treatment and any side-effects, short and long term.

- Ask for any support you need.
- Do not allow yourself to be dismissed. Keep asking your questions until you have received satisfactory answers.
- Ask him to respect the choices that you make.

If there is anything you do not understand during the meeting, ask the consultant to repeat it. If you have any lingering questions or doubts after the consultation, discuss them further with your GP, or ask for another meeting or phone call with the consultant or specialist nurses.

Checking that you are ready to give informed consent

If you are close to consenting to a medical treatment, check that you have fully understood all the ramifications of the treatment by asking yourself:

- What is the treatment (or treatment package) I have chosen?
- What are the pros and cons of this type of treatment?
- How do the statistical benefits of this treatment compare with not having the treatment?
- What are the short-term side-effects of the treatment?
- What are the long-term side-effects of the treatment?
- Am I now ready to give my informed consent to the doctor?
- Do I wish to ask for more time to prepare myself psychologically and physically before commencing with the treatment?

Saying 'No' to Treatment

There is, of course, a distinct possibility that after considering all your options, you may wish to say 'no' to medical treatment – either because the benefits or chances of improvement with your symptoms or prognosis are too small, or because you want to try other things first. If this is the case, be prepared to state your 'no thank you' clearly, assertively and repeatedly, if necessary. Some consultants and GPs are understanding and supportive of a 'no' decision, while others make it seem as if, by so doing, you are committing suicide. Often, the reactions are exaggerated and not in keeping with the statistics. For example, chemotherapy for advanced cancer may offer only a 2–5 per cent improvement in survival time, which equates to extending life by only two or three months, despite four months of gruelling chemotherapy. Statistics like this do not justify disapproving outrage on the part of the consultant.

On the other hand, there are cases where it is foolhardy to say 'no' to medical treatment when the chances of cure are good. For example, medical treatment of a CIN3 (pre-cancerous) cervix, testicular cancer, and some of the leukaemias and lymphomas can be curative.

In general and if possible, it is best to have surgical removal of tumours, even if you are going 'integrated' or 'alternative' overall. You will still need to work hard to change the conditions in your body that allowed the cancer to develop, but you will have dramatically reduced your body's burden once the 'tumour load' is decreased. You will also have lessened the risk of the tumour causing nasty problems locally if it continues to grow, such as breaking the skin, or putting pressure on nerves or blood vessels.

However, if even surgery is too big a step for you, or runs contrary to your chosen system of treatment, try to enlist the ongoing support of a mainstream doctor to monitor your health and the cancer on a regular basis. This way, you will be able to adjust your approach if your current strategy is not working while continuing to maximize your chances of recovery.

If you are contemplating saying 'no' to treatment, please check whether you:

- have fully understood the likely course of the illness without treatment
- are aware what the odds are for the medical treatment giving you a cure or remission of your disease
- are prepared psychologically to take any criticism you may receive from your doctors, friends or family for taking this course of action
- have professional support to follow through with your decision from a counsellor or doctor
- have negotiated with your oncologist, surgeon, GP or a holistic doctor to continue to monitor you so that, should your situation worsen, you have the opportunity to review your decision.

Facing the Downside of Treatment

If the treatment you are going to have will result in your experiencing some physical loss or disfigurement, it is good to face up to this as much as possible before you start it. This might involve having anticipatory bereavement counselling to prepare and grieve for the loss of that part of yourself, be it a breast, an organ or a limb. I have known people who have had special photos or portraits done of themselves to provide a good reminder of how they were before the treatment. I have also known of people who have done a ritual 'letting go' ceremony to prepare for the process. The more consciously the forthcoming loss is embraced and, if possible, accepted before it happens, the less likely it is that you will go into a more complicated grief reaction later.

In relation to the possibility of severe hair loss with chemotherapy, some people like to make a pre-emptive strike by actively shaving their heads before the chemo starts. In some cases, family members, partners and friends have also done this to themselves as an act of solidarity with the patient, though nowadays many people opt for the cold-cap to avoid hair loss. It involves wearing an ice-cold cap during chemo. This makes the scalp so cold that the blood does not flow into it while the drugs are being given and, if the drugs cannot reach the hair follicles, the hair may be saved.

There are specialized support groups for those who have become disabled or disfigured by cancer or its treatment, or who require a stoma after cancer treatment. Over and over again, people have said that there is absolutely nothing like talking to someone who has been through or is facing the same treatment or resulting problem. It may be worthwhile contacting one of the groups mentioned in the support section of the Resources Directory (pages 380–2), or asking your GP or hospital team to put you in touch with others who have had similar experiences.

Looking at how treatment may change your body and your life

Before you undergo treatment, ask yourself:

- In what way will my treatment change my body or my life?
- Do I need counselling before my operation to help me think about, grieve and adjust to this change? If so, what counsellor should I go to?
- Do I wish to find someone else who has been through the treatment I am facing to ask what it was like for them? If so, how will I find this person?
- Do I wish to be photographed, painted or videoed as a record, for myself and my family, of how I looked or sounded before the treatment?
- Do I wish to create a ritual to do with my friends to prepare for the loss I am facing?
- In the case of chemotherapy, do I wish to shave my head as a pre-emptive strike before my hair falls out? Do I wish any of my supporters to do the same? If so, who will I ask to do this?
- Do I want to find a support group or counsellor that deals specifically with the type of disablement or disfigurement I am facing? If so, who can I go to with this problem?

CHAPTER 7

Getting the best outcome from treatment

Both the physical and psychological outcomes of treatment are greatly improved by good mental, physical and practical preparation. It will help you sail through your treatment with minimal trauma and maximum benefits. Complementary therapies can relax and energize you before, during and after treatment (and will be covered in detail in Chapter 8).

Mentally Preparing for Treatment

This involves:

- developing a strong belief in your treatment and visualizing it healing you
- reducing your fear and anxiety levels by:
  - a) getting the information you need about your treatment
  - b) relaxing before the treatment
  - c) expressing your feelings and fears.

Developing a strong belief in your treatment

It is essential that you believe totally in your treatment. Through hypnotherapy, visualization, affirmation or positive thinking, you can develop a positive image of the treatment healing you completely. To help with this process, I have created a CD entitled *Cope Positively with Cancer Treatment* (available from Health Creation, tel: 0845 009 3366 or at www.healthcreation.co.uk) to be used on a daily basis before, during and after treatment. It contains relaxation and breathing exercises to make you feel calmer, and a track to prepare you for treatment by guiding you into the process of forming a positive feeling and association with the treatment.

Dr Leslie Walker's scientific studies have shown that women who visualized chemotherapy curing them while they were being treated had an extra 17.5 per cent survival benefit over women who did not. As the treatment itself had a 15 per cent survival benefit, the effect of visualization was stronger than the chemotherapy, radiotherapy, surgery and tamoxifen combined. Visualization also improves tolerability of the treatment. Many report having only minimal radiotherapy burns when they visualized the treatment only affecting the tumour and not their skin.

It is also effective to visualize cancer treatment as a positive healing force that will completely eradicate the cancer from your body. For example, some people have imagined their chemotherapy as the elixir of life, and their radiotherapy as a beam of pure healing energy. If you find it difficult to 'see' in this way, do it with words instead. Write yourself a script of positive messages such as 'This treatment will completely destroy my cancer' and 'I believe wholeheartedly in the power of this treatment to make me well'. (If this is also difficult for you, you may wish to enlist the help of a transpersonal counsellor or hypnotherapist (see the Resources Directory to find a therapist).

Write down your visualization or the affirmations you intend to use to empower your treatment and take them with you to read before, during and after treatment.

Reducing your fear and anxiety levels

Getting the Information You Need

If you are frightened of hospitals, doctors or treatments, and feel out of control as a patient, it is important to find out as much as possible in advance about exactly what is going to happen to you and how you will get help if you get into difficulties. People who get themselves feeling in control have far fewer symptoms and complications. Often, the nursing staff in wards, operating theatres and treatment centres, and the radiographers in radiotherapy centres are only too happy to show you around or talk you through the treatment in advance. Having the right information will greatly reduce your anxiety.

Before having treatment, make sure that you know:

- who will carry out your treatment, and when, where and how long you will have to wait
- exactly what the treatment involves, how you will feel afterwards, and what incisions, scars, drains or tubes, pain or other symptoms you may have
- how you will obtain pain medication or symptom relief
- whether supporters can stay with you throughout the process and, if not, how you can contact them quickly, if necessary

> • in the case of surgery, when and where you will be taken when you come round. This can vary from a ward, day unit, intensive care unit or high-dependency unit, depending on the nature and seriousness of your operation. Make sure your supporters know where you will be, too.

When you are in full possession of the facts, and feel confident in the team and unit treating you, prepare yourself to let go, trust, hand over and allow the team to do their job.

Relaxing Before Treatment
Relaxation is necessary to take your body out of the sympathetic nervous system 'fight-or-flight' state of arousal that is associated with fear and into the parasympathetic 'self-healing state' so that your body will be best able to withstand and benefit from the treatment. Use the relaxation exercises on the *Cope Positively* CD twice daily before, during and after treatment, and arrange to receive healing, massage or reflexology via your local support group or privately (see the Resources Directory to find therapists).

Expressing Your Feelings and Fears
Try to express any feelings you have, which may have built up prior to treatment, either to a counsellor, a supporter or on your own. Releasing your emotions will also enable your body to better cope with treatment, so do this regularly before, during and after the treatment. In a bath, with candles, bath oils and some gentle music, might be a good place to let go and have a good cry.

Checking that you are ready for treatment
As you come towards your treatment, ask yourself these questions:

> • Am I unclear about any aspect of my treatment?
> • Am I worried about it?
> • Do I feel anxious and out of control in hospital settings?

If any of the answers is 'yes', go back to page 132 and again go through the questions you need to have answered by hospital staff before you feel safe to let go and feel OK about having the treatment. Then ring or arrange to visit your treatment centre to find out what else you need to know.

If you are still unclear or feel frightened, arrange to speak to an integrated cancer doctor, your GP or your cancer specialist to go over your options, needs and treatment plan again. Your treatment will have a far better outcome and fewer side-effects if you can feel in control and create a positive association with it.

Empowering your treatment

In summary:

- Get yourself feeling in control by knowing all the facts about your treatment.
- Create a positive visualization and affirmations (visual or verbal) that the treatment will cure you.
- Do your relaxation exercises two times daily before, during and after treatment until you feel calm.
- Offload your emotions regularly before, during and after treatment.

Physically Preparing for Treatment

This involves:

- good nutrition
- detoxing the body
- raising your energy levels
- resting well
- exercise to tone and oxygenate the body.

How much you can do will depend on the time you have and how physically able you are but, in essence, the idea is to optimize your nutrition by adopting the 'Eat Right' or 'Tough Times' meal plans in Jane Sen's Cancer Lifeline Recipes, available from Health Creation (tel: 0845 009 3366 or via www.healthcreation.co.uk). Also, check whether you have been eating well prior to your treatment and write down the improvements you need to make.

Ask yourself the questions:
- Am I eating plenty of fresh vegetables, fruit and salads daily? What improvements do I need to make?
- Am I eating enough starchy 'energy' foods such as muesli, porridge, rice and potatoes to maintain my weight? What improvements do I need to make?
- Am I eating enough protein (ideally vegetarian, such as quinoa, soya products, beans, lentils with occasional eggs or organic deep-sea fish)? What improvements do I need to make?
- Have I been taking enough essential fatty acids by using olive oil, fish oils or an omega-3 fatty acid supplement (such as linseed oil)? What improvements do I need to make?
- Have I been drinking plenty of good water? What improvements do I need to make?
- Am I underweight or overweight?
- Do I need help from a nutritional therapist to help regulate my weight before, during and after treatment (see the Resources Directory for nutritional therapists)?
- Am I feeling toxic due to excess fats, processed sweetened food, cigarettes and alcohol? (If so, and if you have time before your treatment, you could do several days of detox with the 'Clean Machine' Cancer Lifeline Recipes by Jane Sen.
- Am I taking the correct vitamin/mineral supplementation (see below)? What do I need to get?

Take vitamin/mineral supplements for as long as you can before your treatment starts, and continue taking them throughout treatment, and afterwards.

This is a controversial area, with many oncologists telling patients to stop taking vitamins and minerals during treatment as they may adversely affect the effectiveness of the treatment. The publication of the UK Expert Group on the safe upper limits for vitamins and minerals in May 2003 also led to a widespread reduction in the levels of vitamins, particularly vitamin C, being recommended for cancer patients both during treatment and as prevention after treatment.

However, new evidence from the world's leading authority in this field, Professor Kedar N. Prasad, MD PhD, at the Center for Vitamin and Cancer Research, Department of Radiology, University of Colorado Health Sciences Center, has shown that antioxidant vitamin/mineral therapy enhances the effectiveness of both chemo- and radiotherapy. He states categorically that we should be taking more, not less, antioxidants to treat and prevent cancer.

The conservative regime proposed by most UK integrated medicine doctors and the Bristol Cancer Help Centre is as follows:

Vitamin C Food State	500 mg/day x 3 **or**
Vitamin C as calcium ascorbate	1 g/day x 3
Vitamin B complex	50 mg/day
Beta-carotene	15 mg/day (**or** 1.5 pints of carrot juice daily; NOT FOR SMOKERS)
Vitamin E	400 iu/day (stop taking this two weeks before surgery as vitamin E is mildly anticoagulant; start again after any bruising has settled)
Selenium	200 mcg/day
Zinc orotate	100 mg/day **or**
Zinc citrate	50 mg/day **or**
Elemental zinc	15 mg/day

Reduce all of the zinc doses mentioned above by one-third three months after stopping medical treatment.

Professor Prasad's regime, to be taken during cancer treatment and for four weeks thereafter, is as follows:

Vitamin C as calcium ascorbate	8 g/day (2 g/day x 4)
Vitamin E (as D-alpha-tocopherol succinate)	800 iu/day
Natural beta-carotene	60 mg/day
Selenium	800 mcg/day

Plus appropriate minerals, but not iron, copper and manganese as they interact with vitamin C to produce free radicals.

Professor Prasad says that it is vital to differentiate between dietary antioxidants (such as vitamins A, C and E, carotenoids and their useful derivatives, alpha-tocopherol succinate and the retinoid derivatives of vitamin A) and the not-helpful endogenously made antioxidants such as the SH-compounds glutathione and antioxidant enzymes) as these will modify the effects of X-radiation and chemotherapy.

Professor Prasad also states that the dosage is critical because the effects on normal and abnormal cells are dose-dependent. According to his definition, low-dose vitamins (around the recommended daily allowance, or RDA) do not affect the growth of normal or cancer cells, while high-dose vitamins (doses such as those in his regime and higher) inhibit the proliferation of cancer cells, but not normal cells. They do this by causing more cellular differentiation, proliferation inhibition and apoptosis (cell death), depending on the dosage and type of antioxidant, treatment schedule and type of tumour cells, with no effects on most normal cells *in vitro* (in the lab) or *in vivo* (in the body). Toxic doses are those which affect the growth of both normal and cancer cells, and have no place in cancer therapy (and are in excess of the levels proposed by Professor Prasad).

He has found that the uptake of antioxidants by cancer cells makes them more vulnerable to the effects of both chemo- and radiotherapy. He says:

> *'A treatment schedule with high-dose antioxidants is very important to produce the differential effect on normal and cancer cells. Treatment time of at least 24 hours or more is needed to observe a significant extra reduction in proliferation of cancer cells. Therefore, it is essential that high doses of antioxidants and their derivatives are administered before standard therapy and every day throughout the entire treatment period, and for four weeks thereafter.'*

He also stresses the importance of stopping smoking prior to treatment with antioxidants as the presence of cigarette smoke also changes the activity profile of antioxidants, especially beta-carotene.

Professor Prasad's maintenance regime for prevention of recurrence:

Vitamin C	4 g/day
Vitamin E	400 iu/day
Natural beta-carotene	30 mg/day
A multivitamin/mineral preparation	
Optional: Co-enzyme Q10 and alpha-lipoic acid for optimal health.	

His report 'Antioxidants in cancer care: when and how to use them as an adjunct to standard and experimental therapies' is available from:

Professor Kedar N. Prasad, MD, PhD, Center for Vitamin and Cancer Research, Department of Radiology, University of Colorado Health Sciences Center, 4200 East 9th Avenue, Denver, Colorado 80262-802278, USA, E-mail: KedarPrasad@UCHSC.edu, Tel: + (303) 315 7830, Fax: + (303) 315 8993

Consider your need to detox

Try to stop smoking and drinking alcohol before and throughout your treatment as they both impede the body's ability to heal itself. This may help tip you into better habits after treatment, too. If you are very dependent on either cigarettes or alcohol, you may need nicotine patches or psychological support to be able to stop.

Ask yourself:

- If I plan to stop smoking, what help will I need?
- If I drink alcohol on most days, what support will I need if I decide to stop?

Build up your energy levels

Use healing and energy medicine (see the Resources Directory to find healers, acupuncturists, and shiatsu and reiki therapists).

Consider your energy levels and what energy support you might need. Ask yourself:

- How are my energy levels?
- Do I need an energy boost to get me through treatment and help me cope?

If your energy levels are low, receive healing two or even three times a week, and acupuncture or shiatsu once each week.

Rest well

This will help you to build up your strength before treatment. Cut down your stress levels and do not rush in to have treatments if you feel tired and full of adrenaline.

Ask yourself:

- Do I take enough rest?
- If not, how can I improve this?
- Earlier bedtime?
- Later getting-up time?

- Having rest times during the day?
- Work less hard?
- Delegate some of my responsibility or work?
- If so, what will I delegate to whom?

Take exercise

Exercise as appropriate, to stretch, energize and oxygenate your body. You can use the CD *Heal Yourself*, which I made just for this, which includes yoga stretching and breathing exercises (available from Health Creation, tel: 0845 009 3366 or at www.healthcreation.co.uk).

Ask yourself:

- Am I physically fit and supple?
- Do I take regular exercise?

If appropriate to your current physical condition, try to exercise daily and/or do a 'stretch-and-breathe' exercise at home every day. It is even possible to do breathing exercises and stretches in bed or on a chair. All treatments will be more effective, with fewer side-effects, if your circulation is good and your body is well oxygenated. Try for a mix of outdoor aerobic exercise, stretching and breathing. But be gentle with yourself and do not exert yourself if you feel tired or weak. Take advice from your doctors and nurses after surgery as to when you can start to exercise again.

Practically Preparing for Treatment

This involves:

- Preparing the family by explaining to them fully what you are about to go through, how you are feeling about it, what you will and will not be able to do, and what help and support you will need from them. They too, may need some counselling to help them deal with the feelings they have about what you are going through.
- Being realistic about work and social commitments. Take enough time off work to prepare and convalesce properly. Try not to keep on working and socializing as usual to keep life feeling normal so that you can avoid facing your feelings. It is far better to see a counsellor than exhaust yourself, as cancer treatments can be rather demanding.

- Organizing your support team to look after your dependants, taking over the cooking, shopping and cleaning when you are unwell.
- Organizing your home to feel clean, comfortable and as calm as possible for the days around treatment or for your return from a stay in hospital.
- Overestimate the help you will need and then cut back if you are coping well.

Ask yourself these questions:

- What do I need to do to prepare my family and work colleagues for when I am not able to function normally during or after treatment?
- What do I think I will not be able to do and for how long?
- What do I need to tell them about what will be happening to me, and how I am feeling about it?
- Do I think any of those close to me will need some counselling and extra support to express their feelings about what is happening to me?
- How long will I take off work to convalesce properly?
- What work and social commitments will I cancel?
- What will I ask my support team to do to look after me and my dependants while I am unwell? Who will I ask to help with what tasks?
- What help will I get with:
  - baby- (or granny-/grandpa-) sitting
  - shopping
  - cleaning and washing
  - cooking and juicing for the family and for food/juice I may want brought into the hospital
- What do I need to do (or ask others to do) to prepare my home to be peaceful, clean and comfortable for when I return from treatment?

Once the Treatment Starts

To best address how you can protect yourself and minimize side-effects as you go through your treatment, there are a few basic issues to think about first:

- All cancer treatments are demanding, especially chemotherapy and radiotherapy, so the most important thing is to pace yourself appropriately. This means being very realistic about family, work and social commitments. You may well find that you will decide to cancel everything and make your treatment period a time just for you. This way, you can transform a potentially tricky time into a special self-healing retreat. If you release yourself from normal demands and expectations, then anything you are able to do will be a bonus.

- It is advisable to continue to work with a healer and, ideally, an energy medicine therapist who can raise and balance your energy using such traditional medicines as acupuncture, shiatsu (acupressure) or homoeopathy. This will give you maximum physical, spiritual and energy support throughout your treatment.

- Often, chemotherapy can be a depressant in its own right. People sometimes describe feeling as if they have lost their emotional skin or shell – as if the buffer between themselves and others has gone. This may result in your feeling very sensitive and finding it hard to control your emotions. It is good to know this so that you understand what is happening. It may also help greatly to see a counsellor throughout the treatment period so that you have a safe place to get support and share your feelings as they arise.

- It is crucial that you let your medical treatment team know if you are having adverse reactions, either physically or emotionally, to your treatment so that they can organize the best help and support possible for you, and change your treatment accordingly.

- If you feel that your treatment really is too much for you to bear, it is important that you have the courage to ask your team to stop until you feel better able to cope.

Going to a hospital or a clinic for treatment

If you have taken the advice here on preparing for treatment – you feel relaxed, have a good mental attitude toward your treatment, are taking your vitamin/mineral supplements and are eating well – you will be entering into treatment in a very good state.

While you are in hospital awaiting any treatment, take a portable CD player with you and do the relaxation from the *Cope Positively* CD first. Then, once treatment begins, use the track 'Preparing for treatment' to achieve a positive visualization of your treatment healing you, or repeat your treatment affirmations to yourself.

Preparing for surgery

When going in for surgery, arm yourself with *Arnica* 200X tablets (available from a homoeopath or homoeopathic chemist) and a bottle of *Rescue Remedy*, a flower remedy that is very soothing if you are feeling anxious. Start with one tablet of *Arnica* 200X on the day of surgery, and take one tablet a day thereafter for a week (or as soon as is practical after the operation). This will diminish the effects of the shock and bruising you may experience. This will not be a problem even if you are 'nil by mouth', as the tiny tablet will dissolve under the tongue. If you cannot find the 200X strength, use *Arnica* 30X every six hours or, failing that, take *Arnica* 6X hourly.

Rescue Remedy can be taken at any time, 20 drops in a little water, to help you when you are feeling scared or emotionally shaken. This will also be helpful for your carers, too.

Before surgery, take your vitamin/mineral supplements up to the last possible minute before becoming nil by mouth, and start taking them again once you are allowed to eat food again. It is especially important to make sure you are taking your zinc orotate 100 mg/day (equal to 15 mg/day of elemental zinc). It is a good idea to stop taking your vitamin E for two weeks before surgery, and for a week afterwards, as this can thin the blood slightly, making it harder for surgeons to control bleeding, which can increase bruising after surgery.

A checklist before going in for surgery

When packing a bag, remember to take:

- a portable CD player
- CD of *Cope Positively with Cancer Treatment*
- *Arnica* 200X (or 30X or 6X strength)
- *Rescue Remedy*
- vitamins and minerals, particularly zinc, B complex and vitamin C.

Arrange for someone to bring you fresh homemade vegetable juice and vegetable soup in hospital.
Arrange for a healer to visit you in hospital or send absent healing.
Arrange (if appropriate to your beliefs) for others to pray for you.

Preparing for Radiotherapy

During radiotherapy, as an antidote to the effects of radiation, you can take *Radiation Remedy*, a flower remedy made by Galen (see suppliers in the Resources Directory), one tablet three times a day. Alternatively, you can use the homoeopathic remedy *Rad Brom* 200X, one tablet daily on the days of your treatment and for four days thereafter, dropping to two tablets per week for six weeks after stopping the radiotherapy. This is available from a homoeopathic chemist, some healthfood shops or directly from homoeopathic suppliers such as Weleda (see suppliers in the Resources Directory).

In addition, if you feel nauseated, you may need the homoeopathic remedy *Nux Vomica* 200X or Ipecac 200X. Take these whenever the nausea reaches a peak. If the nausea is less severe, you might try the 30X strength, which can be taken up to three times a day. If you have more of a background nausea, you may prefer to use *Nux Vomica* 6X, which you can take up to one per hour as required. The 30X and 6X strength tablets are also available from homoeopathic suppliers.

Individual radiotherapy treatments are usually over very quickly, but you may wish to take a portable CD player and the *Cope Positively* CD with you to do some relaxation and visualization while you are waiting.

It is important to keep on receiving healing two times a week during radiotherapy with, ideally, weekly energy medicine in the form of either shiatsu or acupuncture to release the heat and energy of the treatments.

Your reaction to food during radiotherapy will vary greatly, depending on the part of the body being irradiated, and the degree of nausea you feel. If you are using The Cancer Lifeline Recipes by Jane Sen, try as much as possible to keep your 'Eat Right' plan going and, if this becomes difficult, try the 'Tough Times' plan. However, if your gut area is receiving radiation, you may need to follow a low-fibre diet as your gut motility may well be affected for a while. In this case, you can derive excellent nutrition from homemade vegetable juices (with all the fibre strained out) and Jane's Banana Body Builder recipe.

Keep taking your vitamin/mineral supplements throughout your radiotherapy. Scientific studies have shown that they improve the outcome of radiotherapy (see Professor Prasad's regime above).

There is also an excellent Louise Brackenbury Radiation Cream that combines anti-burn aromatherapy oils in a very light carrier base. It prevents skin damage from radiotherapy, and should be applied morning and night during radiotherapy treatment and for six weeks thereafter. Most radiotherapy units will advise you not to put creams on your skin at this time. But this cream was designed by aromatherapist Louise Brackenbury, who is also a radiographer, and is safe because it contains no heavy metals that can interfere with the radiotherapy's effectiveness. It should be applied morning and night, and is available from the Bristol Cancer Help Centre Shop (see suppliers in the Resources Directory).

Equip yourself for radiotherapy with:

Your remedies:

- *Radiation Remedy* or *Rad Brom* 200X
- *Nux Vomica* 200X (plus 30X) or *Ipecac* (200X or 30X)
- Louise Brackenbury's Radiation Cream
- vitamin/mineral supplements.

Take a portable CD player and the *Cope Positively With Cancer Treatment* CD into hospital with you in case you feel anxious while awaiting treatment.

Arrange for healing twice weekly during radiotherapy.

Find a good acupuncturist or shiatsu practitioner to work with during and after radiotherapy to help rebalance your energy.

Have a juicer and a good supply of preferably organic vegetables ready to make yourself daily juices.

Preparing for chemotherapy

During chemotherapy, your main problems are likely to be nausea, indigestion, constipation or diarrhoea, appetite loss, hair loss and tiredness.

The most helpful remedies for nausea are *Nux Vomica*, *Ipecac* and ginger.

- **Nux Vomica or Ipecac can be used as described above for radiotherapy**
- **Ginger can be taken either as crystallized ginger or by making ginger tea: grate or slice about an inch of fresh ginger root, then add a mugful of boiling water and a good teaspoonful of honey or three-quarters of a teaspoon of vegetable bouillon powder (such as the Marigold brand).**

If ginger does not work, or you do not like it, applying pressure to the P6 acupuncture point on the wrist can also help. An easy way to do this is to buy a set of Sea-Bands from your chemist. Designed to help people overcome travel sickness, they can also sometimes make all the difference in coping with the nausea caused by chemo.

All of these measures can be used either alongside or as an alternative to the anti-sickness medicine that your medical team will give you.

To help prevent **hair loss**, your medical team may offer you a 'cold cap' (described above). It is also advisable to supplement with kelp during and after chemo. This seaweed is rich in minerals and is reputed to stimulate hair growth. It is available from healthfood shops.

Eating and bowel function may well be a problem during chemo because the drugs can affect the lining of the gut and the gut motility, making it difficult to digest food properly. To offset this effect, it is wise to take aloe vera juice – a minimum of one tablespoon three times a day, or more if you can manage it. Another useful remedy is slippery elm powder. Try to take at least a dessert-spoon three times a day mixed with a liquid, or take one tablet three times a day with food. This will soothe the gut greatly. Even if your appetite is poor, try to keep on eating. It is important to do the best you possibly can to not lose too much weight. This is definitely a good time to turn to the 'Tough Times' recipes in Jane Sen's Cancer Lifeline Recipes (available from Health Creation on 0845 009 3366 or at www.healthcreation.co.uk). If you can manage freshly made fruit and vegetable juices, this will be a good way of maintaining your nutrition. People often find easily digested foods such as porridge or mashed potato and soups very comforting, too. If everything gets 'stuck', reflexology can stimulate the bowel into action again.

The **tiredness** caused by chemo can best be dealt with by resting a great deal and by having healing as often as possible – ideally two or three times per week. Your energy levels will also be raised by either acupuncture or shiatsu.

Remember, too, what has been said about the emotional vulnerability you may experience during chemo, and arrange for a counsellor to be available for your wobbly moments or on a weekly basis.

Equip yourself for chemotherapy with:

- *Nux Vomica* 200X (or 30X)
- root or crystallized ginger (plus honey or vegetable bouillon powder)
- Sea-Bands
- kelp tablets
- aloe vera juice and/or
- slippery elm powder or tablets
- vitamin/mineral supplements
- low-fibre foods
- a vegetable juicer.

Arrange for healing two or three times a week during chemo.
Find a good acupuncturist or shiatsu practitioner to support your energy levels while undergoing chemo.
Find a good counsellor to help you through the chemo if you feel vulnerable.
See the Resources Directory to find therapists and counsellors.

Recovering from Treatment

After surgery

It may take around one to two weeks for primary wound-healing to take place, but up to six weeks for full tissue healing to occur. Traditionally, when life was less rushed, this entire six-week period would have been taken for convalescence – so please don't rush back into activity too soon. Do not forget that you are also convalescing from the anaesthetic as well as the surgery. Do not be surprised if you feel somewhat less sharp mentally than you do usually, especially if you have had two or three operations close to each other. Keep your support systems in place for at least six weeks as this will give you time to convalesce properly as well as allowing you to work through any emotional aftershocks of the surgery with your counsellor and healer. Plan your convalescence well before surgery so that you can completely relax while in hospital and once you return home.

It is helpful to get extra vegetables into you by drinking as much homemade vegetable juice and soup as possible. Ideally, this should be prepared for you by your supporters and brought into the hospital daily. Some units have fridges for use by patients to keep juice cool and fresh. Wholesome soup can be brought in a thermos flask.

Make it a priority to receive healing twice a week for the first three weeks after surgery, and once or twice weekly thereafter until you are fully recovered. Often, healers will come to the hospital to give you healing or will be happy to send you distant healing if you arrange for this beforehand. It may be possible to receive healing free or by donation only. You can find the names of healers in your area and what they can offer from the National Federation of Healers referral line 10–4pm Monday to Friday on 0845 123 2767.

Scientific studies have proved that people who are prayed for during and after surgery have better results than those who are not. So, if it is appropriate to your beliefs, arrange for yourself to be prayed for, too.

After radiotherapy

It is likely that you will have a short-term flare-up of the problems and symptoms that caused you to have the radiotherapy in the first place (especially if the problem is affecting other tissues). This is because the radiotherapy causes inflammation of the tissue that has been treated, creating more swelling for a week or so. Then gradually, the whole area will settle down and the tumour will shrink over the next six weeks. It is therefore wise to wait at least six weeks before assessing how effective the treatment was. The subtler side-effects of radiotherapy can continue even longer than this, so it is important to keep on taking your *Radiation Remedy*, and having the extra support from your counsellor, energy therapist and healer until you are well and truly over the process. Again, plan your convalescence well so that you can recover fully before taking on more.

After chemotherapy

It is likely to take between six weeks and three months for you to feel like your old self again. There may even be the odd surprise in store. Some people find that their hair grows back a different colour or even that, if it was straight before, it is now curly (or vice versa). The most important thing you can do after chemo is to attend to your optimal nutrition as soon as your appetite comes back, and you are able to digest your food properly. When you are ready, resuming the 'Eat Right' plan from *The Cancer Lifeline Recipes* will make you feel heaps better, and your strength will return. If you have lost a lot of weight, it may be necessary to use the Banana Body Builder from the 'Tough Times' recipes between meals until your weight returns to normal.

If after a few weeks you feel better, you may wish to follow the 'Clean Machine' detox eating plan to get rid of the toxicity in your system, and restimulate the immune and tissue-repair mechanisms. You will have to judge the best timing for this based on how strong and what weight you are. If you are more than half a stone underweight, it is not advisable to go on a detox diet. Wait until you are closer to your normal weight. It is also unwise to start if you feel weak or ill. It is always better, if you can, to do a 'spring-clean' diet with the back up of either a holistic doctor or a nutritional therapist. So, if you would like to do the 'Clean Machine' diet, find professional support first so you can decide together when it is right for you to start. It is also a good idea to take detox herbs, whether Chinese or Western, after chemo to cleanse the body (see the Resources Directory for suppliers of these herbs). Chinese detox herbs encourage excretion of the toxins left in the body after chemo by stimulating the organs of excretion. Western herbs work in much the same way and are sold as 'liver herbs'. It is also possible to buy 'lymph herbs', which help to cleanse the lymph system. Carctol also acts as a good detox treatment, and is ideal for this purpose while also providing a long-term cancer prevention strategy.

Emotionally, the end of treatment can be a moment of new vulnerability as, suddenly all the activity, focus, structure and nursing support has gone. This can be the point at which the reality of your new situation hits you. So, it is ideal to have a counsellor available at this point. Now is the time to become proactive about starting a long-term Health Creation Programme. This will give you a new structure for your recovery process, supported by a Health Creation Mentor (covered in more detail in Chapter 9).

CHAPTER 8

Complementary medicine for coping creatively with symptoms and side-effects

The Issues

Both cancer and its treatment can cause a number of troublesome symptoms. Almost universal, though, is the need to raise energy levels, as the treatment of cancer, the associated stress and the illness itself decrease energy levels. (How to raise energy levels is discussed in Section 1 below.)

The second universal need of those with cancer is to be able to enter into a self-healing state through relaxation and meditation, so that the body is freed from the effects of stress and fear that all make healing impossible. (How to do this in covered in Section 2 below.)

The third need is to find natural remedies for common symptoms, so that the side-effects of stronger medical treatments can be avoided. As the treatment of symptoms can cause other problems, it is useful to be armed with a good range of natural approaches to symptom control to avoid falling into vicious cycles. For example, constipation can be brought on by opiate painkillers such as morphine and codeine and, when people feel constipated, they may also feel nauseous and unable to eat. When this happens, there is often weight loss and weakness. In addition, these painkillers can cloud your ability to concentrate, leaving you feeling somewhat depressed. All in all, this can send you into a downward spiral. From this weakened point, it is difficult to muster the strength to fight cancer. So, knowing how to tackle pain more naturally or dealing with constipation with natural remedies can break this cycle or stop it from developing in the first place (see also Section 3 below).

As well as maintaining your energy levels, it is also vital to eat well and maintain your weight. Maintaining a healthy diet can be tricky while going through treatment, but do the best you can to eat healthily. If you are unable to change your eating patterns at this time, wait until you have stopped your treatment before making the big changes. (In Section 4 below, you will find Jane Sen's Banana Body Builder recipe which, unlike most build-up drinks provided by the medical profession, is not full of dairy products.)

The Energy Model of Health and Illness

Raising and balancing the body's underlying energy and vitality is another way of improving our health. In all traditional Eastern medicines such as acupuncture, shiatsu, yoga and tai chi, the aim is to work with the underlying energy or 'life force', ensuring that all the different energies of the body are in balance and that overall energy levels are high. In acupuncture and tai chi, this energy is called '*chi*', in shiatsu, it is '*ki*', in yoga, it is '*prana*' and, in homoeopathy, it is the 'vital force'.

It is actually rather easy, even without Traditional Chinese Medicine (TCM) training, to sense whether a person's energy is basically in good shape or not. All of us make an 'energy diagnosis' when we look at our houseplants, judging whether they are full of life and vitality or not. People with good chi radiate health and are a pleasure to be around, whereas those who are low in energy or whose energy is out of balance often feel draining or uncomfortable to be with.

Nowadays, high-tech photography makes it possible to take pictures of the body's energy field, allowing us to see for ourselves the subtle energy systems on which TCM is based. With new bioenergy measuring and treatment devices, the body's energy levels can be measured and treated at the same time.

Through modern physics, we now know that all matter is fundamentally made up of energy and that all living systems produce electrical fields. The ancient Chinese knew this thousands of years ago, and their ability to detect, assess and rebalance the subtle energies of the body says much about their sensitivity and consciousness. In the West, owing to a combination of poor diet, alcohol, cigarettes, stress, overwork, overstimulation and a sedentary lifestyle, most of us are running on half-empty.

It is often helpful to work out our current energy level (see the graph opposite), imagining that we have a spectrum of energy levels from 0 to 100 per cent. We are usually born with very high energy levels, as all parents of small children will testify! But, over time, our lifestyle can rob us of this vitality, leaving most of us running at only about half our potential energy. At this level, we become susceptible to minor illnesses such as colds, flu and stomach upsets and, while generally able to work, many of us suffer from a lack of energy. The most common complaint seen by GPs is the TATT syndrome, which stands for 'tired all the time'.

Overwork or adverse life events that cause upset, shock or disappointment can bring energy levels down even lower to below a critical level of, say, 30 per cent. At such a low point, people become vulnerable to far more serious illnesses. Any health problem to which a person is susceptible is likely to develop, be it is asthma, schizophrenia or cancer. Even more

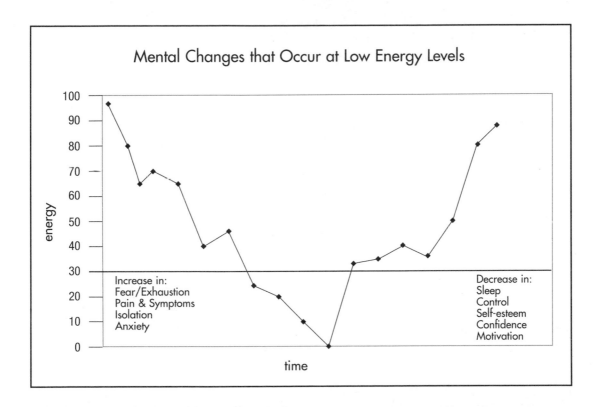

problematic is that when the energy level drops, the mental state drops with it. With low energy levels, self-esteem, confidence and motivation go out the window. People are also likely to become more fearful and anxious, feel pain more acutely, find it harder to sleep and feel their life is out of control.

People in this situation are on a slippery slope. It is hard from this point to take action to help yourself and pull yourself out of the trough you have fallen into. In fact, at this point, people often make things worse for themselves. When we feel things are getting out of control, our response is often to try even harder, causing more stress and exhaustion than before. As a result, people become even more depleted and, at the same time, beat themselves up for failing to make themselves feel better.

A tell-tale sign of being at this low-energy state is when you know what you need to do to increase your energy levels, but feel unable to do anything about it. Many people leading busy lives are in this state. They feel tired, exhausted and demoralized, yet they know they would feel much better if they exercised, relaxed, meditated or had energy therapies, but they do not go to the gym or a meditation group because they are too tired. People in chronically low-

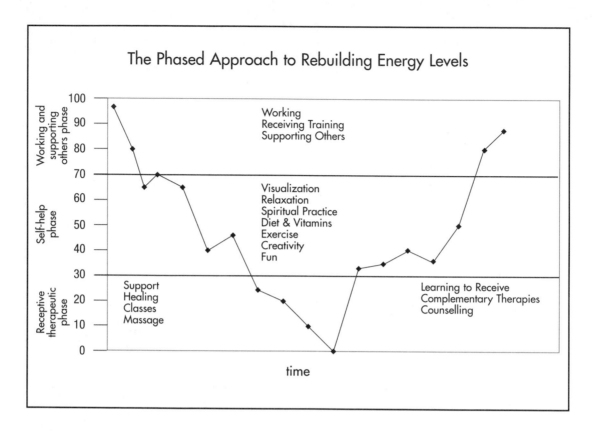

The Phased Approach to Rebuilding Energy Levels

Working and supporting others phase

Self-help phase

Receptive therapeutic phase

Working
Receiving Training
Supporting Others

Visualization
Relaxation
Spiritual Practice
Diet & Vitamins
Exercise
Creativity
Fun

Support
Healing
Classes
Massage

Learning to Receive
Complementary Therapies
Counselling

time

energy states like this are vulnerable physically and psychologically, and will usually not be able to initiate or sustain a self-help programme.

To reverse the energy loss, learning how to 'tune in to' and work with your energy levels, and listen closely to what your body is telling you, is the first step. It is then vital to adjust your behaviour accordingly. The most obvious starting place when working to raise energy levels is to cut down your energy output. But it is also important to learn how to raise energy levels by first passively receiving energy from therapists, then, once you are stronger, building up energy further through self-help techniques.

As energy levels rise, the reverse occurs to our mental state. At about the 70 per cent energy level, psychological health improves dramatically. People feel empowered, as if everything is going their way, and they often start experiencing synchronicity or meaningful coincidences in their life. In other words, as energy rises, so does consciousness. We experience meaningful insights into our own lives, and have a far greater sense of connection to, and support from, life itself. People repeatedly say that, once in this state, the things they want come to them rather than their having to struggle to make things happen.

So, if your energy levels are below 30 per cent, get therapeutic help from either acupuncture, shiatsu or homoeopathy, or especially spiritual healing. Once energy levels are out of the doldrums, and between 30 and 70 per cent, it is possible to keep building-up energy levels through self-help techniques such as relaxation, meditation, tai chi, yoga and exercise. Don't think about supporting others until your energy level is back above the 70 per cent level.

Raising your energy

Healing

If you have never tried spiritual healing or are very sceptical, I urge you to 'suspend disbelief', give it a chance and try it for yourself. You do not need to be religious or have faith in the spiritual healing for it to work.

During healing, the healer meditates and, by placing his or her hands close to your body, becomes an 'energy channel' or a conduit for energy from higher sources. Some healers perceive this energy as Divine, and others, such as reiki or Johri healers, as the life force of nature. Although it is not easy to prove scientifically how this energy exchange happens, it definitely does. The result is a feeling that is extremely nourishing and uplifting. Once tried, even those who were initially suspicious cannot deny that such healing is a lovely experience, with effects that can make a real difference to your vitality and motivation.

The beauty of healing is that you do not have to think, talk or do any work at all. The only thing you have to do is be receptive to the healing energy – rather like lying back and enjoying the sun or soaking in a warm bath. The hard part for many people, however, is the very idea of letting go and receiving from others. This admission of our vulnerability can be difficult at first but, once through this barrier, there is no looking back. If your energy has become depleted, healing may be necessary two or three times a week until energy levels have risen to the point where you can begin to help yourself with yoga, tai chi, mediation, relaxation, exercise and healthy food.

Energy medicines: shiatsu, acupuncture and homoeopathy

Shiatsu and acupuncture are the traditional medicines of Japan and China, respectively. In both systems, the energy state is diagnosed by reading energy pulses. In acupuncture, the pulses are taken at the wrist whereas, in shiatsu, they are taken in the abdomen or *hara*. With this information, the body's energy can be rebalanced. In acupuncture, this is done with needles, while shiatsu uses the pressure of the fingers, hands and even elbows at pressure points throughout the body.

In the East, it is said that people paid their acupuncturists when they were well and stopped when they became ill. This is because these systems of medicine have been used for centuries primarily as prevention, rather than treatment, and this would be an extremely useful practice for us to adopt in the West. An acupuncturist or shiatsu practitioner can quickly tell you what the underlying state of your energy is. You may need several sessions to get into balance and, once this has been achieved, you should ideally go every four or six weeks to maintain a high-energy state to help prevent cancer.

Homoeopathy also raises and balances the vital force, doing this through remedies given in tablet form, which interact with our energy to optimize our state of health and vitality.

To find such energy therapists in your area, see The Resources Directory (pages 354–62).

Freeing the Body and Mind from the Effects of Fear

Relaxation

Relaxation is something most of us have either forgotten how to do or never knew how to do in the first place. We have become accustomed to stress, anxiety and insecurity and, as a result, many people are very tense. As a doctor, when I ask people if they are able to relax, they often say, 'Yes, I can relax really easily. All I have to do is close my eyes and I'm asleep straight away.' But sleep is not the same as relaxation, and what they are is just plain exhausted.

In fact, people who go to sleep feeling tense or anxious often wake up just as tense and anxious. This is because the body continues to make the stress chemicals adrenaline, noradrenaline and cortisol throughout the night. As a result, such people often have anxious dreams, which can leave them feeling ragged and exhausted the next day.

If sleep comes the instant you close your eyes, it could mean you are actually chronically, long-term tired – often because of stress. If this sounds all too familiar, you need to get yourself properly relaxed either by a relaxation therapist, yoga teacher, masseur, healer or by using a relaxation tape. This will allow you to experience what it really feels like to be deeply relaxed, and show you what to aim for when doing relaxation exercises on your own.

Relaxation removes the effects of stress and fear from the body. It also helps the mind to unwind. Whether with a relaxation therapist or on your own, make sure you will not be disturbed and are very comfortable, which means loosening tight clothing, taking off your shoes, spectacles or jewellery, and getting yourself into a comfortable reclining position, preferably with your feet level with or slightly above the head. Relaxation exercises (including those described below) can be found on the *Cope Positively* and *Heal Yourself* CDs available from Health Creation.

To begin with, it is best not to do relaxation on your bed as this is likely to send you straight to sleep. You may also find that, as you begin to relax properly, your body temperature drops, so cover yourself up with a light rug to prevent becoming too cold. If you can, unplug the telephone, put a 'Do Not Disturb' sign on your door, or ask others not to interrupt you for at least half an hour. The next step is to really settle yourself into the chair, or onto the floor or sofa if lying down, and allow yourself to feel very heavy, as if you have completely let everything go. A good relaxation therapist, teacher or tape will then usually invite you to consciously 'unplug' yourself from all your normal activities so that you can switch off completely and relax deeply for the next 15 or 20 minutes.

Start the relaxation exercise with three deep sighs or outbreaths. Then begin by breathing in deeply, all the way to the soles of your feet, and breathe out, making an audible sighing sound as you do so. This instantly tells the body to let go. Thereafter, focus your attention on your breathing, allowing the breath to deepen and the whole breathing pattern to relax. Once you have 'arrived' in this safe, cocooned space, go through each area of the body, releasing tension as you do so. Start at the top of the head and work downwards. Begin at the scalp, allowing it to relax and let go. From here, go one by one to the forehead, eyes, cheeks, mouth, tongue, jaw and throat, letting go of any tension you encounter as you go along.

Some people prefer to tense each muscle group as they come to it, actively squeezing the muscles of each area tightly and then letting go. They find this easier than simply letting go, as it gives extra help in focusing on each part of the body in turn.

With either technique, after the head, attention then goes to the neck, shoulders, arms and chest. In the chest area, pay particular attention to letting go of the ribcage so that breathing can become deeper. Also pay special attention to the abdomen, where an enormous amount of tension and anxiety can be held in the solar plexus and surrounding muscles. Then move on to the hips, pelvis, thighs, knees, calves, ankles and feet.

In theory, by the time you get to the tips of your toes, the whole body should be completely soft and relaxed. But, in practice, if you are just starting to learn this technique, by the time you get to your toes, the head and shoulders may have tensed up again. It can therefore be worth repeating this whole exercise two or three times, if you are a beginner, to make sure you have fully let go of the whole body.

Once you achieve deep relaxation, your body will first feel very heavy and eventually very light – when you will hardly be able to feel it at all. Our sense of position comes from nerve endings in the joints and balance receptors in the middle ear. If there is no movement in the body at all, as in deep relaxation, we may temporarily lose the ability to tell where our body is at all. In this state, breathing will be very slow and shallow, and the heart rate will also be slower.

When you have experienced deep relaxation and learned to achieve this state on your own, you can then start relaxing for 20 minutes a day at home (or even during a break at work). As people become more experienced at relaxing, they can stay relaxed much longer or quickly drop into a relaxed state if they catch themselves being very tense. Most of us put far too much energy and effort into everything we do, getting more and more tense as we go along. When you have mastered relaxation, check every hour or so to see how much you have tensed up again. If you catch yourself feeling tense, make a point of letting go of the tension in your shoulders, jaw and stomach, and start breathing at a normal, deep, slow rate. Over time, the relaxed state will become the norm, and feeling tense will become odd. Try to learn the 'magic of minimal effort', which means putting only the minimum effort required into everything you do. You will soon find that you are doing less, yet achieving more.

Meditation

The single best thing you can do to revolutionize your health is to start meditating. This will make every other aspect of your life easier. As you become calmer with a clearer state of mind, energy levels will rise quickly. Resistance and inertia will melt away, and it will be easier to put all other aspects of life onto a healthier footing. Neuroses lose their grip, and we become more able to 'see the wood for the trees' in our lives.

Learning to meditate does not involve becoming part of a sect or taking up a religion! You can meditate in a religious context, like Buddhism, but it is equally possible to meditate with no religious connotations whatsoever.

Meditation is a process of calming the mind to allow you to experience your pure consciousness and deep peace. Most people go through life without ever experiencing this clear state of mind. Instead, they are totally preoccupied with what is going on in their minds, and therefore experience an ensuing sense of separation from everything and everyone else. Most of us think we are our thoughts, feelings, sensations and emotions when, in fact, these are the contents of our consciousness rather than our consciousness itself.

When we learn how to still the mind and untangle it from these 'contents of consciousness', we discover that the natural underlying state of our consciousness is bliss. This is the reason why all the religions of the world say that the kingdom of heaven is within. As soon as this still and open state of mind is discovered, people quickly realize that it feels much better than the external stimulation they seek or crave. As a result, the continual quest for satisfaction from outside of ourselves diminishes, and what outer contacts we have become greatly enriched.

From here, we become able to do less, but achieve more, as we become more clear, well focused, calm and happy.

Psychologically, the major benefit of meditation is that emotions begin to settle and we become more able to hear our own inner voice or wisdom. This wise part of our self usually knows exactly what we need or do not need in any given situation. As we base our lives more and more on the wisdom of this inner knowing or higher self, a lot of our problems or neurotic behaviour will simply dissolve away.

Physiologically, the chaotic beta brainwaves, associated with intense mental activity and stress, are replaced with gentler alpha brainwaves. At deeper levels of meditation, these may be replaced by the very slow delta or even theta brainwaves. When this happens, the neuropeptide cocktail in the body changes completely, and tissues and cells begin to function optimally.

All people who meditate report a wonderfully enhanced sense of living in harmony with life and feel supported by life, rather than constantly struggling against it. Their sense of separation and isolation is reduced, and replaced with a wonderful awareness of the connectedness of life. Many people are addicted to their chaos, stress and 'emotional dramas', and resist any attempts to quieten down emotionally. However, once the addiction to emotional pain and drama is replaced with real joy, a much deeper and more satisfying sense of emotional fulfilment and pleasure can be attained in life.

In relation to cancer, meditation alone has been shown to heal the disease. In Australia, Dr Ainsley Meares worked with people with cancer, taking them into prolonged states of meditation. In many cases, the deep calming and reactivation of the immune system led to extraordinary examples of remission and healing in a powerful demonstration of the connection between mind and body. Dr Ian Gawler, author of *You Can Conquer Cancer*, had secondary bone cancer in his lungs, but healed himself with meditation. Now, 25 years and four children later, he runs a Cancer Help Centre in Melbourne, Australia, called the Yarra Valley Living Centre.

There are some who say that the cellular chaos of cancer is a reflection of our mental and emotional chaos. And it may well be that, until we sort out our collective fear and disharmony, we will never be able to eradicate cancer from our society. I am sure there is a great deal of truth in this idea if only because of the profound effects of our state of mind on tissue functioning. But, certainly, as individuals we can greatly increase our cancer resistance with daily meditation practice, which deeply harmonizes our mind–body interaction, and optimizes tissue function.

Learning to Meditate
There are many ways to learn how to meditate. The practice always revolves around focusing attention on one thing until the mind becomes so still that it transcends even that focus. The

one thing may be a sound repeated in our heads, or 'mantra', as it is called in yogic practice. It may be an object, or picture such as a 'mandala', a form of traditional artwork that draws your focus to its centre. Or it may be keeping your attention fixed on the flow of your breath. Other forms of meditation involve focusing on loving feelings in the heart, or on generating feelings of love for oneself, the rest of humanity and the world. This is called 'meta bhavana' (pronounced 'meta parvana'). Some traditions focus on the sensation of the skin, which is often used in 'vipassana' meditation.

The best-known school of meditation, using a mantra technique, is Transcendental Meditation (TM), which is a highly effective way of learning the skill. Focusing on the breath is often associated with yogic and Buddhist practices, and teachers can be found through the British Wheel of Yoga and Friends of the Western Buddhist Order as well as other schools of meditation (see The Resources Directory, page 381).

For most Westerners, learning to meditate may seem difficult at first because we have such busy minds and have never learned how to still them. The key to mastering the technique is good tuition, regular practice and meditating in a group. Joining a regular meditation class or group is highly recommended until you are able to meditate for at least 20 minutes twice a day at home by yourself. Initially, meditating in a group will make the whole exercise seem easier, as the stillness and peace generated by a group is 'catching'. Whatever else you do as a result of reading this book, I urge you most of all to practise meditation. It will also unlock your ability to make the right steps towards health, well-being and fulfilment in all other areas of your life as well. If you are not near to a class or teacher, the two meditation exercises on the *Heal Yourself* CD from Health Creation can guide your practice until you are disciplined enough to meditate on your own.

Natural Symptom Control

Most symptoms have three main components:

- the physical symptom itself
- the fear and anxiety that the symptom creates (which can make the symptom feel far worse)
- the emotional upset that builds in response to the pain.

In general, to achieve natural symptom control, first you must work to reduce the fear and anxiety created by the symptom. This can be done through relaxation and breathing techniques, or having massage, hypnotherapy or aromatherapy, or being talked down into a relaxed state by someone calm. Often, through relaxation alone, the symptom can be brought into a bearable range.

The next step is often emotional catharsis, which will often happen spontaneously as relaxation begins. Usually, it comes down to feeling safe enough to cry or become angry about what is happening to you. Once you have managed to let go of the emotion you are feeling, you may find that the symptom becomes more bearable (or even goes). This will permit you to deal with the remaining symptom, using either natural remedies or specific mind–body techniques.

The mind–body approach to symptom relief

Using the mind to help deal with symptoms can be done in two ways.

1. In the first, the mind transcends the symptom. This means that you either distract yourself or learn to rise above it – by using:

- hypnotherapy
- music
- entertainment
- personal visualization
- guided imagery
- a pleasurable stimulus that is stronger than the symptom.

2. In the second way, you go in the opposite direction, focusing fully on the symptom. At first, the symptom may feel worse for a short time. But, remarkably, if you keep focusing on the symptom, it can change significantly. You may begin to feel your way into it, giving it a shape, a colour and even a voice. You can even ask the symptom what it is all about, or what it requires to loosen its grip. Sometimes, 'communicating' with the symptom in this way can bring forth staggering insights into the underlying 'energetics' or emotional dimension of the illness. By doing this with a skilled counsellor or mind–body therapist, the energy of a symptom may be released, bringing a remarkable resolution to the problem.

You can work with symptoms in this way yourself (try track 4 on the *Cope Positively* CD), but it is easier with a trained transpersonal counsellor, who can help you process whatever insights or emotions may be locked into the symptom. In this way, you are treating the symptom as a symbol of the deep mind–body processes you are going through and, by addressing the problem consciously, allow profound healing to occur. Transpersonal counsellors can be found through their head office at the Centre for Transpersonal Psychology in London (see The Resources Directory). Another helpful tool is the tape/CD *Metta: Dissolving Fear Into Love* by Jacqueline Herron, available from Health Creation (tel: 0845 009 3366; not available on the website).

Complementary therapies for symptom relief

Complementary cancer care comprises various forms of therapy in addition to (or as a complement to) orthodox medicine. It is generally used to control the symptoms of cancer, rather than cure it, and can make a huge difference to your morale, comfort, energy levels, symptoms and quality of life.

Here are some examples of therapies used for symptom relief:

Name	Brief description
Acupuncture	Traditional Chinese approach for raising and balancing energy levels by inserting needles into the body's energy meridians
Aromatherapy	Very gentle massage, but using aromatic oils for symptom relief
Ayurvedic medicine	Indian herbs, yoga and special diets to strengthen and detox the body
Chinese medicine	Chinese herbs and acupuncture to balance the body and cleanse it after treatment
Healing	Spiritual energy is channelled by the laying on of the hands to raise energy levels
Herbal medicine (phytotherapy)	Herbs for cleansing, detoxification, re-energizing and symptom control
Homoeopathy	Small doses of natural medicines to increase vitality and reduce symptoms
Massage	Manipulation of soft body tissues to relieve tension and pain

Osteopathy	Relief of bone and muscle problems by pressure and manipulation
Cranial osteopathy	Gentle osteopathy on the head, neck and sacrum to restore circulation of cerebrospinal fluid and relieve symptoms
Reflexology	Stimulation of pressure points in the feet
Reiki	Healing by stimulating and balancing the body's energy fields

Therapies for the relief of specific symptoms include:

Symptom	Complementary therapy
Anxiety and insomnia	Aromatherapy; breathing techniques; counselling; gentle exercise; herbal Valerian-based medicines; homoeopathy; tai chi; yoga
Appetite loss	Acupuncture; herbal medicine; homoeopathy; reflexology
Breathlessness	Acupuncture; breathing techniques; relaxation; pranayama (yoga breathing techniques)
Chemotherapy side-effects	See Nausea below; plus herbal medicines: aloe vera gel or juice, chamomile mouthwash for sores, kelp for hair growth; minerals: zinc lozenges for mouth sores; relaxation; spiritual healing; positive visualizations
Constipation	Herbal medicines: *Psyllium* husks, senna, slippery elm powder; reflexology; if prolonged, enemas or colonic irrigation
Diarrhoea	Herbal medicine: *Psyllium* husks; acupuncture; reflexology
Fatigue, causing loss of motivation	Spiritual healing; reiki; acupuncture; shiatsu
Infertility (see additional notes below)	Reflexology: stimulation of pituitary gland (and ovaries in women); tai chi; chi gong; yoga; Chinese herbal medicine (for detox); good nutrition

Lymphoedema (see additional notes below)	Massage for lymph drainage; raising the affected area above the rest of the body; muscle pumping to stimulate fluid release from the affected limb by exercise; shiatsu; craniosacral therapy
Menopausal symptoms (see additional notes below)	Herbal medicine: including *Agnus Castus* and Black Cohosh; holistic mind–body approach; natural progesterone cream; massage; meditation; relaxation; omega-3 fatty acids
Nausea	Acupuncture; acupressure; Sea-Bands applied at P6 acupuncture point; herbal medicine: ginger root, slippery elm; homoeopathy: *Nux Vomica* 6X, 30X, 200X or more, specific homoeopathic remedies just for you; visualization
Pain	Acupuncture; yoga breathing techniques; craniosacral therapy; mind–body transcendence techniques; music therapy; reflexology; relaxation; shiatsu
Radiotherapy side-effects	As for Nausea above; plus aromatherapy with Louise Brackenbury's Radiation Cream; homoeopathy: *Rad Brom* 200; Flower remedies: *Radiation Remedy*; relaxation; visualization
Weight loss	Nutrition: wholefood build-up drinks such as the Banana Body Builder; herbal medicine: Carctol

More complex side-effects

Lymphoedema

This is swelling of the tissues with lymphatic fluid, which cannot drain away properly because the lymphatic system has been disrupted by either surgery or, more usually, radiotherapy. It most commonly affects the arms after radiotherapy to the armpit (axilla) in the treatment of breast cancer. It can be relieved by lymph-drainage massage; gravity (lifting the affected limb or body part higher than the rest of the body) or muscle pumping of the affected limb – for example, squeezing a tennis ball repeatedly with the hand of the affected arm. Fluid may also build up in the lungs and abdomen and, often, either craniosacral therapy or shiatsu can achieve symptomatic relief. Acupuncture should be avoided in those with lymphoedema as needle punctures may become infected in tissues with poor circulation.

Infertility

This is one of the most distressing potential side-effects of chemotherapy or hormonal treatment of cancer, and it is not always clear whether it will be temporary or permanent. One of the best ways to re-stimulate fertility in women to get the ovaries back into a normal cycle is with reflexology, in which attention is focused on both the pituitary gland, which controls ovulation, and the ovaries themselves. Yoga, tai chi or chi gong is also advisable to help get the body back into optimal balance. Taking Chinese or Western detox herbs after chemo can be helpful if a pregnancy is desired, as can following the 'Eat Right' diet, as suggested in the *Cancer Lifeline Recipes* or the *More Healing Foods Cookbook* by Jane Sen.

Menopausal Symptoms in Women and Hot Flushes in Men

Both chemotherapy and hormonal treatments for breast cancer can induce menopause and the onset of troublesome hot flushes. There are several ways to deal with this, of which the most successful is deep meditation. It appears that hot flushes are triggered by heightened nervous system states, and that calming down the nervous system can reduce their incidence and intensity. Other approaches include taking the herbs *Agnus castus* or omega-3 fatty acids. Argyll Herbs makes a mixture known as Menopausal Herbs that many women have found helpful. Another alternative for women is natural progesterone cream, though this has to be done with the supervision of a holistic or integrated medicine doctor as it is only available by prescription. The cream puts the body into a state of progesterone dominance, making it less sensitive to the lack of oestrogen. However, this is not recommended for those with a progesterone-positive tumour, so it is essential to check your tumour hormone status before starting such treatment.

Some women with hot flushes may be taking too much tamoxifen, so changing the dosage, the way they take it or even the brand of tamoxifen may help to control the flushes. First, try splitting a once-daily dose into a twice-daily dose (i.e. change 20 mg once a day to 10 mg twice a day). If symptoms remain severe, the dose can be reduced slightly, but only if your doctors agree, to 10 mg in the morning and 5 mg at night, or even further, to 5 mg twice a day, until symptom control is achieved.

Some doctors may also prescribe vasoconstrictor drugs to control hot flushes. These stop the dilatation of capillaries in the skin that causes the feeling of heat, and may work well for some men and women.

Maintaining Your Weight

One concern people may have about changing to a healthy diet is that they will lose too much weight. Usually, when people make the change to a vegetable-based diet, they lose some weight initially as refined sugars and animal fats are dropped from the diet. For example, one Mars bar contains the same amount of sugar as about 15 apples. However, people following a wholefood diet would be satisfied long before eating this many apples and so consume far less sugar while getting all the healthy vitamins, minerals, phytochemicals and fibre they need. After a while, body weight usually reaches a new, healthy equilibrium. If it continues to fall, you are probably concentrating too much on fruit and vegetables, and not getting enough carbohydrates and fats. In this case, it may be helpful to seek the advice of a nutritional therapist to find out where you are going wrong.

However, if you are losing weight due to tough medical treatment or your illness, you need to concentrate on actively raising your weight by getting plenty of carbohydrates and vegetable oils. One glass of Jane Sen's Banana Body Builder three times a day with your meals will help you put weight back on again.

Jane Sen's Banana Body Builder
2–6 oz plain tofu (organic fresh or silken)
1 pt (20 fl oz) soya milk
1 banana
1 tbs organic maple syrup
1 tbs slippery elm powder
½ tsp vanilla essence
Blend all ingredients together in a liquidizer until smooth.

Additions and variations:
- *2 tbs ground almonds*
- *2 tbs cooked brown rice (or other cooked wholegrains such as millet or oats)*
- *A little honey*
- *A drop or two of almond essence*
- *1 tbs organic maple syrup or organic sugar*

CHAPTER 9

Long-term
Health Creation

The Road to Recovery ...

Once you have come through the process of cancer treatment, or you are not choosing or able to use medical treatment, what is needed is a well-planned, dedicated approach to recovering your health and well-being.

Inspiring examples of people who have stabilized their health in the long term using natural health approaches can be found in the *Message of Hope* video, available from Health Creation (tel: 0845 009 3366; www.healthcreation.co.uk). Several of these people have managed to stabilize and survive serious cancer against huge medical odds by dint of their own holistic health promotion efforts rather than alternative medicine. Reg Flower, 23-year survivor of secondary melanoma skin cancer, puts his recovery down to an organic wholefood diet and learning how to cry. Zoe Lindgren, 18-year survivor of lung secondary tumours of breast cancer, says it's due to having left her 'fast-lane' lifestyle and becoming a serious meditator.

In the holistic approach to health, the objective is first to harness your creative intelligence and fighting spirit to think about:

- what could have caused the illness
- what may be the 'chinks in your armour' that have allowed the illness to develop
- finding the most effective, appropriate and successful way for you to get well again in the long term.

Many factors are involved in getting cancer, and many factors may be involved in your long-term recovery. The key requirements for getting the body to fight back against cancer are to have:

- a healthy, fully functioning immune system
- excellent nutrition and a fit, well-oxygenated, relaxed body
- a high level of well-balanced energy or vitality
- a calm, clear and highly focused mind
- a strong and clear purpose in living
- strong, loving emotional and spiritual support.

Going beyond the medical model

Once your treatment is over, the aim is to achieve a lasting remission from cancer by producing a 'state shift' in the body to get the body's natural cancer-detection and repair mechanisms working again. The goal is to change the body's state so that cancer cannot recur. In essence, we are promoting health in the presence of illness, however severe, using every known way to improve the condition of the body, mind and spirit to achieve stable, radiant, sustainable health.

To do this, it is important to work on all fronts simultaneously to restore health. However, for each of us, there may be specific causative factors that have damaged or undermined our health, which only we can know. A good starting place on the road to recovery is to think about what may have allowed you to become ill in the first place and then to pay special attention to getting that right.

The causes of cancer are both direct and indirect. Direct causes of cancer include chemical toxins, viruses, inflammatory processes and damaging electromagnetic radiation, all of which can cause damage or mutation of the genes or chromosomes in our cell nuclei. Indirect causes include factors that prevent the body from repairing this cellular damage or removing faulty cells from the body, or which fuel or 'promote' the cancer growth once it becomes established.

The protective mechanisms against cancer in healthy bodies operate on two main levels. The first is within the cell (intracellular), where damaged DNA is identified and corrected. If the damage is beyond repair, then the cell is destroyed, or 'commits suicide' in a process known as 'apoptosis'. The second level is outside of the damaged cell (extracellular) and involves the immune system in recognizing and destroying abnormal cells: in particular, the natural-killer (NK) cells which act like the SAS of the immune system, killing abnormal cells on sight. However, many factors weaken the immune system, decreasing both the numbers and activity levels of the NK cells, leaving the body vulnerable to the proliferation of abnormal cancer cells.

When fighting cancer, it is vital both to eliminate the causes of cancer and restore the intra- and extracellular levels of anti-cancer protection. The intracellular mechanism depends on nutrition, especially our intake of raw plant material in juices, salads, fresh fruit and vegetables. The extracellular mechanism depends on the health of our immune system which, in turn, depends on a complex mixture of factors – nutritional, emotional and hormonal.

Below is a list of the known causes of cancer and of a weakened immune system. See if any of them apply to you. Knowing your areas of vulnerability can help you design a personalized Health Creation Programme to speed your cancer recovery.

However, if you think that none applies to you and you can see no reason why you got ill, then go for an all-round programme that involves immune stimulation and good nutrition as well as raising your energy levels, and strengthening your body, mind and spirit.

What do we know about the causes of cancer?

The chief causes of cancer, according to UK cancer authorities, are:

- **poor diet** (35 per cent), particularly due to overeating and obesity, excess intake of meat and animal fat, and a relative lack of fruit and vegetables
- **smoking** (30 per cent)
- **excess reproductive hormones** (10 per cent), including HRT and prolonged use of the Pill
- **infections** (10 per cent) with viruses, bacteria or parasites
- **excess alcohol** (5 per cent)
- **electromagnetic radiation** (4 per cent), including too much sun, mobile phone use, radiation, electricity in the environment, earth energies and microwaves
- **occupational hazards** (2 per cent)
- **pollution** (2 per cent) at home and in the environment
- **physical inactivity** (1.5 per cent)
- **medical procedures** (0.5 per cent).

This shows that cancer is at least 80 per cent due to lifestyle, according to current estimations of Cancer Research UK. So, think about whether any of these risk factors relate to you and resolve to eliminate these factors from your life by yourself or with the support of a Health Creation Mentor (available via the Health Creation helpline: 0845 009 3366).

However, this list from Cancer Research UK does not take into account other important factors that are now known to weaken the immune system significantly, making us more vulnerable. One of the newest branches of science – known as psychoneuroimmunology (PNI) – has demonstrated that negative states of mind and spirit can have a very pronounced depressive effect not only on the number of circulating white T and NK cells we have, but also on their level of activation. These states (covered more fully in Chapter 2) include:

- prolonged stress over which we have no control
- exhaustion
- loneliness and isolation
- being 'too nice' and hiding or repressing your feelings
- depression and a lack of motivation
- shock and trauma
- grief
- a lack of purpose and will to live.

All of the above can decrease the number of circulating white cells by 10–30 per cent, and the activity of the remaining white cells by as much as 50 per cent. Thus, it is possible to have 70 per cent of the normal number of white cells circulating but, if they are running at only half-power, then the overall immune function will be about 35 per cent of the optimal level.

Conversely, immune function can be improved by:

- emotional support, either one to one or in a group
- emotional expression, or letting go of your feelings
- visualization of recovery, literally seeing yourself well again in your mind's eye
- relaxation and meditation
- care, touch, love and healing
- positive states of mind
- a strong will to live with a clear purpose and goals.

The study of PNI has now given us irrefutable evidence that improving our state of mind and calming our nervous systems can have a profound effect on our ability to resist disease, and survive it if we do fall ill. Science has even proved that love, intimacy and community spirit provide major protection against disease. A very good book on the subject is *Love and Survival* by Dr Dean Ornish, an American cardiologist who demonstrated that it is possible to reverse coronary artery disease if emotional support and stress relief are added to a healthy diet and exercise.

For most of us, there are a number of influences that have caused our health to slip. These negative factors can add up, creating an ever-growing problem of physical and emotional toxicity, low energy, low self-esteem, depression and an increasing sense of struggle. This can leave us badly immuno-compromised and vulnerable to the carcinogens (cancer-causing substances) with which we come into contact.

Your job is to identify any negative influences that may be draining your health and happiness, and replace them over time with what lifts and nourishes you.

Thinking About the Timing of Your Illness

Classically, cancer usually takes two to three years to grow to the size where it starts to cause symptoms. So, it may be helpful to look back around two or three years before your cancer became evident, and ask yourself what was going on in your life at that time. Think about any factors that may have been triggers in breaking down your body's resistance to illness. Perhaps the cancer followed periods of intense stress, exhaustion or a difficult separation or loss? If you are facing a recurrence of cancer, you may wish to consider if there is a pattern in the timing of this secondary cancer comparable to the first. If you cannot find any connection, that is okay, too – we are just looking for any clues as to how your health may have deteriorated to help you create the most effective recovery plan for yourself. The reason for doing this is not to blame yourself or others in any way, but simply to try to understand the kind of factors that may have made you vulnerable to enable you to protect yourself better in future.

The message of illness

It can also be useful to go deep inside yourself and ask whether the cancer has a message or symbolic meaning for you. You can seek help with this type of approach from transpersonal counsellors or those practising psychosynthesis (see The Resources Directory, pages 362–5). After doing a relaxation exercise, go into yourself and try to tune in to your own intuition, then ask yourself: Does this illness have a message for me? If so, what is this cancer trying to tell me? Help to do this is found in the fourth exercise on the *Images for Healing Cancer* CD available from Health Creation.

You may not get the answer in words; instead, you may be given an image, sound, feeling, sense or colour, or insight may come to you in a dream. If your thoughts, feelings or insights do not make sense immediately, write them down. Clarity may come later as you work with your counsellor and see a pattern emerging.

Looking at the possible benefits of illness

Another way of gaining insight into what is going on is to ask yourself what you might be gaining through being ill. This may seem confrontational, but some people have admitted in retrospect that it was only through being ill that they were able to get out of the huge responsibility they had taken on in their lives or that, by being ill, they were given a legitimate excuse to change their life. Sometimes, it is the only way a person can 'stop the world and get off'. Alternatively, it may be the only way to get the attention you need and, sometimes, being ill may be the best technique for getting your own way.

Think hard about the question of what this illness could be giving you.

If you can discover the answer to this, the key is then to learn how to get these needs met without having to be ill to do so. Such a level of self-exploration is best done with your counsellor, who can help you find better ways to define your needs and get them met in less complicated ways.

If you would like to try this exercise, ask yourself:
- What benefit is this illness giving to me?
- What has previously stopped me from getting this before I was ill?
- How can I get this need met without having to be ill to do so?

Getting Well Again

Now that you have had a good think about why you may have become ill, it is time to embark upon your Health Creation Programme to restore your health and happiness, and allow you to feel well again.

In the UK you can do this through residential courses at the Bristol Cancer Help Centre or Cancer Bridge in Hexham.

In the US, contact the Commonweal Cancer Help Center.

In Australia, get in touch with the Yarra Valley Living Centre.

For those not in a position to get to these centres of excellence, I have created an interactive kit called The Health Creation Programme. The aim of this programme is that anyone with cancer should be able to benefit from a holistic health and life revival programme, whatever the stage of illness you have, wherever you are.

The Health Creation Programme

The Health Creation Programme which I have produced on the basis of my twenty years' experience of empowering those with cancer to rebuild their health is available from Health Creation on 0845 009 3366 or www.healthcreation.co.uk. It is a six-month structured self-assessment and self-help programme designed to help you maximize your health and well-being, however serious the illness you are facing. The Programme can be done on your own or with the support and coaching of a Health Creation Mentor – a telephone service that can be accessed from anywhere in the world.

Through the use of the Programme, the accompanying CDs and the Picture of Health exercise, you can assess your state and needs on a monthly basis. The Picture of Health exercise involves answering 10 questions relating to each of the 12 Health Creation Principles: three for body; three for mind; three for spirit; and three for environment. Your score is plotted on a wheel, going from the centre towards the rim. When you have plotted your score for each principle, you then join up the marks and shade in the central area. This represents the part of you that is currently strong and well. The unshaded parts in each quadrant of the circle represent those areas of your health or lifestyle that need work or support to get you really well.

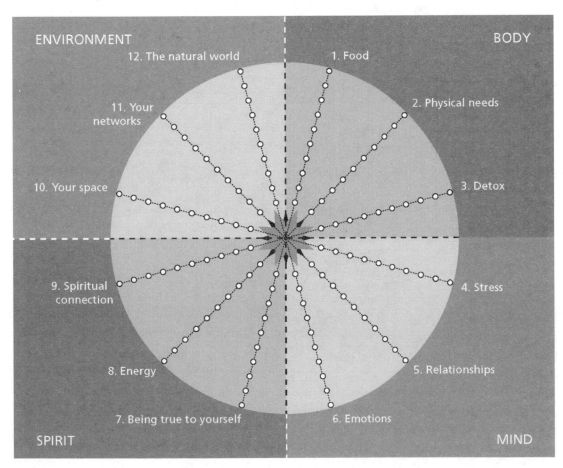

Below is an example of a completed Picture of Health done by a high-powered businessman I've worked with. What is immediately obvious is that while he is highly self-expressed (principle 7) and thinks he is protecting himself by staying really fit (principle 2), he is actually at great risk because:

- he is highly stressed (principle 4)
- with very low energy levels (principle 8)
- an appalling over-rich diet (principle 1) and with very little protective love in his life (principle 5)
- he also has a poor relationship with his community and the environment, and is missing out here, too, on the protection of a sense of belonging locally and making a contribution to society.

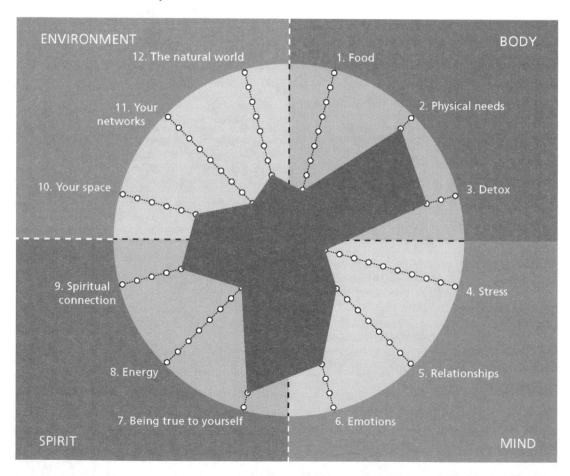

I call this picture 'the heart attack special' because he has all the key risks of stress, an over-rich diet and lack of love, intimacy and a sense of belonging to his community which are the major predictors of coronary artery disease, heart attacks and strokes.

Once this man saw his Picture of Health and understood the holistic health model and science behind it, he committed himself to change.

We started by giving him energy support with acupuncture, as he was too drained to contemplate change without first receiving some energy input. He then chose to have massage and learn relaxation techniques to lower his tension levels.

After three months' regular mentoring, we analysed his stress. Once his energy levels were higher, he then felt able to plan some changes at work, to relieve his stress and free up some time so that he could switch more focus into his marriage. At the four-month point he decided to trade his aggressive gym routine for a combination of cycling and yoga, which he found more calming and energizing.

The final change, in months 5 and 6, was to get his diet on a healthy footing. He now says:

> *This programme came in the nick of time for me, and the real reason it worked was because it was phased well over time, with the help and support of my mentor. It also worked because I got some energy input and relaxation first before I tried to change anything. The truth is I was burnt out and running on empty. I couldn't have changed anything at all if we hadn't started first with the energy boost from the acupuncture and stress relief with massage. The reason I know it will stick is because the mentor went right to the heart of what was driving me, and it turned out to be that I was still running myself ragged trying to win the approval of my dead father! Now I've seen that there is no going back, and now it all starts with the love I feel for my life and my family. Time with them is now non-negotiable!*

Needless to say, this man's life became richer and better by the day and he still feels that he achieves just as much at work because he arrives in a much better frame of mind. His blood pressure has dropped from 150/100 to 130/85, and he has lost a stone in weight.

Once your Picture of Health is complete, you can then create your own Health Creation Goals, and make healthy changes to your lifestyle and stabilize your illness, while being coached and supported by a Health Creation Mentor.

The Mentor will provide the support, encouragement and guidance you need at each step of the way to make the Programme work for you. This is especially valuable to help you keep going if you come up against any setbacks, personally or through illness, or when you feel weak, tired, ill or just plain fed up.

The reason I created the Picture of Health was in response to the many people who have said to me over the years that the trouble with the holistic model is: How do I know where the goalposts are and how will I know when I have reached them? By creating a pictorial representation of your health, you can see within less than an hour each month exactly what state you are in and what needs to take priority. This puts you in charge and, as you work on your health and happiness, each month you will see your Picture of Health grow stronger, too.

By working through the Health Creation Programme, you will be supported and coached step by step to:

- improve your relationship with yourself, learning how to put yourself first to give yourself the necessary time, attention and nourishment to get well and stay well
- work out the current state, needs and pressing issues you must face to get well
- understand the ways in which you may sabotage your happiness and healing process
- live the lifestyle that will allow you to create sustainable health, happiness, fulfilment and peace of mind.

As you embark on this process, you will be helped to:

- develop a strong will to live, getting help to recover enough from previous grief, disappointment or fears
- increase your belief in your own power to self-heal
- learn the relevant factual information backed with scientific evidence to embark on recovering your health
- give yourself permission to receive the necessary therapeutic help you need during this part of your healing journey.

The Picture of Health is available independently as a self-help assessment tool for individuals, therapists and organizations via the Health Creation helpline (tel: 0845 009 3366).

Getting Started Today

There are five vital steps that everyone with cancer should build into their Health Creation Programme and take immediately:

1. Improving Your Relationship with Yourself

Make sure you get the time, rest and nourishment you need.

2. Caring for Your Body

A healthy diet, regular exercise and reducing all sources of toxins in your life – in particular, alcohol, tobacco and household chemicals – are all part of this.

Pay attention to your long-term nutrition:

- Include vegetables and fruit in every meal, at least half of which is raw as a salad or whole fruit.
- Continue to take antioxidant vitamin/mineral supplements, as suggested in Chapter 7.
- Make freshly and drink at least a pint of vegetable juice a day made from alkaline or neutral fruits and vegetables such as carrots, melon, ginger, beetroot, celery and peppers (avoid acid-containing fruit in juices such as apples, grapes, kiwis, lemons, oranges or grapefruits).
- Use the *Cancer Lifeline Recipes* or *More Healing Foods* cookbook by Jane Sen to establish a healthy eating pattern for the rest of your life (available from Health Creation). *The Cancer Lifeline Recipes* come with a sample meal plan to give you an idea of how to eat for the whole day in the Eat Right style. Jane has crafted these recipes especially for people with cancer and with full nutritional needs in mind. Once you have tried these recipes, you may also want to get Jane's videos to see how she produces her own special magic. You may also want to read *Eat to Beat Cancer*, co-authored by Jane and me, and including all the theory about anti-cancer diets
- Take the immunostimulant IP6 (inositol phosphate), 2 g three times a day for three months after treatment, then 1 g three times a day for the next 12 months. Alternatively, take one of the mushroom-based immunostimulants such as *Coriolus*, 4 tablets three times a day, dropping to 2 tablets three times a day after three months (see Chapter 5). Some people like to alternate these immune stimulants on a two-monthly rotation.
- Take anti-cancer herbs such as Essiac, Carctol or Iscador to help prevent cancer recurrence (see Chapter 5). My patients have achieved the best results with Carctol, which makes the body more alkaline to help prevent the regrowth of cancer.

3. Improving Your State of Mind

Reduce stress, improve your relationships and offload toxic emotions by developing strength and peace of mind. Calm your body and mind daily with relaxation and meditation. Create a quiet place where every day you can develop your practice. Make this a special place that is kept beautiful. There are relaxation and meditation exercises on the *Heal Yourself* CD within the Health Creation Programme.

Use the power of your mind to visualize your body completely healed of cancer, and strong and healthy again, using the *Images for Healing Cancer* CD (from Health Creation). This CD offers four types of imaging exercises. You may find that one works better for you than the others, but try to do a different one every day; establish your visualization practice as a regular part of your daily quiet or inner time. Always finish with a visualization in which you see yourself completely healed and strong again. With time and practice, this will become easier and your images stronger. You can even develop images of your own, which will be the most powerful and relevant for you.

The first exercise on the Images CD is a guided visualization of the cancer completely disappearing from your body; in the second, you invite healing to enter at all levels of body, mind and spirit; in the third, you imagine yourself going forward into your life and being present at key events in the future; in the fourth, you are led on a guided journey to find your healing symbols and also to create feelings of tranquillity, uplift and well-being.

Remember, scientific studies of visualization have shown that creating positive mental associations with cancer treatments and visualizing long-term survival can translate into a greater survival benefit than cancer treatment. If you cannot visualize in images, do it in words or affirmations.

Cut out excess stress and overactivity from your life. Be absolutely ruthless in getting out of as many draining commitments as you can. Keep only the good bits of your life that truly excite, nourish and uplift you.

4. Reviving and Honouring Your Spirit

Get a vital lift for your energy and spirit with healing, spiritual practice and living the life you love. Receive regular spiritual healing or reiki at least once a week, and continue doing so even when you think you no longer need it. Call the National Federation of Spiritual Healers (tel: 0845 123 2767) to find a healer in your area. Ideally, visit several healers to find the right one for you, then choose your ideal healer and keep the others as back-up healers in case your regular healer is unavailable.

Use the crisis of illness to live a lifestyle that you really love. Use the illness as a wake-up call to put your life onto a healthier, happier, more authentic footing than before. Take this opportunity to get into an optimal energy and immune state by living out your unlived dreams, fulfilling life-long ambitions and goals, and reorientating your lifestyle and behaviour to reflect your most dearly held values. Shift your motivational axis in life from fear-based to love-based priorities and values, and declutter and simplify your life. You will find that, by becoming fully and authentically who you really are, and learning to express your creativity and uniqueness, you may well feel happier than ever before. The key is to learn to nourish yourself fully at all levels of body, mind and spirit – and most important of all, to have lots of fun.

5. Caring for Your Environment

- Make sure that the places where you live and work make you feel good, and that they are not dominated by the tastes and needs of others.
- Establish good networks with friends and colleagues, and make sure that you feel you belong, and can contribute to your groups and communities.
- Make your own contributions to protect the environment by being environmentally responsible.

The Holistic Approach to Health Creation

As you become more involved with this holistic health promotion approach, you may wish to know more about the holistic model of health on which the approach is based. The word 'holistic' is derived from the Greek *holos*, meaning 'the whole that is greater than the sum of the parts'.

The theoretical basis of the holistic model of health is that:

- our health is something we can influence greatly
- the state of our mind/body/spirit and our environment are all inextricably linked
- illness arises when we have:
  - failed to nourish our physical, mental or spiritual self
  - actively abused our health
  - been saddened or defeated by our life or relationships
  - failed to find any meaning or purpose in our life.
  - lived in a toxic environment.

Working with the holistic approach puts you firmly back in the driving seat of your life and teaches you how to:

- look after and nourish yourself properly
- take charge and improve your physical, mental and spiritual states
- find purpose and commitment to life
- use complementary therapies and self-help approaches to rebuild your health and energy.

Mounting scientific evidence shows that taking personal control of your health stimulates the health creation process, one of the most powerful tools we have for defeating cancer. The key to the holistic health creation process is commitment. The results achieved by this approach are directly linked to the time and effort put into it. The most important step to take in embracing the holistic approach to health and well-being is, therefore, committing yourself fully to life and to regaining your health.

The idea that the body's physical health is related to our state of mind, body, spirit and environment has been around for centuries. However, with the advent of science and Newtonian physics, there was a shift towards a model of medicine where the body was seen as a machine, with parts that could be fixed if broken, or as a collection of chemical processes that could be artificially controlled with man-made drugs. This reductionist approach has been responsible for some astounding progress in medicine, such as hip replacements, cataract removal, organ transplants and the control of many diseases through medication.

However, since the 1960s, there has been much dissatisfaction with the idea of treating only the symptoms of disease, and not addressing the underlying causes. There has been a strong resurgence of interest in the idea that mind, body, spirit and environment are connected and that, each individual is, in fact, connected to the whole of life and, thus, to each other. During the 1960s and 1970s, these 'alternative' ideas were ridiculed and opposed by orthodox physicians. However, in the 1980s and 1990s, hard scientific evidence emerged which has forced people to take seriously the holistic or integrated model of health and illness.

The key message of the holistic approach is that, far from being human machines, we are complex beings, and the functioning of our mind, body and spirit does interact, affecting our health and well-being profoundly. For example, nutrition affects not only our physical health, but also the IQ (intelligence quotient) and mental state. Exercise can radically change our mood while meditation, which calms the mind, has a profound affect on our heart, breathing and immune function. It has also been shown that spiritual healing changes the brainwave pattern from stressed beta-wave activity to self-healing alpha activity, as well as raising the level of immune 'natural-killer' cells that are so crucial to the body's fight against cancer. Perhaps most extraordinary are the effects of prayer and distant healing, shown to improve significantly the chances of survival after a heart attack in scientific trials where the subjects did not even know they were being prayed for!

The Mind–Body Connection

Understanding of the mind–body connection has leapt forward over the last 15 years. From the 1950s to the 1970s, there was only a basic understanding of how stress and fear adversely affected body function. It was known that stress or fear causes adrenaline to be secreted, which 'primed' the brain and muscles for the well-known 'fight-or-flight' response. This means that, when frightened or stressed, activity in the body is diverted away from 'housekeeping' functions such as digestion, absorption, growth, immune response, healing and repair. As a result, when under stress, we are mentally clear and physically strong as preparation to either fight off the current threat or danger or to run like hell!

This short-term stress response is highly advantageous to survival. When being chased by a tiger, digesting your breakfast or warding off infection is not your highest priority. But if stress becomes prolonged or chronic, it can have a disastrous effect on health as vital 'house keeping' functions become compromised in the long term. Most of us these days live our lives in constant anxiety or fear, as if there is a tiger permanently chasing us – albeit in the form of a bank manager, taxman, mortgage company or demanding boss.

In prolonged stress, the body's cortisol and adrenaline levels remain high. Cortisol is the natural steroid secreted by the adrenal glands to help us deal with challenging situations. High cortisol and adrenaline levels directly inhibit our immunity to disease and infection as has been clearly demonstrated both in the laboratory and in real life. Stress has also been shown to have adverse affects on blood pressure, blood cholesterol and fat, not to mention increasing our irritability and dependency on cigarettes, alcohol and drugs, with all their attendant health effects.

Nevertheless, although this understanding of the stress mechanism explained why prolonged stress and high levels of fear are so deleterious to the body, it did not explain why emotions affect our health so strongly. People started to ask, 'Why does falling in love cause eczema or irritable bowel syndrome to clear up?' and 'How can old people die within weeks of their spouse dying, when there is nothing apparently wrong with them?' Neither did it explain why visualization or mind-over-matter techniques have such a profound effect on our physiology.

The real revolution in our knowledge of the mind–body connection came through the new scientific field of psychoneuroimmunology (PNI; covered briefly in Chapter 2). This revolution started in the 1970s with the discovery, by Dr Candace Pert, of a receptor in the brain for a substance similar to morphine. Shortly after this, the substance itself was discovered – called 'endorphin' or 'enkephalin'. The finding of this naturally occurring opiate in the brain triggered an avalanche of over 200 further discoveries of these tiny messenger chemicals, known as 'neuropeptides'. It was quickly realized that these informational substances are not only secreted in the brain and nerve tissue, but in all the other tissues of the body as well.

This made it clear that the old model of a brain and nervous system communicating only through neurotransmitters at the ends of the nerves was completely out of date. A new model was created in which all the tissues of the body are able to communicate with each other through informational substances, based on the fact that receptors for these substances are found in the brain and other tissues of the body. On tracking the pathways of these neuropeptides, it was revealed that there was a feedback communication loop from the brain to the tissues and back again. So, the tissues were 'talking' to the brain just as much as the brain was 'talking' to the tissues. But more than this, it was now clear that the body's tissues could communicate with each other, too. This led to the idea of the 'intelligent body', making it possible to see how visualization and emotions could affect tissue function.

This revolutionary concept has completely blown away the idea of the body as five separate anatomical systems working more or less independently (as was taught in medical schools for the whole of the last century). In fact, communication between all the systems of the body is so complex that even trying to imagine it is difficult. Bearing in mind that computers work on a binary system of two digits, the whole of Western music is composed on a scale of 12 intervals and the English language is based on 26 letters, comprehending the language of a neuropeptide communication system with a minimum of 200 units is hard even to contemplate!

In practice, it has been found that different emotional states create certain patterns of neuropeptide secretion which strongly affect tissue functioning within the body. When people are stressed, depressed, distressed and emotionally repressed over the long term, the most common response is for immune function to be impaired also. This affects both the activity of individual immune cells as well as the number of circulating immune cells.

However, it is not just the immune system that is affected. Studies have shown that red blood cells carry less oxygen when people are depressed or stressed, and a whole range of tissue functions change according to our predominant state of mind. Thus, scientists have begun to work out exactly how the 'mind-over-matter' techniques of visualization and affirmation affect tissue functions. After chemotherapy, low blood cell levels have been found to rise in response to visualizing them increasing in the mind's eye, demonstrating clearly that these techniques have very real physical consequences.

So, where does all this fit into preventing a cancer recurrence?

To date, studies looking at whether there is a link between stress and distressing life events and cancer have had conflicting results – some show definite links while others do not. However, what PNI scientists are now telling us is that it is not stress or distress *per se* that is the problem, but how an individual reacts to it. The concept of 'personality hardiness' describes those who respond to stress and difficult situations positively, seeing them as exciting challenges and sources of potential empowerment rather than leading to a state of anxiety, fear and feelings of powerlessness.

On the other hand, those who have 'learned helplessness' tend to collapse emotionally and, in turn, their immune function collapses when challenged. This is usually because they have repeatedly experienced defeat or domination in early life and, therefore, have a tendency to give up in the face of adversity. Unfortunately, the immune system can mirror the emotional state with white cell levels dropping, too. Nevertheless, this response can be 'unlearned' through counselling or psychotherapy, hypnosis, visualization and affirmation, and you can learn to take control of the mind–body connection and use it to your advantage.

This fits with the observation that people who become helpless and hopeless when diagnosed with cancer fare much worse than those with a fighting spirit. This is why cancer patients who express their feelings in support groups have longer lives, and why visualization can also extend survival time.

It is clear that the state of mind has a great deal to do with the body's ability to defend itself against cancer, but this is not the same as saying that psychological factors cause cancer – nor is it saying that people are in any way to blame if they do get cancer. The bottom line is that the Western lifestyle is extremely stressful, and those who are prone to feeling more anxious, helpless and hopeless or have lost their way in life are likely to be more vulnerable to serious illness, and at greater risk when they have one. But the most important thing is to get going straight away to change these ways of reacting to life, through a combination of psychotherapy, support, self-help, stress reduction and achieving peace of mind and personal fulfilment.

As mentioned earlier in this chapter, the five vital steps to long-term recovery are:

1. improving your relationship with yourself
2. caring for your body
3. improving your state of mind
4. reviving and honouring your spirit
5. caring for your environment

Let's take a look at each one of these in more detail.

1. Improving Your Relationship with Yourself

Answering the following questions will give you a basic idea of what your relationship with yourself is like:

- Do you eat properly?
- Do you get enough sleep?
- Do you exercise regularly?
- Do you walk away from abusive relationships?
- Do you look after your appearance?
- Do you stay out of debt?
- Do you refrain from abusing or harming yourself physically or mentally?
- Do you believe you are valuable?
- Do you believe you deserve attention, love, money and nice possessions?
- Do you believe you are lovable?
- Are you able to spend time alone?
- Do you give yourself time for rest and recuperation?
- Do you love or even like yourself?

If most of your answers are 'yes', then your relationship with yourself is in fairly good shape. If, on the other hand, you answered 'no' to a lot of them, then your relationship with yourself could do with improvement. People who do not have a good relationship with themselves or who do not value themselves properly have low self-esteem. In this case, they are unlikely to put in place, let alone maintain, activities that allow them to become healthy and to fulfil themselves, including implementing any of the advice in this chapter!

So, the first step in your recovery programme is to improve your relationship with yourself so that you learn to value and nurture yourself well.

The relationship each of us has with ourselves is usually based on the relationship we had with our parents or other significant adults in childhood. If we have been loved, cherished, nurtured and encouraged, we will probably be good at doing this for ourselves. If, on the other hand, we have been neglected, criticized, abandoned, abused and shown very little encouragement or affection, this is likely to be how we treat ourselves, too. But it is possible to change your relationship with yourself and begin treating yourself properly. More often than not, however, it takes the experience of a new kind of nurturing relationship with another to create a new template. This is where counselling, psychotherapy, healing and the complementary therapies that employ touch can be extremely helpful.

All of these emotional and physical therapies are based on treating the client with 'unconditional positive regard'. This means that the relationship is based on non-judgemental loving kindness, care and concern. All holistic therapies have, at their root, the aim of enabling you to develop this sort of relationship with yourself so that, when the therapy ends, you can take up this nurturing process for yourself. Once this caring relationship has been modelled for you, you will be able, little by little, to take over and start giving yourself what you really need.

If you feel that your self-esteem is low, you should probably go for counselling or assertiveness training (see The Resources Directory, pages 362–5, for a list of counselling organizations). It is important to have an introductory meeting with the therapist to make sure he or she is suitable for you – not the other way round. If this experience is to build your self-esteem and confidence, then you must feel entirely comfortable with the therapist and feel the person has genuine warmth towards you. It may be wise to meet two or three therapists before making your choice.

If you think you can build a new relationship with yourself without this kind of help, the golden rules are:

- Learn to put yourself at the top of the list of people to look after. If you look after yourself properly, you will be in better shape to care for others and will be giving them a terrific model to follow and apply in their own lives. You will also have a much healthier relationship with your partner. When you are able to care for yourself, you will be far less needy, and less likely to stay in bad relationships just because you are so dependent on the emotional 'crumbs from their table'.
- Get to know yourself and your needs well. Get used to tuning in to how you feel, and react accordingly. This can mean listening to your body's need for food, sleep, sex and exercise; your emotional need for comfort, warmth and support; or your soul's or spirit's need for peace, space, uplift or adventure.
- Learn how to express your feelings and ask clearly for what you need (without being upset if the answer is 'no'). If this is very difficult for you, take a course in assertiveness to learn how to communicate your needs without fear, and to accept a negative response without taking it as rejection.

This advice is particularly relevant for people who are very 'other-centred', who spend all their time and energy looking after others. They may have a particularly poor self-image and low self-esteem. Sometimes, the problem lies in the other direction. If you have become rather self-ish, the need may be to move the other way, learning to think and care more about the needs of others as well as yourself. In general, it is better to err on the side of being self-centred, as people generally take better care of themselves if they have a high opinion of themselves rather than the other way round.

When you have a good relationship with yourself, you could be described as being your own 'good parent'. You cease being at the mercy of your needy, greedy, demanding, rebellious inner child, and are instead able to give yourself what will sustain, nourish and develop you in the long term. This means having a more mature sense of what you really need rather than going for 'instant gratification', or what feels good at the time. This is not to diminish the value of spontaneity or giving yourself treats – it is knowing the difference between treats that will genuinely nurture you and those which may boost you now, but cost you more later.

In the transpersonal model of psychology, these different aspects of ourselves are seen as sub-personalities whose needs have to be negotiated. As you become increasingly self-aware, many sub-personalities may emerge that you can work with, recognize and cater for.

Changing your relationship with yourself does not happen overnight. But, as with every-thing else, having the intention to be gentler, more loving, more permissive and more respon-sible towards yourself is a good starting point. See if you can make this commitment to your-self now, before you go on to read about how to take practical steps to create a healthy lifestyle.

2. Caring for Your Body

Another major factor within the holistic health model is how we look after ourselves physical-ly. Eating properly and exercising regularly will greatly affect our energy, vitality and state of mind. But, it is not just about what food we eat, but also how we eat, where we shop, how we store food and how we cook it. It is also important to make dietary changes that are sustain-able, rather than flipping between periods of healthy eating and binges on unhealthy food.

Combining forms of exercise that build stamina with those that increase suppleness, strength and harmonization of the body, mind and spirit is a good idea. The ideal combination is to take aerobic exercise, preferably outdoors, once or twice a week and do a weekly class in either yoga, tai chi or chi gong as well, with a short daily practice of these disciplines at home.

Healthy eating and cooking

For optimal nutrition, eat an organic wholefood diet that is low in animal foods, acidity, fat, salt, sugar, acid food and drink, processed foods, chemical additives, stimulants (such as tea and coffee) and alcohol. For most people, this will mean dramatically increasing their intake of vegetables, cereals and pulses while reducing total calorie intake, and switching everything 'white' in the diet to the 'brown' unprocessed equivalent. It will also mean drinking herbal teas, vegetable juices and mineral or filtered water rather than continual tea and coffee.

Changing something as fundamental as the food you eat involves a lot of commitment and support. It is essential to make changes in a way that is sustainable. Often, if changes are too radical or too quick, they are abandoned within weeks, especially if the new regime feels like deprivation, leaving you with a desire to binge on 'naughty foods'.

The other ingredients for success are getting the right sort of support to help you make the change, and acquiring the correct information, good recipes and new cooking skills.

Getting Support to Change Your Diet

If you want to start eating in a healthy way, it is vital to enlist the support of your partner, family, colleagues and friends. Also, if you are really serious about making this commitment to yourself, it is good to have 'witnesses' to this intention. The very process of telling people about it will make it seem more real to you. Better still, see if you can get the people you live with to make the changes, too. This will avoid conflicts over how you shop, cook and prepare food, and the more nitty-gritty issue of how the family budget is to be spent. If you can't persuade your nearest and dearest to make the changes with you, then find a 'buddy' or even a small group of friends or colleagues who would like to partner you.

If you can muster several people who want to change their diet, you could then form your own healthy-eating support group, and meet regularly for a few weeks to talk about how you are getting on, and to swap information and creative ideas. I have seen this work in an office environment, where a whole team of colleagues decided to 'clean up their act'. They all supported each other by replacing biscuits and cakes with bowls of fruit, sweetened drinks with mineral water and juice, and tea and coffee with herbal teas. They met weekly to discuss meal plans and their progress.

The group started with a six-week spring-cleaning detox diet to lose weight. This revolved around eating only fruit, steamed vegetables, salads, soup and brown rice for six weeks. Thereafter, new wholefoods were added to the healthy eating plan. The group was delighted with the results, both in terms of weight loss, and the great improvement in energy levels and mental clarity. Also, the feeling of team solidarity was absolutely wonderful, and this rubbed off into how they worked together.

If you know you have a strong emotional dependency on food, you may need more than just family or friends to support you, so going to a counsellor or doctor may be a good idea. Eating less heavy foods, which are sedating, may well uncover anxieties and feelings that have been lurking beneath the surface for years. If this is the case, it is unlikely that you will be able to change your eating patterns successfully until you receive therapeutic help. Counselling can help people offload their emotions and change the way they deal with their feelings. (Organizations through which you can find counsellors are found in the Resources Directory, pages 362–5.)

Gathering Information

Acquiring information on how to cook healthy food is getting easier and easier. Healthy eating is talked and written about frequently these days, and there are many excellent cookery and nutrition books available that offer step-by-step advice on what to do. I recommend Jane Sen's videos, books and recipe cards; she has spent 12 years developing vegan recipes which are perfectly balanced to help prevent cancer.

The sort of information you need is:

- dietary advice explaining what and what not to eat
- a clear idea of what healthy foods are available and what you should buy
- a meal plan to take you through the first few weeks
- nutritional information to ensure that what you are eating is balanced and healthy
- a good set of recipes
- professional advice if you have special dietary needs as a result of illness or disability
- information on how to store and cook food for maximum nutritional value.

This information is explained, step by step, below. But if it all seems too much, it can be made much simpler by going to Jane Sen or a nutritional therapist for one-on-one help in successfully making the change. A nutritional therapist is not the same as a dietician. Most dieticians are trained in the standard Western diet and how to adjust this for certain illnesses or conditions. In general, they will happily recommend a diet based on meat, dairy foods and refined carbohydrates. Nutritional therapists, on the other hand, look at the role of food itself as a cause and treatment of illness, and tend to advocate a healthy, wholefood diet. Planning changes to your diet with a professional can make all the difference to your success and so is highly recommended (see the Resources Directory for information on how to get a consultation with a nutritional therapist or Jane Sen via www.janesen.com.)

Dietary Guidelines

The key guidelines for a healthy diet include:

- Eat non-acidic fruit and/or vegetables at every single meal. Include a high proportion of raw fruit and vegetables every day, either on their own, in salads or in homemade vegetable juices. (Commercially-made fruit and vegetable juices have to be pasteurized by law. This involves heating the juice, which destroys the health-giving plant enzymes, so the homemade variety is much better.) You will need a basic juice extractor, which can cost around £50, or a high-quality juice press such as the Champion Juicer, which costs around £250. Tomatoes and citrus fruit, plus other fruits which are unripe or sour, should be avoided until the body's pH is alkaline. You are aiming for a pH of 7.5. Test your saliva and urine with litmus paper (available from Health Creation).
- Get as much variety in your diet as possible and try different pulses, fruits and vegetables. This will ensure your getting the full spectrum of minerals, vitamins and vital plant (phyto-) chemicals necessary to prevent cancer.
- Replace refined and processed foods with the wholefood, unprocessed equivalent. This means replacing white bread with brown, white rice with brown rice, white pasta with brown pasta, ordinary cheese biscuits with oatcakes, sugary cakes with wholefood cakes, normal breakfast cereal with muesli or porridge, sweets and chocolate with nuts, or dried or ordinary fruits, and sweetened drinks with mineral water or homemade vegetable juice.
- Replace red meat and farmed chicken and fish with organic, free-range eggs and vegetable proteins from beans, lentils, peas and quinoa. If you cannot bear to live without animal protein, treat yourself to the occasional deep-sea fish, wild salmon or trout, free-range organic chicken and game or, occasionally, organic red meat.
- Replace most animal fats with vegetarian equivalents – except for fish oils, which are healthy as they contain essential omega-3 fatty acids. These are found in oily fish such as mackerel, herring or salmon (organic), or can be taken as supplements. Otherwise, replace milk with vegetable milks such as soya, oat and rice milks. Porridge can be eaten without milk, and flavoured with fruit concentrates, dates or maple syrup.
- Replace cheese with vegetable patés using olives, aubergines, avocados (guacamole) or mushrooms. Check that these patés or pastes are not full of 'hidden' cream cheese.
- Replace animal cooking fat with vegetable oils – preferably cold-pressed olive oil or ground nut oil. Use speciality raw oils, such as sesame oil and walnut oil, for flavouring salad dressings or cooked vegetables.

- Replace cream with soya cream, and ice cream with soya ice cream.
- Replace normal yoghurts with soya desserts and yoghurts (such as Provamel).
- Replace butter with vegetable equivalents such as olive oil-based spreads. Many margarines are unhealthy because they are highly processed, and contain hydrogenated and trans fatty acids – a by-product of excessive heating of the fats during the production process. Margarines free of hydrogenated fatty acids include Vitaquel and Granose, which are another alternative to olive oil-based spreads.

Faced with this advice, some people panic that they will not obtain sufficient protein and calcium for healthy growth and bones. At this point, I usually remind people that massive creatures like elephants and cows are vegetarian. They have no problem whatsoever maintaining their huge bone structure and health with their plant-based diet.

In reality, most people in developed countries eat far too much protein every day. We only need 40 grams (just over an ounce) of protein a day, to replace the wear and tear on our joints and muscles. Excess protein acidifies the body, increasing cancer risk. All the basic vitamins and minerals we need are available from a varied vegan diet. Over the years, the meat and milk marketing boards have done a good job of convincing us that good health depends on our intake of dairy, meat and eggs. But just bear in mind that most degenerative health problems in the West are due to overeating, acidic tissues and particularly the excess consumption of animal fats and meat. To reduce acidity in the body, cut down on wine, vinegar, yoghurt, tea, coffee and all acid fruits, fruit juices, fruit teas, jams and tomatoes. Good non-acidic fruits are bananas, melons, papayas, dates and figs.

Buying Healthy Food

If wholefood is new to you, the best thing to do is visit a good healthfood shop and see what is on offer. You will be amazed at the huge selection of raw ingredients as well as the many pre-prepared vegan and vegetarian meals that are now available. Of course, many of these healthy foods, such as pulses, seeds, nuts, dried fruit and wholefood cereals, can be found in supermarkets, too. But, as most supermarkets only stock a small selection of healthy food, which is distributed between rows and rows of processed foods, it is worth going to a speciality wholefood shop first to see the full range of what is available and familiarize yourself with it. Supermarkets are now taking on board the healthy-eating message, and are launching more healthy-food ranges as well as stocking organic fruit and vegetables. So, once you know what you are looking for, it may well be possible to return to your usual supermarket for your groceries.

Recipe Books

Healthfood shops often have a book section, where you can choose from a range of both European and East Asian vegetarian cookbooks. Quite often, getting into Indian or Middle Eastern vegetarian cookery is the saving grace for those who are used to an elaborate diet and can tend to find vegetarian food rather boring. The main problem is that the intensity of flavours and the variation of textures involved in traditional cooking can, at first, seem hard to replace by more basic vegetarian meals. However, Jane Sen's recipes, and a variety of Asian cooking methods and ingredients can fill this gap. Any good high-street bookshop will also have a vegetarian section in the recipe and food department and, often, healthfood shops will have a particularly good selection. Jane's books include *More Healing Foods*, *Eat to Beat Cancer* and the *Cancer Lifeline Recipe Cards*, available from Health Creation or Waterstones bookshops.

Wholefood Shopping

On your first trip to a wholefood shop or good supermarket, your basic shopping list would include:

- brown rice, pasta and flour
- beans
- lentils
- sugar-free high-quality muesli and porridge oats
- good-quality organic wholemeal bread
- nuts, seeds and dried fruit
- vegetable paté or hummus (ground chickpeas)
- herbal teas and mineral water
- wholefood biscuits and cakes
- soya, oat or rice milk
- soya yoghurt or desserts
- olive oil-based spread, Granose or Vitaquel margarine
- olive oil
- tamari or soy sauce for flavouring foods (as an alternative to salt)
- herbs and spices
- vegetable bouillon powder.

Building up a selection of herbs, spices and specialist ingredients is a good way to flavour vegetarian food in more interesting ways. Useful ingredients are garlic, ginger, balsamic vinegar and chilli sauce as well as unusual options like chestnut puree and coconut cream. It is also possible to buy soya mayonnaise that has less fat than ordinary mayonnaise. Excellent green and red curry pastes from Thailand are available as well as many delightful herbs such as lemongrass, star anise, Chinese five spice, and basil, coriander, rosemary, thyme and bay leaf as fresh herbs. Soya deserts mixed with fresh fruit can be more interesting if the soya is marinated with vanilla pods and star anise along with some honey or maple syrup. Green salad served with freshly chopped basil, olive oil, garlic, salt and pepper is an absolute delight.

Maple and date syrups can be used to flavour sauces, desserts and cakes, as can dried fruit soaked with herbs. For example, soaking Hunza apricots with bay leaves and cardamom before cooking can transform a dish into a completely magical, gourmet experience. Soak the apricots overnight with the bay and cardamom; the next day, bring them to the boil and simmer for 5–10 minutes, and leave to steep for a further 24 hours before serving, as this thickens and enriches the juice. Served with soya or nut cream, you will find that eating healthily can be just as rich and delicious as more conventional food, and does not equal deprivation at all.

An Introductory Meal Plan

The better the structure of a new diet, the more successful it is likely to be. A week's meal plan is a good idea to begin with, and it can then be repeated or changed at the beginning of each new week. You will find meal plans within Jane Sen's *Cancer Lifeline Recipe Cards*.

Breakfast should include some of the following:

- banana, melon or papaya
- healthy cereals such as muesli or porridge, which can be made from many grains as well as oats
- brown toast with honey
- the occasional organic, free-range boiled egg
- vegetable juice or herbal teas.

Decide whether your main meal will be lunch or dinner, and swap the following meal plans accordingly.

A light lunch could include a choice of:

- vegetable soup
- fresh green salad, bean salad, rice salad, coleslaw or other grated vegetables
- wholefood vegetarian pasty, pie, samosa or falafel
- wholewheat bread or toast with vegetable paté, and salad
- a banana.

For a main meal, you could choose from:

- pasta with mushroom or pepper sauce
- vegetable curry and dahl (lentils) with rice
- lentil or bean shepherd's pie with vegetables
- stir-fried vegetables with rice
- vegetable stew, baked or stuffed vegetables
- nut roast
- the occasional fish, game, organic chicken or red meat
- a wholefood dessert.

Your lunch and dinner should be accompanied by a fresh green salad and/or steamed vegetables.

A healthy, balanced diet includes a good balance of:

- protein
- carbohydrates (starch and sugar)
- essential fatty acids
- plenty of fruit and vegetables.

Vegetarian protein comes from beans, peas, lentils, nuts, seeds and the delicious cereal quinoa (which contains all 21 amino acids we need).

Carbohydrates are available from bread, pasta, potatoes and other root vegetables.

Essential fatty acids are obtained from nuts, seeds, vegetables and fish oils.

With all these foods, make sure you have as much variety as possible. These healthy wholefoods have a different balance of vitamins and minerals and, for optimum health, it is best to vary your intake and experiment with new pulses, fruits and vegetables. Jane Sen says that an easy way to be sure you are getting the full range of nutrients is to include vegetables and foods of different colours in one meal. If you are worried about getting the right nutritional balance, especially for children and the elderly, the best advice again is to invest time with a nutritional therapist or purchase a good wholefood nutritional textbook. The most important thing to remember is that you *can* get all the nutrients you need from a vegetarian diet.

Specific Anti-cancer Foods

All vegetables, nuts, seeds and pulses contain some vital cancer-preventing phytochemicals, so eating the widest range possible of these foods is essential. However, some foods are particularly high in the protective plant chemicals, and you should make sure your cancer-prevention diet includes lots of these foods. Nutritionist Suzannah Olivier has compiled the following list of anti-cancer foods:

- alfalfa
- almonds
- apples
- apricot
- arame
- arugula
- beans
- beetroot
- blackberries
- black walnuts
- bok choy
- broccoli (and sprouted broccoli)
- Brussels sprouts
- burdock root
- cabbage
- cantaloupe melons
- carrots
- cauliflower
- chives
- citrus fruits
- dulse
- flaxseed oil
- garlic
- ginger
- grapes
- horseradish
- kale
- kohlrabi
- laver bread
- leeks
- linseeds
- liquorice
- mushrooms (*maitake*, *reishi* and *shiitake*)
- nettles
- olive oil
- onions
- parsley
- pecans
- peppers (yellow and red)
- pineapple
- potatoes
- pulses
- radish
- rice (brown)
- seaweeds (kombu, kelp, nori)
- soya products
- spring onions
- squash
- sunflower seeds
- swede
- sweet potatoes
- tea (black and green)
- tomatoes
- turmeric
- turnip
- wakame
- walnuts

However, if you are trying to reduce your acidity, avoid apples, grapes, red and black berries, pineapple and tomatoes.

To check your acidity, obtain litmus paper from Health Creation and test your saliva first thing in the morning. You are aiming for an alkaline pH of 7.5. Once you are alkaline, you can try adding back a few acidic foods, but continue testing your pH to ensure you stay alkaline.

(The full list of phytochemicals they contain is found in The Resources Directory, pages 321–4). For a detailed explanation of the scientifically researched properties of these phytochemicals, I thoroughly recommend Suzannah Olivier's book, *The Breast Cancer Prevention and Recovery Diet.*

Learning New Skills

Changing to a wholefood vegetarian diet will inevitably involve acquiring new culinary skills. You may be fortunate enough to have access to a wholefood cookery class with Jane Sen, or through a local college of further education or cookery school. Local nutritional therapists may also teach or know about courses on wholefood cookery, as may the staff at your local healthfood shops, restaurants or natural health clinics. Also, a good wholefood recipe book will offer ideas and essential guidance on how to master the basic skills. But the simplest thing you can do is to find someone who already eats healthily and who can teach you the first steps, including learning how to:

- cook brown rice, pulses, grains and cereals successfully
- stir-fry and bake vegetables
- make a variety of salads using raw vegetables, seeds, nuts, fruit and cooked pulses as well as the usual salad ingredients
- make vegetable soups and juices
- make wholefood cakes, biscuits and desserts
- make basic sauces and dressings using healthy ingredients.

Sustainability

To maintain the changes you make, the golden rule is to start adding healthy foods to your diet before you take other things out. For example, try to have fruit or vegetables with every meal first. Once you get into this habit, the next step is to replace all processed 'white' foods with 'brown' equivalents. As these foods are so much more sustaining than 'white' foods, you will begin to experience fewer dips in your blood-sugar levels, reducing the desire to eat sweets and savoury snacks between meals. Once this starts to happen, your appetite will level out, and it will then be possible to drop the richer and heavier foods such as meats and animal fats. In a short time, you will feel so much better that you will wonder how you survived for so long eating in such an unhealthy way.

Healthy Cooking

Cooking methods to avoid are barbecuing, smoking, deep-frying and microwaving (especially meat and meat fats), as overheating oils, and the smoke from barbecues and smoked-food processes, produce dangerous free radicals which can cause cancer. So, keep clear of barbecued, smoked and chargrilled meats and fish, and restrict frying to a minimum. When you do fry food, always use new oil, and avoid heating it till it smokes as this is a sure sign that the fat is beginning to superheat and break down into free radicals. Boiling food in water is not ideal either, as many minerals leak into the water and are lost when the cooking water is discarded.

The best cooking methods are:

- steaming
- stir-frying
- stewing
- roasting
- baking.

Steaming and stir-frying mean that foods are cooked quickly and lightly, thereby retaining much of their natural texture and nutrients. Baking, roasting and stewing are gentler ways of cooking than frying or grilling, allowing flavours to melt into one another at lower temperatures. Believe it or not, it is actually possible to 'fry' food in a little water. Heating a small amount of water in the bottom of a frying pan will cook the food as if it were being fried. Good-quality cold-pressed oils (like olive, sesame or walnut oils) can then be added at the end of cooking for flavour and nutritional value, or to help put on weight after treatment. Cooking this way is safer, and you can also appreciate the flavour of the oil far more than when it is overheated and broken down in frying.

When stir-frying, a minimum amount of oil is used – just enough to stop vegetables or other foods from sticking to the wok or frying pan.

Steaming is the healthiest method of cooking because the food then retains maximum flavour and texture. As there is a loss of minerals into the water if food is being boiled or steamed, it is advisable to recycle the cooking water into other recipes such as soups, stews and sauces.

One culinary skill worth mastering when you change to healthy eating is how to make really good and varied salads. In Britain, people are brought up with the idea that a salad comprises lettuce, tomato and cucumber. In fact, the range of possibilities is enormous. What works particularly well is to grate raw vegetables and mix them with conventional salad foods and sprouts. For example, grated carrot, beetroot and finely chopped courgettes or broccoli mixed with sprouts, watercress and rocket make a stunning salad. Experimenting with pre-cooked beans in salads is another good idea. For example, red kidney beans with finely chopped peppers, parsley, a little chopped onion and a good garlic dressing makes a nutritious and delicious meal.

You can also make salads with grains such as rice, quinoa, bulgar wheat and couscous, and vary the dressings you use. Most of us get locked into oil and vinegar dressings, but wonderful non-acidic dressings can be made with other ingredients – for example, try blending a good olive oil with basil, garlic, tamari, pepper and a little honey.

Equipment

As you will be preparing more vegetables and salads, it is worth investing in a good food-processor. This will chop and grate vegetables quickly and easily. Also, invest in a juice extractor or, better still, a press to make pure vegetable and fruit juices both for drinks and for making delicious sauces and soups. A small collapsible vegetable steamer that fits inside an ordinary pan is also very useful. These are circular, with petals that open like a flower, so they can fit different sizes of pans, and are available from all good cookware shops. If you have a large family and are likely to be doing a lot of steaming, you might invest in a more elaborate, multilevel steamer, which allows you to cook three types of vegetables simultaneously at different levels. A hand blender is also invaluable for making vegetable soups or purees in the pan in which they've been cooked.

Another handy skill to acquire is sprouting seeds and pulses in jam jars or other glass containers. The secret is first to soak the seeds or pulses in double their volume of water for the first day, drain and rinse them on the second day, then leave them damp in the jar to germinate. Rinse them again each day until the sprouts are ready to eat. The best seeds and beans to sprout are alfalfa, mung, aduki and chickpeas.

For stir-frying, it is worth investing in a Chinese wok, which is what the Chinese use for most of their cooking. It looks like a frying pan, but has a gently curved shape and a long wooden handle. It's been designed this way to make it easier to keep gently tossing the contents of the wok during cooking, to ensure that everything in the pan is cooked quickly and evenly without burning or overcooking. A good set of knives is helpful for peeling and chopping vegetables, and another handy tool is a small mandolin-style vegetable peeler (which peels vegetables much quicker than the standard peeler). It is also worth having a dedicated electric coffee grinder or a mortar and pestle to grind seeds, nuts and spices.

An added bonus of changing to a healthy, cancer-prevention diet is that other illnesses you may have will start to clear up. The most common improvements are seen in asthma, eczema, arthritis, migraine and gut complaints. Many of these illnesses are caused by allergies to animal or processed foods, or a lack of the right minerals, vitamins or phytochemicals, which are rectified with a healthy, vegetable-based diet. People also have far less mucus, and the throat, ears and sinuses become much clearer, which means fewer infections, too. Other benefits are an increase in energy levels, clarity of mind and healthy skin. In fact, most people who make these changes ask themselves why on earth it took them so long to do so as they feel lighter, clearer and so very much more alive.

By drinking at least two large glasses of freshly prepared vegetable juice every day, you ensure that your supplements are optimally used by the body. It will allow all the naturally occurring cofactors and enzymes from the vegetables to support the body's uptake of extra vitamins and minerals.

In any good healthfood shop you can find antioxidant products such as 'Wholly Immune', designed with cancer prevention in mind and containing a good range of phytochemicals, vitamins and minerals known to be helpful. Usually these are either powders or liquids to be taken daily. There is no doubt that these products can make you feel fantastic as well as provide excellent protection. Of particular value are plant supplements containing catechins, the elements found in green tea that are so protective.

Exercise

Exercise is a vital element of cancer prevention as it cleans out and nourishes the tissues of the body. When we exercise, blood flow increases to all parts of the body, bringing oxygen, nutrients and white blood cells to the tissues. This, in turn, promotes the flow of blood and lymph away from the tissues, taking with them toxins to the kidneys, liver, skin and lungs for excretion from the body. As already mentioned, in Traditional Chinese Medicine, disease is believed to develop in areas of 'stagnation' in the body. Acupuncture and shiatsu see this as stagnation of energy or *chi*, but the concept can just as easily apply to physical stagnation – when the tissues and joints become 'silted up' with toxins from our diet, and the by-products of alcohol, drugs and cigarettes. Fats, acid, calcium, heavy metals and organic chemical residues from environmental pollution are deposited directly in the tissues, as are the breakdown products of radiation. So, it is easy to see how tissues become more and more toxic.

This creates the ideal environment for cancer to develop, so it is not surprising that exercise lowers cancer rates. Certainly, women who exercise are 10–20 per cent less likely to develop breast cancer than those who do not. This shows that exercise represents a very significant contribution to the overall protection against cancer.

The question is: what sort of exercise should you do? In the holistic approach to health, forms of exercise such as yoga, tai chi and chi gong are favoured. This is because they are intelligently designed to involve every tissue, joint and organ, bringing blood and vital energy to every part of the body. In addition, these practices incorporate elements of relaxation, deep breathing and meditation, all of which provide strong benefits through the mind–body connection. They can also generate a harmonious and respectful attitude to life, laying good foundations for the development of a spiritual practice.

Yoga is a multilevel process in which learning the postures, or *asanas*, is only one of seven paths to complete health, happiness, 'right living' and, ultimately for the masters, spiritual enlightenment. Of course, it is up to you as to how far you wish to take your study of yoga but, even at the most basic level – attending a weekly class that combines *asanas* with relaxation, meditation and breathing exercises, or *pranayama* – the benefits to health and well-being are phenomenal. You can find a reliable teacher through the British Wheel of Yoga, which has an excellent training programme and high teaching standards (see Resources Directory, page 369).

Tai chi, meaning 'energy flow', is what you may have seen in films being practised in a park early in the morning or in the evening. Again, the benefits are profound, and its practice is highly recommended as a form of cancer prevention.

Chi gong – which means 'energy work' – comes from the same roots as tai chi, but is used more specifically, often when people are already ill. The practice is usually tailor-made to the needs of the individual to help rebalance and strengthen the mind, body and spirit to overcome a particular health problem. In the West, as most of us have allowed our physical health to degenerate, chi gong is just as beneficial as yoga and tai chi, and is even more relevant if you already have some health problems (see The Resources Directory, page 365).

There is also an important role for regular aerobic exercise such as running, dancing, swimming or other sports. Try to take some of your aerobic exercise out in fresh air. A daily stretching routine is found on the *Heal Yourself* CD from Health Creation. Swimming regularly also exercises every single part of the body and can be a relaxing form of exercise. The ideal regime would be to attend a weekly class of yoga, tai chi or chi gong, and to do at least 15 to 20 minutes a day of stretching or exercising in one of these disciplines at home. This would then be complemented by one or two sessions of aerobic exercise a week, one of which is done out of doors.

In addition, try to walk whenever you can, rather than taking the car, and make sure you do some form of stretching every day. If you do not do yoga, tai chi or chi gong, then do your own routine: stretch your arms up above your head to extend your spine; do side bends to stretch your waist and try to incorporate a spinal twist, too.

If you have difficulty with mobility, and all this seems beyond your reach, think again – it is possible to do yoga stretches even while sitting in a chair or in bed. Ask a yoga teacher to help you adapt some postures to your physical state. There are also hydrotherapy exercise classes in most good swimming pools for those who are physically limited. And if your mobility is limited, it is then even more important to take up some form of physical exercise or, if this is not possible, have a weekly massage. A good massage technique called lymph drainage can also help shift toxins out of the body.

3. Improving Your State of Mind

Stress, anxiety and overwork

Stress, anxiety and overwork are usually connected in a horrible, vicious cycle. If you are anxious about money, work performance or making a good impression on others to get a promotion, affection or bonuses, then you are likely to push yourself harder and harder at work, at home or in social situations. This is further exacerbated if you are also the sort of person who takes on more and more without thinking through the cost to you in terms of finances, time, energy and personal compromise. If, in addition, you are a perfectionist, workaholic and have high integrity but poor self-esteem, the demands you make on yourself can become ridiculous.

Stress can be a form of excitement or a healthy response to a challenge or threat. In fact, in the early stages, stress can improve performance greatly. A healthy stress level can bring out the best in people, helping them to break through inertia or laziness that can make them underachieve. However, the greater the anxiety, the more pressure and the greater the fear of failure, the higher stress levels will go – to a point that is beyond optimal performance. When this happens, people work harder and harder, but achieve less and less. At this stage, there is a serious risk of 'burnout'. Individuals will begin to display the tell-tale signs, such as inappropriate emotional reactions, bad decision-making and failure to meet deadlines, will feel an ever-increasing sense of panic, despair and helplessness as the situation gets further and further out of control.

Sometimes this is accompanied by physical exhaustion, which can prevent people from working harder. But, if their stamina is good, individuals will often respond to these feelings by driving themselves even harder until they are forced to stop because of a mental breakdown or physical illness.

In Western society, high stress and anxiety levels are reaching epidemic proportions. The cost of living, and the complexity of the roles, demands and expectations we all face, combined with a personal tendency to drive ourselves very hard can put our health and well-being at grave risk. And this is before we take account of the personal tragedy of discovering that you have managed to squeeze all the joy, fun, creativity and, often, love out of your life through stress and overwork.

Various studies have shown that stress puts people at greater risk of cardiovascular disease, high blood pressure, heart attack and stroke. But what has not been so clearly emphasized is the effect that this kind of stress has on the immune system by predisposing it to cancer and infections at one extreme, and allergic and autoimmune disorders at the other.

If you recognize that you are in a spiralling stress cycle, take action immediately. This applies as much to people in formal work as well as those who are not. Many of those who are out of work, or who stay at home looking after small children, become just as stressed as individuals with important jobs and high positions. In fact, it has been shown that, when stress is linked to power, the negative effects on health are not as great as when stress is associated with powerlessness. Caring for sick relatives, elderly parents or small children, and juggling all the tasks and priorities that this involves, combined with the personal sacrifices, frustration and lack of personal space and time to achieve your own goals, can make a person severely stressed. Indeed, any situation in which there are deep and complex conflicting emotions can trigger stress in the same way that overactivity can.

Stress has two major components:

External stress comes from your environment and your relationship to it. This covers everything from the stress of heavy work deadlines, trying to drive across a busy city at rush hour, living or working in a hostile environment, getting married or divorced, having a bereavement or even going on holiday, to the need to raise enough money to pay the mortgage and bills each month.

Internal stress arises as a result of your relationship with yourself. Most people are conscious of external stress, but are largely unaware of the ways they stress themselves. Internal stress tends to mirror our early life experiences and upbringing. Our relationship to ourselves often reflects the type of relationship we had with key adults in childhood. So if, for example, you had a harsh, critical, judgemental parent, then the chances are you will have adopted these qualities in your own personality and relationship with yourself. If so, you will then be very likely to criticize yourself mercilessly, and push yourself harder and harder to achieve the kinds of results that this harsh parent would have found acceptable.

Perhaps even more often, people who have not received the love and affection they needed will stress themselves interminably in trying to prove their worth and win love and approval from others, putting themselves through all kinds of hoops in the attempt. Quite often, our relationship with ourselves and our past history will determine the level of external stress we experience. Where we live, how we work and the demands we make on ourselves and others will often come from an underlying sense of who we are and what we should be doing with our lives. So, if you were brought up in affluent surroundings with a public-school education, foreign holidays and designer clothes, you are much more likely to put immense pressure on yourself to maintain this type of lifestyle.

To this extent, many of us are victims of a large number of relatively unconscious forces that push us into living a life that makes us miserable. This whole issue of our deeper relationship to ourselves and how to change it is addressed later in this chapter. Meanwhile, we focus here on how to become aware of your stress levels and make practical changes to bring them under control.

Looking for Signs of Stress

Most of us know when we are stressed – we feel anxious, irritable, miserable and pressured. Physical signs include a rapid, racing heartbeat, palpitations (where the heart misses a beat or jumps about), shallow breathing, indigestion, diarrhoea or constipation (sometimes accompanied by piles). As stress levels become severe, we become less effective in everything we do. This may be difficult to own up to, but it is better if you can spot it before it is pointed out to you by others – especially at your workplace.

At this stage, people often say, 'I feel like I am running as fast as I can, but I just can't keep up – in fact, I feel like I'm going backwards.' This may be followed by feelings of complete despair because they are already working as hard as they can and, in fact, are facing collapse. With such severe stress, it becomes impossible to distinguish between key tasks and trivia. People are often only able to deal with the tip of the iceberg – coping with what is immediately in front of them, answering phone calls and letters, but failing to do any strategic thinking or planning to make life or work run more smoothly and efficiently.

Another alarming symptom of severe stress is 'thought block', when you can't remember what it was you were talking about mid-sentence. When stress levels are really high, this may be full-blown panic attacks. Ordinary anxiety spirals into terror, and people become so paralysed by fear that it is impossible to think clearly. At this point, medical help is often required.

If you have any of these symptoms, or are driving colleagues or family members into such levels of stress with your behaviour, it is crucial to stop now and address these issues to help prevent cancer and other serious illness.

Dealing with Stress

There are two fundamental approaches to deal with stress in a practical way. Before you even begin, however, think of stress as an addiction which you are now really determined to give up. The first practical step is to tackle the symptoms of stress through relaxation, exercise and meditation. The second way is to reorganize your day – at home or at work – to remove any unnecessary sources of stress, prioritizing only those activities that are absolutely necessary. Practical ways to analyse your stress and reorganize your priorities are covered in Principle 4 of the Health Creation Programme available from Health Creation.

Nine times out of 10, reducing stress means simplifying your life and letting things go. People who are stressed almost always have needs, commitments and expectations that are beyond their ability to 'deliver', whether at work, or financially or emotionally. A life so out of balance is nearly always a sign of displaced emotional needs combined with the sense that everything will be all right if only 'X' can be achieved, sorted out or bought.

When stress has become severe, most people need a break of two to four weeks with support and therapeutic help to allow the body to regain its balance. In this case, it is wise to start a programme of relaxation, counselling and physical therapies such as massage, aromatherapy, reflexology and spiritual healing to reestablish equilibrium and recover from exhaustion. Counselling is usually necessary because, as people become more stressed, emotion is often suppressed or, indeed, it may be suppressed emotion causing the stress in the first place, putting great strain on the heart.

If these options are not available, then try to let yourself sleep and rest as much as possible. Spiritual healing is often an invaluable source of support at these times (and is often free or inexpensive). You can find a healer through the National Federation of Spiritual Healers (see The Resources Directory, page 358). If you cannot get to a healer, you might want to arrange for them to send you distant healing.

In the furthermost reaches of stress and burnout, it is usually not possible to think clearly enough to reorganize your priorities and simplify your life. So, do not even try until your stress levels have fallen after a period of rest and therapy. Part of the problem of stress is that people can no longer 'see the wood for the trees', which makes it difficult to prioritize sensibly.

Once stress levels have come down, a good idea is for you, either alone, or with your family or work team, to sit down and address the problem. There is no doubt that if you are feeling stressed, then those around you feel stressed, too. By getting a grip on the situation, you will thus be doing everyone in your immediate circle a favour. This may, at first, make you feel vulnerable. But, if you can get this type of support, it will ultimately be a helpful and bonding process. Explain to your family and colleagues that you are radically reappraising the way you live your life. If you can get them on your side before you start, you should meet with far less resistance while gaining solidarity and creative solutions.

At work, you may need to seek the help of an external consultant to manage organizational stress, or see where you are losing efficiency and building stress into the system. You may also need to work with a Health Creation Consultant to learn new, more effective ways of running your working life. In your personal life, a stress or debt counsellor may be necessary to help you sort out your problems, priorities and goals.

Be aware that this simplifying or 'letting go' process will inevitably involve some disappointment as you give up things you have been struggling to achieve. However, what you may discover in the longer term is that, paradoxically, the less you do, the more you start to achieve.

This may be clearly seen when you start to meditate properly. Once a meditation routine is established, life becomes easier, and whatever you have planned or visualized starts to come to you, rather than your having to struggle to make them happen. It is remarkable how, when you start to 'get yourself out of the way', the underlying process of life begins to support you as well.

Getting Out of Severe Stress

When trying to get severe stress under control, the golden rules are:

- Take a good two- to four-week break from all normal activity, and combine this with a stress-busting programme of rest, relaxation, massage and exercise to lessen the grip of stress on the body.
- Start counselling to unburden yourself emotionally.
- Do not start work or activity again until all the physical and mental symptoms of stress have gone for at least a week.
- When preparing to go back to work, go through your diary and cancel every engagement or meeting for the next six months that is not absolutely vital.

When you are able to start thinking clearly again, analyse your personal and work objectives, and aim to cut your load by half. This may sound drastic, but half of the extra time you gain must be spent on yourself, and the rest on doing the things you are committed to doing properly, without rush or struggle. It will also leave room for the inevitable expansion of your activities until you need to do a major pruning exercise again.

List all your regular commitments at home and at work, and calculate the percentage of your time given to each, including the time spent on:

- your important relationships
- carer roles for dependent relatives or friends
- your social life
- clubs or societies you belong to
- projects you are involved in at work or at home
- changes going on at home, such as moving house, building work, getting divorced, weddings or bereavements
- activities with your children or partner.

Remember to also include time spent for:

- rest, exercise, relaxation and recreation
- unstructured time just for yourself
- work commitments.

When you have worked out the amount of time you normally devote to each area, this may well be an eye-opener and highlight where the imbalance has crept in.

Most people in stress find that their work dominates the majority of their time and energy. Another major stressor is looking after other people's needs. But probably the main reason why most people become stressed is that they simply forget to put time aside for themselves, leaving no time for rest, recuperation, reflection, creativity or processing or 'digesting' what is happening in their life. Over time, failing to take time to be nourished, and find meaning and pleasure in life, makes people feel bored, unsatisfied, empty and depressed. To fill this emptiness, people then often resort to food, alcohol or drugs to feel better. Alternatively, these difficult feelings may cause people to give even more of themselves to others, thus draining themselves even further.

The next step is to reorganize your priorities, allocating the correct amount of time to key areas of your life.

The underlying essence to this process is to be clear about your core values and what really matters to you. Another vital element is to simplify life radically so that you can bring real energy to the areas of life that you love. But the foundation stone of all this is to make time for yourself. This must take the highest priority on your revised list. Ideally, this should include totally unstructured time as well as time to relax, meditate, exercise and seek the help of support groups, counselling or complementary therapists. It should also include at least one creative activity, which may mean reviving an interest in art, music, literature, theatre or dance, for example. Creating unstructured time means leaving space for yourself each week to just potter, rest, reflect or read. If you live with others, you must guard this space fiercely and make sure the people in your life respect your special time alone.

This will encourage them, in turn, to do the same for themselves, which is a particularly helpful message and example to give to children. Many adults 'programme' their children for stress in later life. They organize their children's lives without leaving any space or 'down time' for them to be alone with their inner world. It then becomes increasingly difficult for them to be quiet or on their own which, in turn, is why so many adults have problems being on their own and sustaining an inner life and are continually chasing the 'buzz'. It is, therefore, important to start right from the beginning with children, allowing them space and time to unfold in their own unique, inner-directed way.

At work, reducing your goals by half will take a great deal of clarity, courage and discipline. But taking the stress off yourself in this way means you will achieve better results in whatever projects you are working on. However, if this is impossible to do with your job situation, it may well be time to change it, or seriously challenge your manager (or yourself) about your job description. Usually, however, it is we who make the jobs we do impossible – by being either too ambitious, unrealistic or incapable of saying 'no'.

Ultimately, you may need to challenge the belief in yourself that 'more is better'. Many of us think we will be considered virtuous or more lovable if we are high-achieving. But, the tendency to take on more and more can also be seen as a form of greed. It may look virtuous or altruistic but, often, it is driven, just like overeating, by an underlying hunger for, in this case, more power, money or recognition. These needs, in turn, ultimately stem from an emotional or spiritual hunger that can and must be filled in much less destructive ways. When addressing these underlying needs, most people need the help of counselling and of a sustaining spiritual practice.

If you are suffering from stress that is not so extreme, it is still important to get your own stress-reduction programme going. This should involve a mixture of relaxation and self-help techniques alongside your normal work. You can then streamline and reprioritize your home, work and social activities, as described above, while making sure that there is plenty of time for you.

Sleep, rest and relaxation

To become really healthy and avoid cancer recurrence, addressing the need for proper sleep, rest and relaxation is vital. Think of life as the shape of the infinity symbol (the Greek omega) – we move out on one side of the loop into activity, arousal and achievement, then flow back again to the opposite side of the loop of rest into relaxation, letting go and regeneration.

The Indian Ayurvedic physicians believe that the body goes through a series of four-hour cycles around the clock – at 2, 6 and 10 a.m. and 2, 6 and 10 p.m. At the end of the evening cycle (from 6 to 10 p.m.), we naturally feel sleepy and ready to rest. However, if we resist this urge and stay up beyond this point, we go into a new, more fiery type of energy cycle that will often keep us up late into the night. If we then need to get up early to work or look after children, we are burning the candle at both ends, failing to get the restorative rest and sleep we need. Most people do feel sleepy at around 9:30 to 10 p.m., and could easily go to bed then, but they overcome these feelings to try to achieve more or play harder.

In the Ayurvedic system, the best time to get up is soon after 6 a.m. with the dawning light. Try to get your life more in harmony with these natural cycles of the body. You must also make a cut-off point for all work-related activity as you walk through the door of your home after work. If this is not possible, then make an absolute deadline of about 8 p.m., after which all the rest of the time is spent relaxing and nourishing yourself in creative ways.

Start settling down from around 9 p.m., whether by reading, meditating, reflecting, writing down your feelings in a journal or making love. All these things will deepen your connection with yourself and your loved ones. Make sure this gentle time is absolutely sacrosanct in your home life. Then allow yourself to sleep from 10.30 or so. Achieving this balance will make your life instantly richer and far healthier. Your immune system and tissue functioning will recover, and the risk of cancer will diminish greatly.

Improving your relationships

The usual keys to improved relationships are better communication, a good relationship with yourself and clarity about your needs. But it is sometimes necessary to heal the wounds of the past, especially if there has been abuse or neglect, before it is possible to establish a truly nourishing relationship with yourself and others.

If you find yourself trapped in bad relationships, there are a number of sources of help, including the agency RELATE, and the many forms of counselling available. But a surprisingly helpful source is the study of Tantric Yoga. Through this teaching, old wounds can be healed, and a new template for loving, pleasurable and honouring relationships with yourself and others can be established (see The Resources Directory for help in finding Tantric Yoga teachers).

Letting go of your emotions

Many people are simply too frightened to express their feelings, but these feelings have to go somewhere. A feeling produces chemical neuropeptides in the brain and body. As feelings are expressed, these neuropeptides are discharged or metabolized, thus restoring equilibrium. The neuropeptides found in tears of rage are completely different from those in tears of grief or heartbreak. If these chemicals are not released, these 'molecules of emotion' will affect the body, causing physiological changes which may, over time, cause illness. In effect, 'What the mind represses, the body expresses.'

It is useful to define 'feelings' as what we feel as something happens. When feelings are not expressed, they turn into emotions in the mind and body that are memories of our feelings that are retained over time. Sometimes, people are comfortable expressing one kind of feeling, but not another. For example, some of us find it easy to cry, but are never able to get angry whereas, for others, it is the reverse – they can erupt like a volcano, but would rather die than cry in public.

The most common feelings that people hang on to are grief, disappointment, bitterness, envy, guilt and anger. When these become lodged as emotions in the body, Eastern energy medicine observes that they can have specific effects on different organs. For example, grief tends to affect the lungs and throat, anger affects the liver and gut, bitterness affects the pancreas, and disappointment the kidneys. Although these are broad generalizations, it is surprising, in my medical practice, how often these associations are true. All of these effects occur through PNI (psychoneuroimmunology) or mind–body mechanisms.

Emotions also have major effects on the blood and immune systems. It has already been mentioned that stress and upset can reduce the number and activity of circulating immune cells, and the amount of oxygen carried in the haemoglobin of red blood cells. If you are burdened with a lot of old emotion from upsets, losses or frustrations in the past, then it is essential for both the health of your immune system and your ultimate protection against cancer to heal or offload these emotions.

The most common way to do this is through counselling or psychotherapy, when a person is taken back into the emotional memory and allowed, in a variety of ways, to discharge or clear out the energy or emotion felt at the time which they are still embodying. Another route of release is through the body. Good-quality massage or shiatsu and sometimes powerful sex can reach old emotions, which can then be expressed in the presence of loving support. Spiritual healing can also unlock these emotional doors and allow emotion to flow.

A different way to clear toxic emotions is by forgiving and letting go of old hurts or wounds. This can be achieved through Brandon Bays' Journey work (see The Resources Directory, page 328). People often hang onto or even nurse old grievances, bearing grudges and resentments even after the others involved have died. Not only do these harmful emotions silt us up, but also part of our vital energy is then trapped and inaccessible to us for living. The message is clear: we need to detox emotionally as much as we need to detox physically.

4. Reviving and Honouring Your Spirit

If you have become dispirited, or your spirit has been crushed or broken by life as a result of a combination of disappointment, grief, frustration or simply not finding a way to fully express yourself, then this can have a depressing or even devastating effect on the immune system. A clear example is the case of the elderly person who dies within six weeks of losing his spouse. This clearly illustrates that when the will to live has gone, the physical body can very quickly give way.

Sadly, many people nowadays live in an unfulfilled state, having little sense of purpose or meaning in their lives and no genuine sources of spiritual nourishment or emotional well-being. Often, people live their lives according to the expectations and demands of others, with little excitement or passion to enliven and vitalize them. Certainly, in the field of integrated cancer medicine, it is clear that, when someone has lost the will to live or has no exciting creative focus into which to channel their energy, then no medicine – orthodox or complementary – will get them well. On the other hand, if this sense of purpose and passion is rekindled, people can rapidly get well from the 'inside out' as their immune system comes back to life.

To free and heal your spirit, it is often necessary to work on several fronts at the same time. To start with, it is important to attend to your 'emotional hygiene' as described above.

Once you start to tune in to this concept, it is easy to see what emotions people are hanging on to. Look closely at people and you will find that their body language, breathing patterns, eyes and facial expressions say it all. We actually 'embody' the feelings we can't let go of in our posture and breathing pattern. Shedding old emotion and, more important, learning how to express rather than repress emotions are crucial steps on the path towards good health, lifting depression, freeing our spirit and reactivating our immunity.

The next step is to identify what drives your behaviour and change fear-based motivation to life- or love-based motivation. Often, we are programmed from childhood to push ourselves relentlessly to prove ourselves worthy, be successful, win approval, love and affection, or achieve the perfection we think is expected of us. This means that, most of the time, we behave the way other people want us to be, and our own unique spirit becomes submerged. This is often linked to low self-esteem and a tendency to take care of others while neglecting or abandoning ourselves. Having identified these slave-driving, perfectionist, workaholic or approval-seeking sides of yourself, the task is then to replace this programming with kinder, more encouraging and supportive messages to allow the real you to emerge and flourish, thus lifting your spirit. (Help with working on the identification of what is burdening your spirit is found in the Health Creation Programme Principle 7, 'Becoming True to Yourself', and on the *Know Yourself* CD within the programme.

Again, the key here is to put yourself first. It is staggering how many people put themselves at the very bottom of the list of those to care for. Most people look after their houses, cars and pets far better than they look after themselves. Getting the relationship with yourself right also lays the foundation for everything else to fall into place. If you take time to listen and respond to your own needs, making these as important as the needs of others, then your life, health and relationships will be transformed beyond recognition.

Finding meaning and purpose in life

To take this process further, the next step is to learn to trust your own inner wisdom. Spend time either in retreat, meditation, counselling or supportive group work to quieten down and listen to your inner voice. Discover what your core values and needs truly are. It is vitally important to be involved in things that truly express you and give you a sense of purpose and meaning. Over time, try to work towards living in the right place, in the right way, with a lifestyle, home and job that reflect who you really are.

It is also important to ensure that you can both express and receive the love you need. This may be through personal relationships, or through meaningful links with community or spiritual groups. By redefining your core values on a regular basis, you will be able to organize your life to reflect these values, giving attention, priority, energy and time to the important things in your life rather than the trivia.

Closely linked to this is ensuring that your personal spiritual needs are being met, and that you are receiving the nourishment and uplift you need. It is important in our own unique way to take our hearts and minds out of the hurly-burly of everyday life, and into communion with our own spiritual nature and into connection with the spiritual side of life. People suffer from, often without even realizing it, a deep spiritual malaise and a longing to touch into the world of Spirit and 'the kingdom of heaven which is within'.

For many of us, everyday hassles can be transcended simply by being in places of great natural beauty or in contact with nature. For others, music can lift them out of their normal preoccupations, or the essence of love tapped into through their relationships or by service to others. Creativity and self-expression are other major sources of joy and spiritual well-being. Spiritual connection and uplift can also come through meditation or religious practices. Some may have a more immediate or gnostic sense of spirituality, enabling them to feel palpably the presence and love of the Holy Spirit. Others may have their relationship with Spirit through religious beliefs and the faith these generate.

Certainly, many with whom I have worked to restore health have said it was the recognition of their spiritual nature and prioritizing of their spiritual needs that was responsible for their healing. The profound personal transformation you can undergo as a result of opening up to your personal spirituality can result in a wonderful new relationship to both living and dying, and can catalyse remarkable physical recovery as well.

If you are prepared to prioritize your peace of mind and spiritual well-being, your life will become both simpler and more enriched at the same time. You will feel as if you have come home to yourself in a profound and meaningful way. Most of those who go through this door, choosing peace and joy above all else, say they feel more alive and happier than ever before.

Attending to the State of Your Spirit

Phase 1

Unburden yourself of:

- toxic emotions you have been carrying for a long time such as hate, anger, resentment, disappointment, bitterness, jealousy and guilt
- disabling attitudes or limiting beliefs you have picked up in earlier life
- roles you play or personas you project which do not represent who you really are
- dominating presences or forces in your life that stop you from being yourself.

Phase 2

Discover who you really are by becoming true to yourself, which involves:

- eliciting your core values in life, particularly what it is that gives your life purpose or meaning
- finding ways to express yourself in the world, which includes thinking about your job, the environment in which you live, the relationships you choose, the expression of your sexuality and outlets for your creative or physical side.

Phase 3

Attend to your spiritual nourishment, lifting your energy levels and consciousness through:

- beauty, as in fine art or music
- religion
- meditation
- spiritual retreats
- developing your personal spirituality
- dedicated service to others
- sharing spontaneous fun with others
- creative activity
- giving and receiving love.

Not only does their health improve greatly, but they also start to feel younger, too. This slowing down of the ageing process is noticeable in people who are free and fulfilled spiritually. This is an authentic phenomenon, which can be put down to the effects that a positive state of mind and spirit have on our immune and tissue function as all the body processes begin to work optimally. In essence, this is all about you – the unique being you are – becoming enabled and empowered to reach your full potential. This has nothing to do with competitiveness, however, but is rather about your being allowed to flourish and grow, and express your true nature, irrespective of anyone else. This will enable you to live fully and happily in the present, and experience real joy and freedom in living.

Going deeper into freeing your spirit

Changing Difficult Attitudes and Limiting Beliefs

As well as forming the basis of our relationship with ourselves, early life is also the source of many underlying attitudes and beliefs about life and our abilities. As children, we are trusting and tend to believe what adults tell us. We are also equally affected by what they fail to tell us. If we get the message that we are not good enough, this will become our belief and, as adults, we will tend to give up even trying to get the things we want. If we do not get the attention and encouragement we need, we will believe we are unlovable, and constantly strive for approval and attention.

If our environment as a child has been hostile and abusive, we tend to believe the world is a dangerous place, and are then driven by a constant sense of fear and insecurity (even if, to others, our situation seems secure). If we have had a harsh, critical, judgemental parent figure in our early life, we often become harsh and judgemental of ourselves. If we have been told that children should be seen and not heard, it becomes difficult for us to be spontaneous or exuberant. If we have been told off every time we got angry or cried, then it will be extremely difficult to express emotion. If we have discovered that the way to get attention is by being sexually provocative, we may be sexually manipulative as adults.

While these survival codes may have worked in childhood, as adults, they may be severely limiting our pleasure, fulfilment and ability to reach our potential. The worst situation is when people pick up the message that they do not deserve good things to happen to them and so would rather push good things away than experience the discomfort of receiving. Those who give too much often have such an underlying belief. They may be very generous towards others, but it is almost impossible for them to accept anything from others. Most of us have many limiting beliefs, such as that we cannot have the love, money, power or enjoyment that we really want and need. As a result, we live in a semi-depressed state the whole of our lives.

To turn this situation around, start identifying the underlying attitudes that are affecting your behaviour or curbing your expectations, and replace them with healthier ones. This kind of work can be done with the help of a transpersonal counsellor (see The Resources Directory, pages 362–5). Once you start recognizing them, it becomes easier to change these beliefs.

The way to replace them is to challenge yourself every time you find these attitudes coming into play. Another way is to make a list of your attitudes and limiting beliefs, then make a separate list of statements that reverse them. For example, if you believe 'I am unlovable,' write on a clean piece of paper 'I am lovable.' If you believe 'I do not deserve to be wealthy,' write on the new list 'I deserve wealth and abundance in my life.' Once you have made a list of reverse statements, you can use them as affirmations and repeat them to yourself on a daily basis, say, after meditation. You can also repeat and affirm the healthy belief to yourself whenever you find an old limiting belief is 'running you' in a given situation. For example, if, while being interviewed for a job, you are thinking 'I'll never get this job; I'm not nearly as good as the other candidates,' replace this with 'I choose to get this job. I am fully qualified and experienced for the post, and they would be lucky to have me.' Just watch the effect this will have once you allow the power of your new, positive affirmations to sink in.

This will replace, over time, the negative messages and beliefs with positive ones. Eventually, you will behave according to the new positive code and not the old one. Although it is easier to do this work with a therapist than on your own, it is certainly not impossible to do it yourself, especially if you use the 'belief-busting' page in the Health Creation Programme. Add to your list as you discover new ways in which you are limiting or compromising yourself, then flip them over into positive affirmations. This exercise really works and your life will change positively when you give this your attention.

Shedding Unhelpful Roles and Personas

Our roles or personas in adult life are also an extension of the attitudes and beliefs we have adopted from childhood. For example, if the desire to win approval has extended into your professional life, you may well have chosen a well-respected role such as doctor, nurse, vet or vicar. If you have grown up believing the world is a frightening place, you may have built your life around trying to control others by becoming a politician, teacher, member of the armed forces or policeman. This is not to say being a carer, politician or a policeman is not the perfect role in life for some. It will largely depend on whether you are doing this job from your strengths rather than weaknesses, your wholeness or your wound, or 'shadow' as it is known in Jungian psychology.

The simple questions to ask yourself are:

- Do my roles genuinely reflect who I am, and give me excitement and energy?
- Are my roles driven by my underlying fear or the secondary gains the role brings with it?

An example of a role or persona that is 'shadow'-driven would be the seemingly generous person who is actually giving out a great deal because of their own immense emptiness and need. By behaving in this way, such a person is actually showing other people how he would like to be treated, but is too afraid to ask. By overgiving in this way, a person becomes even more depleted and is likely, ultimately, to go into some form of burnout or depression. This has its foundations in the anger such a person feels inside at not being treated properly. Again, it is easier to examine these things with a therapist rather than on your own.

A good example of this is a colleague of mine who had breast cancer while being a schoolteacher and 'executive wife', producing endless immaculate dinner parties for her husband's high-powered business associates. In a period of soul-searching after her diagnosis, she realized that none of this activity was really who she was and that, at heart, she was a 'creative' who adored nature, crafts and natural medicine. She had become drained by this persona which did not reflect her true nature. Over time, she gradually withdrew from her previous roles and allowed the gentler aspect of her personality to emerge. She now lives as a potter, organic gardener and spiritual healer, and is wonderfully well 20 years on from her initial diagnosis with breast cancer.

Getting Free of Dominant Presences or Forces in Your Outer Life

Another reason why people may fail to express themselves properly is because someone or something is dominating them to the extent that they don't know how they feel or what they want. We talk about being 'possessed' by the dead, but people can be just as 'possessed' or dominated by the living! Some people were completely dominated as children by the emotional needs of their parents or siblings. As a result, they are then permanently in a state of reaction to the needs of other family members. This can also happen in school or at work, such as when a dominant character organizes all the attention around him- or herself, manipulating others (including you) in the process.

This happens in partnerships, too, where one person's needs are always considered more important than those of others. Of course, powerful needy parents can continue to control the lives of their offspring until a ripe old age, if the pattern is not challenged and broken early on. Such a pattern set early is hard to break. Indeed, later relationships may well be chosen on the basis of finding someone else to occupy this very dominating role in your life as such a way of being has become your 'comfort zone' – however much it may undermine you. The problem is, when you are being dominated in this way, it is hard to know yourself or what your needs really are.

Extensions of this phenomenon can be found at different levels. For example, we are all dominated by the high-tech marketing-led world in which we live, which itself is dominated by materialistic values. We are all subjected to left-brain achievement-orientated education systems, and we are also ruled by reductionist medicine. Those of a gentler, more spiritual nature often find themselves 'on the back foot', overwhelmed by these types of social pressure. It can be difficult for such people to assert their own values and lifestyle, leading to chronic compromise at many levels of life.

If people are very sensitive, the atmosphere or energy of a building or area in which they live may dominate them, too. There may also be problems if people are forced to live in a country where the dominant cultural values around them are in conflict with their own underlying values or nature.

Without realizing it, we may be using a lot of energy to resist the dominant forces around us. The key in this case is to recognize the phenomenon in the first place. The minute you recognize you are subject to the power of another person, value system, situation or place, you can begin to do something about it.

Very often, people who allow themselves to be dominated themselves become, in other circumstances, very dominating. Taken to the extreme, this can mean that those who have been abused can become abusers themselves. This realization can be shattering, and it often requires a therapist to help break the cycle. If you have been chronically abused over time, it may take some time to rebuild your sense of who you are, once you are no longer being dominated. However, once embarked upon, this process of 'reclaiming your power' will enrich and strengthen you, and eventually provide you with an enormous sense of relief. This, in turn, will mean that your energy and will are not being sapped, and you will have much more energy for your own healing and self-defence.

Caroline Myss, the spiritual teacher and author, tells us that our ability to be well is directly proportional to the amount of spiritual energy we have available to ourselves rather than trapped in past wounds, relationships or memories of other times. This must be taken seriously, and we must all free ourselves from domination, past or present, to be truly well.

Reorientation to your true self

As you stop being the way others want you to be, the question of who the real you is almost inevitably arises. You may never have had a chance in your whole life to think about the answer to this question. People are constantly on the receiving end of pressure from parents, teachers and society to live up to their expectations, to be the way they want them to be, to take 'good' advice or simply 'play the game'.

Discovering Your Core Values

To find out what would be a fully authentic life for you, it is a good idea to take some quiet reflective time in a loving supportive environment. This could be on retreat, or with a therapy group or good friends who know that you need the time and space to reorientate yourself. You can also achieve this by doing the 'Becoming True to Yourself' and 'Seeing Yourself in Your New Lifestyle' exercises in the Health Creation Programme.

Start with a relaxation exercise, and then focus your attention on your heart area. Concentrate on generating loving feelings in your heart towards someone close to you or towards yourself, or feel a more general sense of compassion towards others. When you achieve this loving 'heart space', ask yourself:

- What is really the most important thing to me in life?
- What really matters to me?

Write down your responses, and repeat this exercise on different days. You will probably find that, as the days go by, you are making an archaeological journey into deeper and deeper levels of yourself to discover your innermost values.

Checking Your Will to Live

Another major key to knowing the state of your spirit is to take a really truthful look at your will to live. We may be fighting cancer because we are frightened, but after looking more deeply within yourself you may find that you are rather ambivalent about life and not really that keen to go on living at all. A part of you may even be longing for death. Don't be afraid or embarrassed if you discover this. As already mentioned in Chapter 2, Freud asserted that all of us have equal and opposite urges – *thanetos*, the urge towards death, and *eros*, the urge towards life. Normally, people move back and forth between these poles, but some of us have a much stronger longing for death than others. We may be so frightened of dying that an enormous amount of our energy is taken up trying to avoid even thinking about death, even though, underneath, we may have lost our will to live.

Therefore, a helpful part of getting into a deeper relationship with yourself is to examine your feelings about death and dying to discover where your true motivation lies. It is said that people can only truly embrace living fully when they can also embrace the reality of dying, and when the desire for death has been worked through to a point where we can genuinely choose life.

Most therapists working in the holistic field do not view death as 'failure' or even necessarily as the final end, but more as a transition. When dealing with this profound territory, you could ask yourself whether you really do have the will to live, or whether it has been beaten or squashed out of you by the hardships of living. If you are ambivalent about life, deeply soul-weary or just plain lost, it is time to seek a combination of spiritual healing and transpersonal psychotherapy to help rekindle your commitment to life and find the joy in being alive.

If you feel that your main purpose for living is your children or partner, then it may be worth exploring whether there are unexpressed areas of yourself that need to emerge just for you. Your personal needs and desires may have been abandoned as life became focused on others. Although our dedication to our nearest and dearest is absolutely right and wonderful, living out your life through others is not a good way to be. It can make you totally dependent on them and them on you, making it harder for them to have their own lives. It can also limit your own potential for self-realization and growth.

Living Life with Purpose and Meaning

Once you have a clear sense of what really matters and excites you in life, the task is then to make sure this is reflected in the way you spend your time. If the best bits of your life are squashed into a tiny fraction of your time, your soul or spirit will inevitably suffer. Once you know where your priorities lie, try to change the balance in your life step by step, and watch your health and happiness blossom as you become more and more fully alive.

C. G. Jung, one of the most significant psychologists of recent times, said that there is one state above all others that will surely kill a person – living a life without meaning. For some, this meaning may come through their inner life, creativity, relationships or spirituality. For others, it may be from a concrete focus such as helping the homeless or protecting the environment.

Increasingly, people are finding meaning by trying to understand and become conscious of their souls' or spirits' journey through life. People with a spiritual inclination often see themselves as 'spiritual beings in physical bodies'. While anticipating the ultimate release back into the spirit dimension at the time of death, they seek to understand the purpose of this physical incarnation and try to heed the lessons they are learning as they progress along their life path. This is consistent with the Eastern view of sequential reincarnation until we have learned enough to not need to come back again.

Whatever your belief, the important thing for the immune system is to be as happy, excited and committed as possible in life. Psychologist Lawrence LeShan described this as 'singing your own song' – feeling full of excitement when you wake each day, and full of gratitude as you go to sleep. For many people, this is a very long way from how they currently feel. Our goal must be to seek this kind of happiness, breaking where necessary the addiction we have to our suffering and the comfort of staying stuck in our previously safe, but unsatisfying, rut.

Encouraging Self-expression

One of our great 'soul' needs is for self-expression and recognition of who we are. We are all unique and different, and encouraging our own personal forms of expression is fundamental for the health of both the individual and society. Unfortunately, the Victorian ethos and schooling that most of us received tend to encourage the reverse, squashing individuality and encouraging uniformity. The educational process, by and large, tends to push all students through the same courses so that they achieve the same standards in the same subjects at the same age. At the age of 15, we are allowed to make some choices towards different career paths. But, by this time, it is estimated that the school system has lost the interest of six out of seven children. This is because the way we are taught at school is only one of seven key learning styles. The vast majority of children being put through the educational system will never come close to being able to reach their full potential or express themselves well in life, having not been 'met', engaged with or taught appropriately in school.

It is important for our health that we redress these inhibiting influences of our schooling and make strenuous efforts in all other areas of society to reverse this trend. It is essential that, whether at school, home, work and in the community, we enjoy how different people are and how unique are the skills each person can bring to a situation. Most particularly, we must learn not to be prejudicial and discriminating towards those who do not follow the conventional path. For yourself, check that you are expressing your true self in your chosen job, the place you live, the people with whom you maintain relationships, and your sexuality, creativity, physicality and appearance.

If you dress to please others, I suggest you stop immediately and start dressing the way you like. If you make love in a way you think is expected of you or that your partner likes, think again and start finding out how you would like to express yourself sexually. If you live in a house that is full of your parents' old furniture, which you have kept out of duty, think again about your own style. Start defining your own taste, hanging on to only one or two key things for historical and sentimental reasons. If you are a physical person who loves to dance, run or climb mountains, but have forgone these activities because of advancing age, get your body moving again.

If you feel limited or inhibited in your relationships, make a stand to change the pattern of the relationship and be exactly the way you are. The other person will have been aware that you have not really been yourself, and will be losing respect for you because of it. There is nothing more off-putting than someone who is being inauthentic in this way. If someone does not like or want to be with the real you, then it is definitely time to leave the relationship anyway.

If you feel too vulnerable to let go of such a 'false' relationship, then seek the support of a counsellor with whom you have built up a relationship so that he can 'hold you' emotionally through the period of transition. On the other hand, if it is a long-term committed relationship which you do not want to break, then seek counselling for yourself or jointly with your partner through RELATE (the relationship-counselling charity) or a good counsellor to help you change your relationship patterns (see The Resources Directory, pages 362–5).

If your job is not really you, try to find a different job that will reflect your core values more closely. Your work will then be much more fulfilling.

If you think you are too old to make these kinds of changes, let me assure you that it is never too late to 'come home to yourself' and start leading an authentic life. I have witnessed thousands of people who, at all ages, have made key changes in their lives when in a health crisis, and have literally come back to life in body and mind in the process, restarting their lives on much better foundations.

Spiritual nourishment

The next vital step is to find ways of nourishing your precious and beautiful spirit. Having read the last few pages, your spirit may already be jumping for joy at the thought of getting some recognition and attention, and having permission to be fully expressed in your life.

Many people grow up thinking that spirit equals religion, which is seen as repressing rather than freeing their spirit. The sad thing about religious practice in the West is that, historically, spirituality has been something acknowledged perhaps once a week, on a Sunday, rather than continuously throughout our lives. His Royal Highness the Prince of Wales, in his Millennium Reith lecture, urged people to 'rediscover or reacknowledge a sense of the sacred in our dealings with the natural world and with each other'. By doing this, we will live our spirituality rather than keeping it in a separate compartment in our lives.

Buddhists and yogis believe that the material world and even our emotions are an illusion, and that it is the spiritual dimension that is reality. They maintain that it is our preoccupation with the material world and our sense of self that stops us from understanding the true nature of this reality, and experiencing its associated bliss and freedom.

Recognition of the spiritual dimension of life is growing in our culture at this time. Those who are changing from material to spiritual values are often described as being 'in transformation'. It is obvious when you meet people who are no longer in the grip of material values and the anxiety that goes with it. Invariably, they say that now they live in the present moment and that, when this can be given full attention, life becomes truly happy.

I have witnessed this transformational process over and over again with my patients as the shock of a cancer diagnosis awakens them to the reality of their spiritual nature. For others, fleeting glances of this spiritual nature and connection to life can come at moments of intense joy, pain or beauty, through sexual union with another, while meditating or through experiencing true communion with God or the Holy Spirit. Some people reach this state under the influence of consciousness-raising drugs. What is crucial is to recognize that each of us has our own way of experiencing our spirit and the spiritual dimension, and finding ways of exploring this for yourself is the key.

As we explore our spiritual life, we are presented with the paradox that, on the one hand, we seek to be fully individual and express our true nature whereas, on the other hand, we seek to transcend our ego state so that we can 'let go and let God'. Being fully in the world while retaining our sense of the greater spiritual reality and our ability to see into the bigger truth is the challenge of 'being in the world, but not of it'.

Appreciation of these different levels of reality comes from a shift in our perception or consciousness. In our everyday consciousness, we need the ego, for a strong sense of self and the will to live out our unique purpose. But, from time to time, we also need to 'rise above the clouds' and see the greater reality, appreciating the tiny part we play in the vast process of life. From this perspective, the pressures and priorities of our own existence become much less all-consuming. Once you have experienced this other perspective, you will not let your life become so driven or stressed, or lose yourself in your own 'personal drama'. You may even stop taking yourself quite so seriously!

When developing your individual spirituality, it is also important to be completely authentic. People can spend years going to church or sitting in meditation groups, following other people's 'recipes' for the spiritual life, but gaining absolutely nothing at all. If you are doing this, I suggest you stop now and do something more profitable with your time.

Watching people unfold into their own sense of Spirit and spirituality, I have been aware of recurring themes. One universal source of spiritual uplift is to bring more and more beauty into life, whether through nature, your home or clothes, art or music. In Japan, the Johrei Society has the fundamental philosophy that health depends on three things: respect for the environment and eating organic food; daily spiritual healing within the family context; and the central need for beauty in life. The more I think about this philosophy, the more I agree that beauty in our lives is essential for spiritual health. If people live in an ugly concrete jungle, they can become starved of the uplift that natural beauty offers. Making time to catch a sunrise, to climb to the top of a mountain or to visit the woods in autumn can be incredibly uplifting to the spirit.

Another key to spiritual nourishment is simply making time and space for yourself, which has been mentioned over and over again. The spirit often longs for simplicity and time to 'be' rather than 'do'. If you find it impossible to rest or have space in your own home, it may be worth going on retreat. More and more centres are making it possible to have time to yourself in a loving atmosphere, either with or without spiritual guidance. Regularly taking time to 'come home to yourself' in this way and deepening your spiritual connection is profoundly healing and nurturing, and the best possible preventive medicine you can take.

If you already have a strong sense of Spirit or a religious belief, you may wish to seek a context that supports these beliefs. But there are also plenty of atheist retreat centres for those who wish to explore their own sense of spirituality (see The Resources Directory, pages 390–1). Many retreat centres allow people to study about or improve their meditation techniques. Doing this in a dedicated way with the support of others can make it easier to maintain the practice at home.

The most fundamental spiritual value of all is the need to give and receive love – both in our personal relationships and in our relationship with the Divine. For some, their spiritual problem is having a great deal of love to give, but no way of expressing it, whereas others feel desperately in need of love and attention. If your ability to give and receive love feels blocked, or you have been deprived of love through social circumstances, you may wish to start, through therapeutic relationships, support groups or spiritual healing, finding ways of giving and receiving love in a safe context.

Many self-development groups offer courses based on a strongly supportive, loving ethos. It is amazing how people on these courses can be given such high-quality love and support from people who were strangers only a few days earlier. People tend to get stuck on the idea that, to be meaningful, love must come from a partner, close friends or family. Happily, as more and more contexts in which to develop trust and meaningful connection with others appear, a much more open sense of being part of a universal family is developing. Good feelings can be generated in yoga groups, meditation classes, support groups, tantric yoga groups and a whole host of other psychological growth and developmental workshops (see The Resources Directory, pages 366–9). As with finding the right therapist, it is always wise to assess group facilitators for their skill, experience, warmth and professionalism, taking note of their reputations, before signing up for such courses.

For many, an important outlet for loving and caring is voluntary work. If, for example, you feel frustrated because all your children have left home and you are without a partner, it can be deeply satisfying to work with those in need of loving care within the community. However, remember to balance the love you give out with the love you give to yourself and receive from others.

A completely different way of generating and expressing love is through the Buddhist meditation called 'meta bhavana' (pronounced 'parvana'). This involves sitting in meditation and focusing attention on the heart area, and generating loving feelings towards someone who is easy for you to love, such as a child, parent or partner. Then, gradually visualize extending this love out to a wider circle of family and friends. Next, extend the loving feeling to your colleagues and associates, then on to the whole community or town you live in, then to your county, country and so on. If you are able, you can even extend this feeling of compassion all around the world until you are holding the world in your heart. As you become more comfortable with this practice, you can consciously include those whom you dislike or are feuding with, and hold them in your heart until you can genuinely extend warmth towards them too. It is also a good opportunity to include yourself in this process as a recipient of your own love. (This meditation is found on the *Heal Yourself* CD in the Health Creation Programme.)

Developing a sense of compassion for yourself and others will make forgiveness and living in harmony easier. When you work on this inner plane, you are changing the template or programme on which you live the whole of your life. Once you start to hold your enemies in compassion, your relationship with them will also change. In addition, holding yourself in this compassionate way is the quickest way to develop a better relationship with yourself, which will make adopting all the health-promoting changes suggested in this book that much easier.

Raising your energy levels

Another key to achieving optimal health is to become aware of what you do with your energy – how you spend it and how you build it. Most people are like a seriously overdrawn bank balance – they spend energy recklessly without giving much thought to how they will replenish it. In fact, a tendency to overspend money often goes hand in hand with a tendency to overspend energy. Overspending, like overeating, can be a compensation for inner emptiness, caused by a failure to nourish ourselves emotionally and spiritually. Others may find themselves depleted of energy because they simply do not have enough support to cope with their commitments to children, elderly relatives, work and home life. This is then exacerbated by failing to ask others for help.

Start looking at where you are expending, or even haemorrhaging, vital energy. Many of us spend vast amounts of energy getting caught up in the affairs of others or simply battling our way through shops or roads when they are crowded. We often try to sustain full social or work lives while remaining involved in extremely draining relationships. On a more subtle level, we may also be living or working in places which drain our energy. Some people and places are like 'black holes' – a phone call from such an 'energy vampire' can leave you severely depleted. Or you may be losing energy simply because you are putting too much energy into everything you do.

Some people are so much more energy-sensitive, so tuned in to the energy of others, that they lose track of how they themselves feel. Such people can become 'symptom carriers' for their family or close friends, as they are often highly empathic types. These 'energy chameleons' tend to soak up the unpleasant, inharmonious energies around them in an attempt to 'clear' and harmonize the atmosphere. They can become especially compromised if they fail to make space for themselves. If this is you, be extra certain that you spend plenty of time on your own, and around healthy energy such as in forests or by waterfalls. Learn to recognize the people, places and activities that drain or build up your energy. People often say their energy levels are raised dramatically by trips to the countryside, working in the garden, beauty, music, meditation, or just spending time alone being still or doing something creative.

Once you start thinking about it, you will begin to recognize exactly what feeds and drains your energy. You may find you are being propped up by the energy of another person, which may be because you are not taking responsibility for building up your own energy levels. It is important to change this pattern and raise your energy levels in healthier ways. Make a list of the things that feed and drain your energy. (For help in doing this, see Principle 8 of the Health Creation Programme, which uses a balance sheet to compare the debit and credit elements of your energy account.) If it is evident that you are pouring your precious energy into many non-productive areas, then start to gradually eliminate the draining activities, and replace them with things that raise your energy. Avoid draining phone calls, difficult relationships, unnecessary shopping trips and other non-productive 'busy' behaviour, and replacing all this 'doing' with just 'being'. Your energy levels will rise dramatically.

Take care over the issue of energy and exercise. Sometimes, exercising hard when you are low in energy can reduce energy levels even further. However, exercising when your energy levels are beginning to rise will strengthen you and raise your energy even more. You need to be aware of the effect exercise is having on your energy levels. This is also relevant to rest – once you are more aware of your underlying energy state, you will stop overriding your body's signals that you are tired and take the appropriate rest.

Cancer is much less likely to develop when the body is in a high-energy state. It has been shown that, with more energy, immune and enzyme activity increase at the cellular level. High energy levels wake up tissue repair and defence mechanisms so that abnormal cells can be identified and eradicated from the body.

Remember that feeling excited, enthusiastic or passionate about life will have the most profound effect on your energy and vitality. When we find love, become fully expressed in our life and work, or open the door to our spirituality, energy levels can leap to the top of the graph.

5. Caring for Your Environment

Once you are healthier and happier, with a strong immune system and good nutritional protection, you will be at much less risk from environmental causes of cancer. Nevertheless, you still need to learn to take good care of yourself, protecting yourself from the sun, chemicals, medicines and electromagnetic radiation and, of course, from unprotected sex.

Make sure that your home and place of work reflect your nature and needs, and that you are not being adversely affected by geopathic stress or electromagnetic radiation.

Become environmentally friendly and consciously develop a 'green' lifestyle both at home and at work. This will protect you and others from the effects of toxic chemicals.

A Clear Intention

At this stage, you may be feeling rather daunted or overwhelmed by the number of things you can do to prevent cancer recurrence. However, to summarize, the most important things to address first are eating healthily, stopping smoking and drinking too much alcohol, taking exercise and reducing stress.

Start by having one clear intention, and finding all the necessary support you need to help you make the necessary changes. As you progress, tackle the next area and carry on, step by step, until you are in a state of positive health.

Remember the emphasis throughout this book – that if you are currently low in energy and emotionally vulnerable, you will need emotional support and an input of energy through healing or energy medicine before you can make any changes at all.

If you lose your way, do not be too hard on yourself.

You may wish to seek the help of a Health Creation Mentor, who has been trained to guide and support you through the process of regaining health. Also, Integrated Medicine doctors like myself and others, who specialize in the holistic treatment of cancer, will be more than delighted to provide the necessary support, encouragement and guidance for anyone who wishes to form a personal cancer-prevention programme.

Most of all, give yourself permission right now to live fully and passionately in the moment, to enjoy yourself thoroughly and bring yourself fully alive through the exciting healing journey that lies ahead of you.

The call to action

When you have recovered your health, may I please encourage you to become active politically and environmentally to stop the cancer epidemic we are witnessing at this time. It is vital that each of us involved with this subject becomes vociferous as regards the adoption of anti-cancer policies in all areas of life. You could join the charity CancerACTIVE set up by Chris Woollams (www.iconmag.co.uk), of which I am a patron, and help us work together to make sure that our children, and the generations to follow, can live safely without cancer.

We must ensure that the next generation eats balanced healthy diets, has access to safe, nutritious food, and lives in a smoke- and pollution-free environment. Let us go together, step by step, determined to clean up our environment, and restore the health of all people as well as this beautiful and extraordinary planet we share.

We cannot wait for governments to act, and those of us who have been affected by cancer must resolve, as a matter of urgency, to make thinking about and eradicating cancer one of our most urgent priorities.

In tackling this issue, we will be confronting many of the problems that wreck lives and cause immeasurable human suffering. Let us all commit ourselves to becoming involved in cancer prevention today – first in your own life, and then as part of a wider cancer-prevention movement so that our grandchildren may one day be able to look back on cancer as a nasty bit of history, as we now do on tuberculosis.

Never has there been a clearer indication that we have drifted off course in relation to nature and our biology as one in three people in 'developed countries' are getting cancer. Never has there been a greater imperative to act now to restore our health and balance in all aspects of life.

So please, become active today to protect yourself and all who will follow you in this glorious adventure of life on earth.

CHAPTER 10

Help for carers

Caring for someone close to you who has a life-threatening illness can be a stressful and harrowing experience, but it can also be profoundly rewarding, deeply enriching your relationship with the person you are caring for.

Your first aim will naturally be to want to be as helpful and effective a carer as possible, and this chapter contains many useful ideas to help you achieve this. But sustaining the carer role has much to do with how well you can identify your reactions and needs, and get the support and help that you, too, will require. Ultimately, your ability to help will depend very much on how well you are able to deal, on the one hand, with your own feelings about illness, doctors, hospitals, disability and loss and, on the other hand, how good you become at looking after yourself.

The aim of this chapter is twofold:

- To help you be the most effective carer you can be
- To help you understand your own reactions and needs, and to help you plan and source the help you will need.

The ideas and thoughts in this chapter come from talking to many carers over the years as well as from being myself a professional and personal carer of people with cancer. However, these ideas may not exactly fit your experience; they serve only as a framework to get you thinking about what you are going through and how to begin identifying your own needs.

We will start with a description of the initial emotional reactions frequently experienced at the beginning of the cancer carer's journey, and the range of reactions people have to these emotions. This may help you to feel less alone with the experience you are going through. We will then describe the strategies and ideas for the most effective caring, and consider the major changes that the diagnosis of cancer in someone close to you is likely to initiate. This includes changes in your relationship to that person, your relationship to yourself, your role, your life plans and lifestyle and, of course, the impact that the diagnosis may have on your health – both physical and mental. We will then consider the longer-term reactions that frequently arise and, finally, move on to the crucial question of how you are going to take care of yourself.

You are invited to identify your emotional state, your reactions and the needs you currently have. We offer you guidance in finding the personal support you need to help you create your own survival strategy for both short-term crisis management and the longer-term ongoing role of carer. We also invite you to consider using this cancer crisis as an opportunity to embark on your own Health Creation Programme with the person you are supporting, and to journal the whole experience. The Resources Directory (pages 386–90) also has a section on psychological support services for carers to make the task of finding help easier.

The Cancer Shock

No one is ever prepared to receive the news of a diagnosis of cancer in a loved one. We always think that cancer happens to other people – and not to us, or our families and friends. But the stark reality is that, in developed countries at this time, one in every three people will be diagnosed with cancer – which means that almost everyone in the Western world will, at some time or another, have to care for someone with cancer.

Many of our reactions as carers at the time of diagnosis will be similar to those of the one with cancer: complete shock, tremendous grief and a feeling of disbelief that this is really happening. The diagnosis can be just as stressful and life-changing for you as it is for them but, sometimes, it can be even worse. The first reason is that the person with the illness will be receiving a lot of attention, support and direct sympathy. You, on the other hand, may receive very little. Second, the person who is ill has a legitimate reason to take time off work or cancel social commitments. Yet, despite your being equally upset, shocked and tired, your workload and pressures may easily be doubled as you take on many of the roles and responsibilities of the person you are looking after in addition to your own. The third reason is much more subtle. Often, for the person who is diagnosed, there may come a genuine sense of calm, like being in the eye of the hurricane while everyone else is swirling about in complete emotional chaos.

So, for the carer, there is a wide mix of emotions, depending on how close you are to the person diagnosed. If it is someone you love dearly, there will be alarm, concern and perhaps anxiety or panic. It can feel as if your world is crashing down around you. Inevitably, there is fear – of the disease, of loss and change, of suffering and disability – and all the feelings that the thought of the person becoming dependent on you may raise.

Anticipatory grief

The level of grief you experience will, of course, depend on the nature of your relationship with the diagnosed person. If it is a stable relationship with a family member or long-term partner, a life-threatening diagnosis may well put you into profound grief.

Frequently, people have said that the diagnosis made them feel as if the person had already died. We are plunged straight into imagining what life would be like without them because of the huge uncertainty that comes with the diagnosis. It may feel too emotionally risky to remain engaged in the relationship, so a typical reaction is to withdraw as a form of protection. This can put a distance between you and the person you are caring for. The result of this reaction is that the person with cancer will sense your withdrawal, and may feel abandoned or isolated at the time they need you the most.

Fear of responsibility

On the other hand, if it is not a fully committed relationship, it is possible to feel trapped or overwhelmed by the sense of responsibility that the diagnosis brings. Again, there can be a strong urge to withdraw, which can be very distressing for someone who is newly diagnosed and in need of support.

Wanting to help

The usual reaction is to want to do anything within your power to comfort, console and support the person you are close to. Our natural desire is to ease the blow, lessen the anxiety, share and soothe the pain, and do whatever we can so that everything will turn out well.

It is important not to feel guilty about the feelings you have – most people in your situation experience the full range of feelings described above at some point or another when helping someone with cancer.

Going through your feelings

Intense emotions, shock and grief can seriously affect our ability to function professionally and socially. It is also likely that, while you are going through your initial reaction to the diagnosis, the person diagnosed needs you the most – both emotionally and practically to help in general and with gathering information.

Take the time you need to go through your feelings. Ask yourself:

- Do I feel that I need to take time off work or cancel other engagements to go through my emotional reactions and come to terms with what is happening?

- Would it be helpful to talk to someone about these feelings and, if so, who?
- Would it be helpful to seek professional help from a:
  - counsellor
  - GP
  - nurse
  - spiritual guide or minister?

Fight or Flight

The classic response to every stressful situation is known as the 'fight-or-flight' response. We are hard-wired to quickly assess, in any dangerous or threatening situation, whether it is best to stay and fight or to run like hell. It is, therefore, entirely natural and completely predictable that this is the response, or dilemma, that most carers have initially, or even at later stages in the cancer journey if things get difficult. Of course, it is not necessarily so clear-cut – as carers, we can experience both urges in the same day or even hour. But how you deal with these feelings, and whether or not you act upon them, will greatly affect the person you are caring for.

The first question, then, is whether you can really 'be there' to help and support the person you love or care for. The second question to ask yourself is what you are realistically able to offer.

Balancing your own needs with the needs of the person you're caring for

As you look at your feelings and assess realistically what you may be able to offer, you may well discover that your needs are in conflict with the needs of the person you are caring for. There may be major issues to confront in terms of how much you are actually able to take on, and how the diagnosis may be affecting the relationship.

In this situation, there are no right or wrongs – the bottom line is that you have to do what is right for you as too much self-sacrifice can damage your health as well as the relationship. However, if possible, try to stick to the basic code of behaviour, which says that you:

- wait until the person with cancer is out of acute crisis before you express your needs or withdraw any level of support that they have counted on from you
- try to make sure that other support is in place before you withdraw any support that is being counted upon
- remember that you can remain in a close relationship even if you are not able for any reason to perform all the 'carer's duties'

- remember that you can remain a very good carer or part of the overall support team even if the primary nature of the relationship between you has changed.

Take time to review your feelings and how you will act on them because your feelings will inevitably change. Be patient with yourself and the one for whom you are caring, and err on the side of waiting before acting rather than taking precipitous action when there are questions in your mind.

Being honest with yourself

A good starting place is becoming clear about how you feel yourself. For some carers, there is no ambivalence whatsoever. They know clearly that they wish, and are able to, stay and help the person they love or care for without reservation. For others, they may be complex, mixed feelings.

Perhaps this is a new relationship, to which you have not yet fully committed. The diagnosis of cancer may well make you question whether you feel able to care for someone you are still unsure about.

Perhaps you have always been the one in the relationship who gets looked after. Seeing the person you normally depend on become ill and unable to provide the care you need may be very threatening to you.

Perhaps you have a lot of fears about illnesses, hospitals or doctors and feel much too squeamish to help. Perhaps you yourself are suffering from illness, anxiety, stress or depression, and this situation feels like the last straw.

Or perhaps you are so overwhelmed with your own emotional reaction that the person who is ill will have to look after you.

Maybe the problem is even more fundamental than this. You may not feel able to bear being around someone who may suffer pain, anxiety, confusion and grief. These feelings may make you feel too uncomfortable to cope. More basic still, you may simply feel unable to be in a partnership with someone who is or may become disabled, disfigured or unable to fulfil your needs – whether emotional, sexual or social.

Take time now to think about what you do feel about taking on the carer role – it may be very positive but, on the other hand, it may not.

Please take care not to rush into sharing these raw feelings with the person who is ill. It may be too much for them to deal with at present. Wait until your initial reactions have settled, and you feel clearer about what you can realistically offer.

How are you going to deal with your feelings?

There are four fundamental ways in which people tend to deal with their feelings:

1. They keep their feelings to themselves without expressing them, bottling them up or even hiding them from themselves
2. They share their feelings with friends or family, which can include the person who has cancer
3. They may talk to a counsellor or spiritual guide about their feelings
4. They may talk about their feelings in a support group.

One thing is certain – the quickest way to change and lighten the way you feel is to start talking. Hiding your feelings from yourself and others or bottling them up is the fastest way towards depression, stress or self-harm. Self-harm can take the form of excessive drinking, smoking, use of drugs or food to cover up feelings or can, in extreme circumstances, manifest as an attempt at suicide. Of course, there is also the risk of stress-induced illness, which can range from infections, high blood pressure and autoimmune disorders to heart attack, stroke or even cancer further down the line.

Talking to friends is natural and can feel good, but may also feel risky if you are having doubts and feel like giving up or 'running away'. You may well find yourself censoring what you say to avoid shocking others or being judged by them, or for fear that what you say may get back to the person you are caring for.

Talking to the person with cancer about how you feel can be immensely liberating, but what you are able to say will depend on the previous level of honesty you had in your relationship with them. It will also depend on how seriously you both take your day-to-day feelings. In reality, the fact that you feel strongly one way one minute does not mean that you will continue to feel that way or need to act upon your feelings. As already mentioned, the quickest way to change the way you feel is by talking about it. In a mature relationship, it may be possible to 'empty out' and say all the worse things you feel, and have it bring you both closer together than ever. However, honesty can also backfire on you both.

It is likely, therefore, that you would benefit most from the opportunity to talk about your feelings first to someone completely neutral, such as a professional counsellor or spiritual advisor, who will keep the contents of your session completely confidential. Talking to a counsellor will give you the opportunity to express and explore your difficult feelings before you talk to others about them. This, in turn, will help you become clearer about whether these are just initial reactions or something that you really do need to share and act upon.

Working out what you are able to offer

The next thing that you need to be clear about is what you feel able to offer the person you are caring for. He or she will have a wide range of needs and, unless you are some kind of super-hero, it is unlikely that you will be able to meet them all. At this early stage, it would be helpful for you to think about the sort of shape you and your life are in, and what will be possible for you to give realistically.

Ask yourself:

- Are you happy to take on the carer role?
- What do you feel able to give emotionally?
- What might limit your ability to give emotionally?
- What do you feel able to do practically to help
  a) with hospitals and doctors?
  b) on the home front?
- How much time are you able to give to the carer role?
- How much energy do you have to give to the carer role? (How much of your energy are your current commitments taking?)
- Are you well enough to give the help needed? What might physically limit your ability to help?
- Are you reliable enough to help when it is needed? What might prevent you from being reliable?
- Are you able to offer financial help? What financial help can you offer
  a) towards therapies, supplements and other medical needs?
  b) towards the living expenses of the person you are caring for?
- Are you able to help with fact-finding and information-processing? Are you good at using the Internet, or reading and understanding medical information?
- Are you good at dealing with doctors and nurses?
- Are you good at arranging fun events and creative distractions? If so, what might you like to arrange?

Will you be able to cope?

Having looked at your feelings and thought realistically about what you are able to offer, it may perhaps be the time to look at the bigger question of whether you think you can cope with the carer role. Do you need to back away from the role? Will you need serious help to be able to cope?

There are a few important things to say at this point.

If you have identified a lot of difficult feelings about the situation and feel that you have relatively little to offer, then being honest and clear about this means that either you or the person with cancer will be able to face this, and arrange for other sources of help and support.

If you feel you have no choice, but have to stay around and 'do the right thing' for the person with cancer, you may have withdrawn emotionally – and the person with cancer will know this. So, if you are unable to give him or her what is needed, then it is better to stop pretending and set about finding other ways to 'bring in the cavalry' to help both of you to cope.

If you can recognize your limitations as well as the areas in which you would be good at providing help, then you may well be able to divide and share the helper/carer role with people who are stronger in your areas of weakness.

If being the carer in a medical situation is difficult or abhorrent to you, you may still be able to maintain your relationship, but delegate the medical aspects of the carer role to others better suited to give the help that is needed. Conversely, if the diagnosis and illness have changed the relationship forever, then you may need to acknowledge this clearly, and go through the individual and combined reactions to this change to ultimately become a good practical carer.

So, to clarify your feelings further, ask yourself:

- Should I divide up the carer role and share it with others?
- Which elements of the role do I need to delegate or share with others and, if so, who could share:
  a) giving emotional support?
  b) providing practical help with:
  - hospital visits?
  - help around the home?
  - financial help?
  - help with finding out information?
  - helping to arrange fun events and creative distractions?

In more extreme situations:
- Do I need to delegate the practical element of the carer role entirely to other people to save my own relationship?

- Do I feel the diagnosis of cancer has changed my relationship irrevocably? And am I still happy to be a good practical carer?
- Do I feel it would be better to withdraw from the situation completely to either protect myself or let the one I care about find better help than I am able to give?
- Do I feel wholeheartedly able to commit myself to both the carer role and deepening the relationship that I already have with the person I am caring for?

It may well have put you through a lot to be so honest with yourself. If so, take the time to feel your feelings and, if you are in difficulty, talk to a counsellor or spiritual advisor about what you are feeling now.

Congratulate yourself for being prepared to be this honest. It will help you AND the person you are caring for.

If you think there is no one else who can help with the caring, think again. There are a vast number of support groups, healers, and community and church volunteers who may be keen to help, not to mention the local health and social services professionals. An important aspect is not to isolate yourself in the role, but to build up a support network from the beginning both for you and the person who is ill.

Mapping the support resources in your area

Find out what support resources there are:
- in your local oncology centre/unit
- from Macmillan and Marie Curie nurses
- from the local hospice (even if the diagnosis is new)
- via your GP surgery
- by contacting Cancer Link within Macmillan Cancer Relief to find out about support groups in your area
- by checking what charities and support groups may be available for the particular type of cancer or resulting disability that the one you are caring for may have (see The Resources Directory, pages 376–82)
- by contacting your local Citizens' Advice Bureau
- by contacting your local Social Services
- Find out about private counsellors in your area via the Centre for Transpersonal Psychology, the Centre for Psychosynthesis or the British Association of Counselling

(see The Resources Directory, pages 362–5). Transpersonal or psychosynthesis counsellors are trained in a holistic approach, looking at issues from the perspective of mind, body and spirit, and using a right-brained imaging approach as well as more conventional counselling techniques.

- Find out about healers in your area for you and the one you are caring for through the National Federation of Spiritual Healers (tel: 0845 123 2767). Get the names of at least three healers so that you have back-up if your chosen healer is away or unavailable.

Setting up a support network

You may have already discovered in assessing what support you can offer that there are gaps in what you can provide as well as times when you may not be available. There may also be times when you are too upset or tired to fulfil the needs of the person you are caring for. For this reason, it is essential to set up a support network as soon as possible after diagnosis. (This is covered in detail in Chapter 2; it may prove helpful to read this again and work through it with the person for whom you are caring.) You may both need to get over any embarrassment you may feel at asking for help, but experience has shown that those who care will want to help and will depend on both of you for a clear idea as to how best they can help. It will encourage you to read Veronica's story on page 34.

Forming a personal support group

Recruit a group of six or eight friends into a support network, and find out from each one what he or she feels able to offer in terms of the framework posed in Chapter 2, page 35. But be sure to discuss this fully with the person you are caring for so that you are sure this is what he or she wants and that you do not duplicate efforts or invite the wrong people to help. You also need to decide whether or not to convene this support group at regular intervals to discuss the care needs for the coming month. Encourage the person for whom you are caring to be bold in terms of what he or she asks for. Remind him or her that people appreciate the opportunity to express their care and love, and may have far more resources at their disposal to share than you realize.

Strategies for Being a Great Carer

Here are some ideas gathered from the experience of others to help you move forward positively as a carer.

First of all, it is helpful to know when you will be needed most. There are many moments of extreme vulnerability for a person who suspects or actually has cancer. Such vulnerable times include:

- waiting for test results
- getting test results
- facing treatment
- going through treatment
- finishing treatment
- getting a re-diagnosis
- being told there is no more treatment available
- being told that they are dying.

Try to be even more available than usual at these times, and bring in extra help if you are not yourself able to cope.

Giving emotional support

If you are the person closest to the person with cancer, the likelihood is that the primary and ongoing need he or she has from you is for emotional support. As discussed in Chapter 9, your ability to give this support depends on three main things:

1. how upset you feel yourself
2. how able you feel to stay close rather than distancing yourself or running away
3. how able you are to cope with the shift the diagnosis has caused in the relationship because the other person has suddenly become so much more dependent on you.

Of course, the bedrock need of the person with cancer will be for love, encouragement and hope, laced with plenty of enthusiasm, energy, bright ideas and a jolly good sense of humour!

When first going through the shock of diagnosis, the most likely support that will be needed is for you to be able to listen and hold or contain them as they go through their feelings. At this most insecure time, they will most likely need you to be there for them, giving them time to talk, cry, rant and express their feelings.

The Power of Listening

Often, we tend not to be good at either expressing our feelings or listening to the feelings of others. We either bottle-up our feelings and engage the proverbial 'stiff upper lip' or, when others start to emote, we quickly shut them down with handkerchiefs, murmurings of 'there there' and quick-fix solutions. Between a person's own inhibitions and our tendency to try to stop them from crying or expressing their feelings, we do a good job of repressing emotions. These emotions then stay in the body and lead to stress reactions. Therefore, the first and most important skill to learn and cultivate as a carer is being able to listen in a supportive, non-judgemental way, without trying to 'fix' or 'shut down' the other person.

When listening with empathy, what we are effectively trying to do is to give our completely undivided attention to others, helping them to know that we are listening by making good eye contact and responding with reassuring sounds such as 'aha, mm, yes, I see what you mean.' It can also help make people feel really well listened to if you are able to reflect back to them the odd word or phrase they have said at natural pauses in their flow, or to paraphrase the content of their thoughts back to them at suitable intervals. This may seem odd or unnatural at first, but it is profoundly helpful. Resist the urge, when in listening mode, to attempt to calm them down, to try to find solutions, or to distract them in any way from what they are saying or feeling. Also, avoid talking about your own feelings at this time, and give them plenty of time and space to unravel or 'empty out'.

You may be able to help them further to express their feelings by asking open questions like 'How did that make you feel at the time?' or 'How are you feeling about it now?' You may also be able to make encouraging comments like 'Don't be embarrassed,' 'It's all right, I'm here for you,' 'Please feel free to let go of your feelings – it's fine with me if you need to cry or get angry,' 'I really want to know how you feel' or 'Please go on and tell me about your feelings – I'm sure it will help you to feel better.'

After a while, the need to talk or express feelings will naturally begin to subside, and a point will come where you can begin to move from listening mode into helping them to define their needs by asking questions like 'What do you feel you need?' or 'What would make you feel better?' or 'What can I do to help?'

Eliciting the Needs of the Person You Are Caring For

Once the emotion has subsided and you have asked these questions, the big challenge is to avoid deciding yourself what you think they need and telling them. The most helpful thing of all for people being cared for is accessing their own sense of knowing or authenticity. This, in turn, will help them feel that they are regaining control of the situation and are being helped to discover their own truth and what is absolutely right for them.

Often on asking these questions, the first answer may be 'I don't know.' Again, resist jumping in with solutions and, instead, try breaking it down into enquiring:

- what they feel they might need emotionally
- what they may need practically (medically, at home and at work)
- what time they may need from you
- what financial help they may need
- what help they need with gathering medical facts and information about sources of help
- what help they need to realize their own self-healing potential and to put their Health Creation Programme into action
- what help they may need to get out of themselves and have fun.

When they are ready, it may be helpful for you to work through this list with them to work out what they need.

Getting Distress Out of the Family, Social or Relationship System

While reading the advice on the power of listening above, you may have felt that there is no way that you can provide this type of listening help. Neither may it be possible for the one you are caring for to be able to provide the support needed to listen to what you are feeling either. It may, therefore, be profoundly helpful for both of you to have your own counsellors to help each of you to express your feelings and fears, rather than trying to perform this role for each other, especially when you are both upset, and your feelings and fears have such a direct effect on each other.

Often, people with cancer say they do not need a counsellor because they have such a good listening ear at home. However, feelings discharged to one family member often have a funny way of ricocheting back to you like a ball in a pin-ball machine. The expression of your loved one's distress can end up leaving you feeling bad. You then end up taking it out on one of the children, who will then pick a fight with another sibling so that the person with cancer may end up having to sort out and re-harmonize the situation.

Emotional giving

If you both have your own counsellors, then much of the distress and difficult feelings you are having can be released from the family, or social or relationship system, into the neutral counselling environment, leaving you and the person you are caring for free to share the more positive aspects of giving and receiving emotionally. Once you are both unburdened of your distress, you can then focus on giving and receiving love, affection and making gestures of care like filling the house with beautiful candles, flowers or scented oils, giving each other a massage or finding your own ways of making uplifting, loving gestures. If the other person is your partner, this can also mean enjoying more loving sexual contact or, alternatively, just holding each other in a loving embrace.

In essence, try to find ways of releasing 'toxic' emotions outside of the family relationship or social environment where possible, leaving yourselves free to enjoy each other and the positive feelings you both share.

Maintaining Good Communication

When talking to people with cancer and their carers about the issues and difficulties they have with each other, the most commonly mentioned problem is that which can develop with communication over time. The most common problem of all is the tendency of both parties to try to protect the other from what they are feeling or thinking. This, of course, is done out of love, and the desire to stay positive and upbeat, but it may result in a 'protective double-bind' that can lead to a major communication problem between the two of you. The key here is to keep your communication as open and clear as possible, taking care to listen for cues, for what is being said 'between the lines' or even to what is not being said. If this feels too scary for you to deal with, it is always possible to seek the help of a third party – a friend who loves or wishes to support you both, or a professional counsellor.

Even if it means changing the habits of a lifetime, get used to clearing the air on a regular basis by having a good two-way dialogue about what is happening to both of you. If you can do this every day, so much the better, but even if this means a regular, weekly fixed time to share your feelings, desires, hopes and fears, this will keep the relationship stronger and communication clearer.

Telling Others

It is important to decide, with the person you are caring for, who you are going to tell what to. You may be able to act as a buffer by taking on the role of message-bearer, thereby protecting the person with the diagnosis from the initial emotional reactions. Questions to ask each other and thoughts about telling others are found in Chapter 2.

Helping with treatment decisions

Helping to Elicit the Values and Choices of the Person You Are Caring For

You could be enormously helpful by finding all the information needed to make a treatment decision, as described in Chapters 3, 4 and 5. But a point will come when the person you are caring for needs to make their own final decision about their treatment and self-help plan. At this point, it is often useful to consult an integrated medicine doctor, who is skilled in providing medical counselling to help people with cancer decide upon the best treatment option, which may often be a combination of the best of all worlds: orthodox, complementary and alternative.

Often, cancer doctors who are either purely orthodox or alternative tend to have a polarized view, steering the individual towards their type of treatment only. This may undermine the potential of the person with cancer to have a truly integrated approach to their cancer care.

The medical profession often assumes that all those with cancer will want or 'should' have conventional medical treatment, and that they will want to know the results of any tests taken. However, this may conflict very much with the values of the person with cancer, who may feel very strongly against having any conventional cancer treatments. This may be for many reasons, such as that the person:

- may believe that the benefits of the medicine are not enough to justify enduring the rigours of treatment, and the loss of quality of life that these may bring
- may feel that these treatments are too harsh and may damage the body's ability to fight cancer or heal properly
- may feel unable to cope with the medical treatment either physically or emotionally
- may not want to know all the facts.

To best help the person you are caring for, try to elicit what his or her values and preferences are in terms of treatment before meeting with the consultant to discuss the subject. This will help to direct you both in your research and in the questions you ask of conventional, complementary, holistic and alternative doctors and practitioners.

Working through the following questions with the person you are caring for, before you see doctors or practitioners, will help greatly.

- How much information do you wish to have about cancer in terms of:
  - the degree of severity of the illness?
  - the course of the illness if left untreated?
  - the likely prognosis (survival time) with medical treatment?
  - the likely prognosis without medical treatment?
- What information do you wish to have about standard medical treatments?
- What information do you wish to have about frontier medical treatments?
- What information do you wish to have about alternative cancer treatments?
- What information do you wish to have about complementary approaches to symptom control?
- What information do you wish to have about holistic mind, body and spirit approaches to healing cancer?
- Do you wish to have the help of an integrated medicine doctor to help you make decisions about your treatment plan?
- What are your feelings about undergoing conventional medicine for the treatment of your cancer?
  - if it may cure you
  - to help prevent recurrence
  - to palliate (improve) symptoms.
- What degree of benefit would you require the medicine/treatment to have before agreeing to it?
  - 75–100 per cent
  - 50–75 per cent
  - 25–50 per cent
  - 10–25 per cent
  - 0–10 per cent.

Once you have understood all the treatment options and have worked out the person's health-care values with him or her, you can ask:

- Do you wish to receive orthodox cancer medicine?
- Do you wish to have alternative medical help instead of conventional medicine?
- Do you wish to find complementary help for symptom control?
- Do you wish to work with integrated mind, body and spirit approaches to promote your health and fight your cancer?

The key issues to remember in information-gathering and treatment-plan decisions are that:

- The person with cancer may very well not retain what is being said in consultations. You can, therefore, provide invaluable support by taking notes during all consultations, and organizing this information for the person to read and evaluate when they are feeling less stressed and upset.
- The person's values and preferences may be very different from your own. You may well feel considerable frustration in wanting to pursue options that seem right and helpful to you, but in which the person with cancer has no interest whatsoever. Be totally clear that it is their choice, and not yours, that matters. Try not to enter into conflict or to push your own views if your way is clearly not the way the other person wishes to cope with the situation. If the disagreement is intense, you may need to see a counsellor to express your frustration or even grief at the choices the person with cancer is making, especially if you believe that the choices being made will limit or shorten his or her lifespan.

Taking Time to Make a Treatment Decision

Usually, when a diagnosis of cancer is made, the medical profession and the processes that are set off seem unstoppable, rather like an express train. This often means that you are both having to deal with the shock of a cancer diagnosis, the choice of difficult treatments and the potential loss of a limb or organ, all while in a state of profound shock. It is a very bad idea to make important decisions or receive medical treatment while in such a state, so it would be helpful for you to support the person you are caring for to take the necessary time to make a decision that seems absolutely right for them. The outcome of the treatment will be far better if the person feels they have taken their own choice in the matter and is therefore completely behind the treatment they are having.

Researching the Options and Gathering Information

Once a diagnosis of cancer has been made, there follows an intense period of information-gathering so that:

- the best choices are made about medical treatment
- the best complementary help is found to prepare for and continue during the treatment
- the best alternative options are found if medical treatment is undesirable
- the best support options are found.

When someone is diagnosed with cancer, the state of shock often makes it nearly impossible for him or her to take in information either orally or in written form. At the best of times, it is calculated that people only retain an eighth of what they are told in medical consultations but, when there is shock as well, a person can come out of a consultation and not remember a single thing that was said.

The important issue here is that people are expected to make decisions about treatment that may affect them for the rest of their lives at precisely a time when they are unable to take in and evaluate the facts, and the short- and long-term implications of the treatment they are being offered, or assess the range of options available to them.

So, a hugely important role of the carer is to help slow the other down and help in gathering and organizing the information that the newly-diagnosed person is being given.

The relevant necessary information, both about the cancer itself and the available treatment options, includes:

- **the degree of severity (staging and grading) of the cancer. You may also wish to enquire about the natural progression of the illness if left untreated**
- **the medical treatment being offered by the cancer consultant. This may include the surgical options from a surgeon, the chemo- and radiotherapy options from an oncologist, and the control of symptoms of advanced cancer from a palliative-care consultant or anaesthetist.**

Make sure you understand the possible benefits, and the short- and long-term side-effects, of the treatment and, if this is an issue, the possible consequences of not having treatment. Be very clear as to whether the percentage benefits claimed refer to survival or to extension of the 'disease-free interval' (the period of time that a person is free of symptoms).

Chapter 3 on cancer medicine covers all the questions you will need to ask, and also offers an idea of what is going on at the frontiers of medicine. Alternatively, you can ask the Cancer Options team (tel: 0845 009 2041) to make a report for you of all the frontier treatments available worldwide for the relevant type of cancer.

Alternative Cancer Treatments

The range of alternative cancer treatments currently available are found in Chapter 4, and contact details for alternative cancer doctors and clinics through the UK and the rest of the world are found in The Resources Directory (pages 331–51).

Complementary Cancer Care

Complementary help for the symptoms of cancer and side-effects of treatment are described in Chapters 7 and 8, and can be obtained through complementary health centres or at supportive care units within some oncology centres and many hospices.

Integrated Medicine

Integrated medicine to get the best of all possible worlds can be obtained from integrated medicine doctors, therapists and centres (see The Resources Directory, pages 331–51).

Health Creation Resources Directory

The database from which The Resources Directory in Part 2 is derived is held on the Health Creation website. This is updated regularly so, if you have problems with any of the contacts listed in Part 2 and want to check for any alterations, log on to www.healthcreation.co.uk and go to the contacts section.

Preparing for and going through treatment

Chapter 7 includes a section on preparing for, going through and convalescing from treatment that involves looking at all the practical, emotional and physical steps which can be taken to be well prepared, to minimize the difficulties of treatment and maximize the benefits. Your role here is to help take the person with cancer through this process, helping to buy the necessary supplements, herbs and homoeopathic remedies needed to minimize side-effects. You can also help by supporting them in the self-help techniques of relaxation and visualization prior to and during treatment as well as finding them the emotional counselling support for facing any fears. Another key form of support is to help them take enough time off from the usual home and work duties to allow them to get enough rest after treatments, and to convalesce properly after the treatment process is over.

Assess and Delegate Roles and Responsibilities

Assess which of the roles and responsibilities of the person you are caring for will need to be delegated to you or other members of the support team, both short and long term. Inevitably, the illness, its treatment or a holistic Health Creation Programme will take up a lot of time, so that the person you are caring for will most likely need to shed some of his or her roles and responsibilities. This need will vary over time as people with cancer often go through rough periods, followed by long periods of being strong and well again. The key here is to have both flexibility and sensitivity to the times when they wish or are able to take up all of their roles and responsibilities again, as well as to the other times when they need to be dependent and cared for.

There are a number of questions to answer at this point:

- Which roles or responsibilities does the person wish to delegate in the short term because of health problems or treatment?
- Who will pick up these roles or responsibilities?
- Which roles or responsibilities does the person wish to drop or delegate permanently as part of a long-term Health Creation Programme?
- What changes or arrangements will you need to make to find the space or time to give practical help to the person you are caring for throughout their treatment period?
- What arrangements will you need to make to give practical help throughout the treatment period?

Embracing Change

One of the most challenging aspects of being close to someone who has a life-threatening illness is the loss of the sense of certainty you had before in many areas of life. As humans, we need to build up a sense of security and permanence to create a sense of stability in our lives.

However, the true nature of reality is that everything is changing at every second. Indeed, the only thing we can be certain of is that everything changes. What a diagnosis of cancer does is bring us closer to the true nature of this reality. The same can be said about our relationship to death and dying. Most of us live with a sense of immortality, never considering how vulnerable we are, and how completely and utterly inevitable death is for all of us at some point in life. Cancer puts us in touch with this reality and gives us a clear perception of the fragility of life. This can throw us into pain and panic but, if the mind can be stilled and the fear transcended, what remains may be an extremely poignant and enhanced sense of appreciation for life, and all the things that we normally take for granted.

So, rather than resisting change and trying to keep everything the same, the best approach is for both you and the person you are caring for to embrace change. Learn to lean into the process of discovery, growth, humour and healing that the challenge of illness can bring, discover the learning that each new situation brings. Allow yourselves to evolve and grow even closer through the process. This may mean, for those of you who are partners, embracing the fact that eventually your relationship may change from being a caring lover to being a loving carer. But, in either relationship, the essential love you share can grow deeper and stronger day by day.

Your changing relationship

We have looked at the difficult or ambivalent feelings that may be caused by the diagnosis of serious illness in someone close to you, but let us look now at the positive changes that can come out of the new situation.

Think about what aspects of the carer role you are enjoying, and how it is enhancing your relationship with the person you are caring for. Perhaps there are things that you have not said before or for a long time, and would now like to express?

What sensitive and caring new ways can you find to express the love or positive feelings you have for this person? What treats or surprises would you like to arrange for the person you are caring for? What are the things that you know the person really loves which will give him or her pleasure or uplift? Can you arrange it so that he or she can enjoy his or her favourite people, music, sacred or beautiful places, films, plays, scents and foods, for example?

Supporting the evolution of the one you are caring for

Think about what you are learning about this person through the process of caring for them. In what ways could you support the development of his or her inner strength and peace of mind? How best can you support his or her full enjoyment? How best can you support the life changes he or she is planning to make?

Embracing changes in sexuality

If it is your partner who is ill, think about what reassurance he or she needs to engage in and enjoy sexuality? How does he or she need to be held or made love to now that illness or its treatment has changed his or her body image?

If your loved one has lost confidence physically or sexually, what help is needed to regain this confidence?

Embracing the challenge of more serious illness

If illness progresses, then many new feelings may be arising in you – most typically, hopelessness, inadequacy or impotence. It is extra-important for you to receive counselling at this time to help yourself to grieve about the changes that are happening, and to relieve yourself of any inappropriate sense of responsibility you may have for making everything better, or saving the other person's life.

If possible, once you have explored your own feelings, try to assess the hopes and fears of your loved one in terms of progression of the disease, any new treatments being faced and what he or she is going through.

Facing death and dying

If you can be brave enough to face together your feelings regarding the possibility of death, you can then find out his or her fears, needs and desires, and be prepared to give what is needed, in the way in which he or she needs it, if and when your loved one becomes compromised at a later date.

The most important thing to remember is that death is not a failure of either one of you. Death is a natural process that we all will have to face. Death is also a sacred process that brings with it a great deal of spiritual energy and grace. The spiritual teachers tell us that as much as we may struggle to understand it, the ultimate timing of each person's death is perfect – it means that they have accomplished what their spirit or higher self came here to do, however strange the timing may seem to us.

Even if your loved one is early on in the illness, facing the worst and exploring these feelings can enable you both to feel much lighter and, paradoxically, far more able to carry on living fully and happily again.

Your changing relationship with yourself

As surely as the process of illness will change your relationship to the person you are caring for, so it will also change your relationship to yourself and life in general. Ask yourself what is changing in your relationship and life. In what ways do you perceive a need for your relationship to yourself to change?

It is also important to take a good look at the effect the role of carer is having on you.

- Are you taking enough time for yourself, or is all your time now being given to the person you are caring for?
- Do you feel you are neglecting yourself and, if so, what do you need to do about this?
- Is the role of carer affecting your health and, if so, in what way?
- Are you showing signs of exhaustion such as continual tiredness or frequent infections?
- Are you showing signs of stress such as irritability, feelings of panic or anxiety, physical symptoms such as a racing heart, palpitations or tummy problems?
- Do you find yourself feeling increasingly angry about the situation?

- Are you showing signs of depression such as feeling emotionally flat and waking up early in the morning?
- Have you lost your joy in living?

If the answer to any of these questions is 'yes,' it is time to take better care of yourself by creating and implementing your own survival strategy. More seriously, if you have ever considered self-harm or suicide, *please* see a GP, counsellor or psychologist immediately.

Embracing your changing roles

It is very likely that the illness has caused the person you are caring for to give up or change some roles for the long term. This may well have had a rebound effect on you. One of the most stressful situations reported by carers is suddenly finding themselves the family breadwinner, the main provider of emotional and practical care, as well as the social secretary, housekeeper, gardener, childminder and all other stations in between. On the one hand it is good to feel useful, but on the other you may be setting yourself up for resentment or collapse if you try to absorb all the roles of the person you are caring for over the long term.

In this situation, it is worth considering the tale of the hare and the tortoise. It may be possible to withstand a super-human load and effort for a brief sprint during acute illness but, if the situation is likely to be ongoing, you may then have to start making some well-considered decisions as to what is practical for you to take on over time and what you both need to let go of.

If the illness becomes more serious, ask yourself the following questions:
- Which of their usual roles does the person I am looking after need to drop at this time?
- What help do they need to come to terms with this?
- What extra roles am I taking on at this time?
- What help do I need to come to terms with this change?
- Are the new roles I am taking on realistic for me on an ongoing basis?
- What could I delegate to others to lighten my load?
- Could I employ help in certain areas to make things easier?
- Is there help available from charities, Social Services or the NHS that could lighten my load?
- Are there any roles, either professionally or socially, that I should consider shedding altogether and, if so, whom do I need to tell?

- Is financial stress affecting me as a result of a loss of income either because of being the carer or because the person being cared for no longer has an income?
- Do I need help with looking at the work and financial issues? If so, see The Resources Directory (pages 392–5) for how to contact the carer's agency 2 Higher Ground.

Embracing Positive Changes

It is possible that the experience of caring for someone with a serious illness has begun to change your priorities and values for the better.

Ask yourself:

- What possibilities has the illness created for radical changes in my lifestyle?
- What change has the illness precipitated in my life plans?
- What possibilities has the illness created for me to embark upon something new and exciting with the person who is ill which I might not have previously allowed myself to do, or kept continually on the 'back burner'?

Creating Your Survival Strategy

In working through this chapter, you have been giving a lot of thought about the changes – both positive and negative – that the role of carer has brought upon you.

Just as you have helped to elicit and cater for the needs of the person you are caring for, it is now time to do the same for yourself. You need to form a plan so that you will be able to continue to be an effective carer, and to protect yourself against the long-term effects of stress and emotional upset.

Carers do have an understandable tendency to put the other first on all occasions, pouring all available time and resources into the well-being of the person being cared for. However, this will not work in the long run as being the carer is widely acknowledged to be one of the most difficult and testing roles we can possibly have, especially when it goes on for a long time. It is vital that you do not put your own life on hold or stop pursuing your own activities. More than ever, you need to work on finding your own sources of fun, enjoyment, uplift, sanctuary, rest, energy and nourishment. You may also need a regular 'debrief', when you can talk through what you have been doing with a counsellor, nurse or doctor. This may serve solely for you to let off steam, but you may also need to do this with one of the medical team to check that what you have been doing to help with the nursing has been going as well as it can.

You may also like to consider embarking upon the Health Creation Programme I have created. It is not only for people with cancer, but for anyone who would like to take the opportunity produced by crisis, or simply through a desire to prevent illness, to work towards optimal health and well-being. It would be ideal if you feel inspired to do the Programme alongside the person you are caring for to protect yourself and to grow through the opportunity created by this illness. This way, you will understand the health creation process he or she is going through and will be able to support each other better in making the positive changes necessary in your lifestyles and health.

The Health Creation Programme lasts for six months (in the first instance), during which time, you are fully supported by a Health Creation Mentor who will help you with the regular monthly assessments of your state and needs. The Health Creation Programme can be obtained via the Health Creation helpline (tel: 0845 009 3366) or website (www.healthcreation.co.uk). The Mentors provide telephone coaching to encourage support, and guide you every step of the way. They will empower you to follow through the changes you have decided to make. Taking this step is a great way to protect yourself and potentially to transform your situation into a genuine opportunity for happiness and self-development.

Meanwhile, ask yourself:

- What improvements do I need to make in my nutrition to protect my health?
- What vitamin and mineral supplementation do I need take to withstand the stress of the carer role?
  - Minimum recommended daily supplements to combat stress include:
  - Vitamin C (500 mg/day)
  - Vitamin B complex (50 mg /day)
  - Multivitamin (one daily)
- What exercise do I plan to do daily?
- What exercise do I plan to do weekly?
- In what ways will I detoxify myself to protect my health?
  - Will I give up smoking and, if so, what help will I need?
  - Will I cut down drinking alcohol and, if so, what help will I need?
  - Will I cut down my intake of excess food, particularly animal foods, sugar, sweets, crisps and fried foods?
- In what ways could I cut down my stress levels?

- What self-help techniques could I learn to help reduce stress?
  - ◆ Relaxation
  - ◆ Meditation
  - ◆ Tai chi
- Do I need complementary therapies to energize or relax me? Would I like to have any of the following therapies?
  - ◆ Acupuncture
  - ◆ Shiatsu
  - ◆ Reflexology
  - ◆ Massage
  - ◆ Aromatherapy
  - ◆ Reiki
  - ◆ Spiritual healing
- Do I need a counsellor to:
  - ◆ offload my emotions?
  - ◆ help me to re-prioritize my life?
  - ◆ counsel me for specific problems such as relationship problems, financial problems or legal problems?
- If so, which counsellor will I contact?
- Do I need spiritual help to explore the big questions of living and dying?

Taking 'time out'

Another key survival strategy is to take regular time out from your role of carer – by getting out or even going away for a few days. If the person you are caring for is very ill, it may well be possible for him or her to go into a hospice for a few days for respite care. Alternatively, another member of your support group or family may be able to stay for a while to let you have a complete break. But try to time-table special time for yourself into your diary. Make appointments with yourself to meditate, go for walks, visit friends or go out. Treat these dates as seriously as you would a date with a friend or colleague.

Support and guidance

You will have read this chapter at a particular point in your experience of being a carer for someone with cancer. Your reactions, needs and answers to many of the questions will change over time, depending on the course and nature of the illness of the person you are caring for.

The role of carer is a noble one. It is an act of enormous love and service, which goes largely unrecognized by the medical profession and society as a whole. It is very important that you keep looking regularly at the question of how you are doing and what you need. Make sure that you make a formal reassessment of your state at least once a month. You may well be able to do this by re-reading this chapter and making new notes in a notebook. However, please know that I feel for you keenly in this role. I urge you to get Mentor or counselling support to receive the support and guidance you need when the going gets tough, or even to have a listening ear to help revive your spirit and your ability to keep giving as a carer.

Meanwhile, I wish you all power in your carer role, and that it may be a rich, rewarding and deeply creative time for you in which you benefit as much as the one for whom you are caring from the holistic approach to health and the energizing self-help programme you will create together.

It is helpful to make a journal of your experience to keep note of the changes that take place over time. Record your feelings and the precious insights you will have during the intense process of being a carer. Though difficult, these are very special times when you will learn a huge amount about yourself, your loved one and your relationship to life.

To ease your path a little, always remember throughout this time that the other person's illness and life is not your responsibility. You may be a companion on the journey, but his or destiny belongs only to him or her.

The essence, then, of both life and love is learning to be able first to 'take hold tightly and then let go lightly' – being able, on the one hand, to hold on passionately and fight for the life we adore and, on the other hand, when the time comes, being able to let go, allowing the spirit to fly free on the glorious journey homeward.

This is the greatest challenge of all, but one that is helped the most by developing a strong meditation practice and a deep spiritual faith. The best advice that I can give you is to learn to go inward and practice detaching yourself from all around you through regular meditation. This will nourish your spirit, enabling you to develop inner strength and a safe, still, insightful place to go when life is difficult or disturbing, or if we are facing loss.

Finally, may I wish you all power and send love to you, as you embrace the challenges and pleasures of being a brilliant carer and companion, on this wonderful path of compassion and service. It is a truly great role you are playing, and I commend you highly for your kindness, bravery and care.

And please remember that telephone support, guidance and coaching are available for carers too from my Health Creation mentors (tel: 0845 009 3366).

PART TWO

The cancer resources
directory

Introduction

This Directory will provide the reader with a comprehensive set of resources, with information and guidance in the areas of:

1. Frontier orthodox cancer medicine (page 257)
2. Pioneer hospitals offering integrated cancer care (page 264)
3. Alternative cancer medicines (page 266)
4. Alternative cancer doctors (page 331)
5. Alternative cancer clinics (international) (page 336)
6. Integrated medicine doctors and services (page 351)
7. Complementary medicine organizations for finding therapists (page 354)
8. Counselling organizations (page 362)
9. Self-help organizations for finding classes or teachers (page 365)
10. Support services (page 369)
11. Retreats, spiritual development and holistic holidays (page 390)
12. Cancer care and practical help: nursing, social, financial, insurance (page 392)
13. Cancer prevention (page 396)
14. Product suppliers and diagnostic centres (page 414)

This Directory contains primarily UK-based organizations, but worldwide resources are included in the frontier orthodox and alternative cancer sections (1, 3, 4 and 5). It is produced and maintained by Dr Daniel's organization, Health Creation. To ensure the ongoing high quality of the information, please give us your feedback on these resources and any others we may have missed so that we can continue to develop and upgrade it. It is particularly important that you let us know if any entries are wrong, or if you have had especially good or bad experiences with any of the resources listed.

Please send any comments, updates, ideas and corrections to admin@healthcreation.co.uk (using as your subject line: Cancer Resources Directory Suggestions).

The continuously updated version of the Directory is found at www.healthcreation.co.uk in the section 'Contacts and Links'. Please check there if you are having difficulty finding a listed resource, or call our helpline (tel: 0845 009 3366).

Many thanks for your help.

1. Frontier Orthodox Cancer Medicine

1.1 Websites for Medical Information about Cancer and its Treatment – Recommended by Professor Karol Sikora

www.cancerbacup.org	The best UK information site on all aspects of cancer, with great links to other sites
www.cancer.gov	The website of the US National Cancer Institute in Washington, it is also the largest cancer website in the world
www.oncolink.org	The excellent site of the University of Pennsylvania Cancer Center, with good links to other US sites
www.oncology.com	The website of the American Society of Clinical Oncology, treatment protocols and drugs are well explained
www.cancerhelp.org.uk	Smaller, very manageable site from the University of Birmingham
www.cancerresearchuk.org.uk	Britain's Cancer Research Charities site
www.macmillan.org.uk	Site of the Macmillan Fund, with useful contacts especially for palliative care
www.cancereurope.com	European School of Oncology site with good links to other cancer sites in the EU

1.2 General Cancer Information (including Research Bodies)

American National Cancer Institute site	Probably more information provided here than at any other site on types of cancer, treatments, research, trials; search engine for cancer literature and research. Information on treatments is clear and informative, with outcomes of treatment trials; information on	www.nci.nih.gov

	complementary medicine also included	
American Society of Clinical Oncology	ASCO patient-information website; treatment protocols and drugs explained	www.oncology.com; www.asco.org; www.peoplelivingwithcancer.org
BBC Online	Very good site with lots of information on cancer, treatment, helplines, organizations, support, prevention	www.bbc.co.uk/health/cancer
Breakthrough Breast Cancer	Fighting breast cancer through research and awareness	www.breakthrough.org.uk
Canceradvice.co.uk	Managed by Dr Nick Plowman, a leading oncologist in London; site offers support groups, cancer links, opinions and advice, current issues, leaflets, etc.	www.canceradvice.co.uk
CancerBacup	One of the most extensive sites for cancer information and support for patients, carers and health professionals; eight freephone lines staffed by cancer nurses; booklets, factsheets, videos, audiotapes, CD-ROMs, and newsletter available; also a section on complementary therapies	Helpline 0808 800 1234 Mon–Fri, 9 a.m. – 7 p.m. www.cancerbacup.org.uk

Cancereducation.com	Good information and definitions to help you understand cancer from the medical perspective	www.cancereducation.com
Cancerhelp.org.uk	Cancer research clinical trials as well as information on specific cancers, prevention and health checks, living with cancer and healthy eating	www.cancerhelp.org.uk
Cancerindex.org	US guide to Internet resources for cancer, has over 100 pages of links to cancer-related information by disease, country, treatments and other topics; also has a useful page about the quality of cancer information on the Internet	www.cancerindex.org
Cancer Options	Personalized information about orthodox and alternative cancer treatments	Tel: 0845 009 2041 www.canceroptions.co.uk
Cancer Research UK	UK's leading cancer-research organization information service	Tel: 020 7269 3142; www.cancerresearchuk.org
Cancersource.com	US site run by Cancer Treatment Centers of America; information on complementary and integrative therapies	www.cancersource.com

Cancer-UK	An independent non-profit site aiming to provide an overview and a gateway to UK-based cancer resources: information, e-mail discussion groups	www.cancerindex.org/
European School of Oncology	Good links to other cancer sites in the EU	www.cancereurope.com
Integrated Cancer Care	Information, support and follow-up integrating the care of those patients using non-conventional or alternative anti-cancer therapies back into the conventional NHS system; telephone helpline, and an e-mail advice and support service are available for those unable to get to the centre; video-conferencing between practitioners and patients also available	Tel: 01483 406 618 www.integratedcancercare.org
Jonathan Chamberlain's website	A survival guide for fighting cancer; has lots of information on holistic approaches and offers sensible advice; also, some interesting reflections on certain complementary therapies and many useful links	www.fightingcancer.com

Leukaemia Research Fund	Information on research currently underway for leukaemia	www.lrf.org.uk
Medicinenet.com	General medical site including a very good search feature for medical terms; a medical dictionary is available as well as search engines for diseases, tests and procedures, and medications	www.medicinenet.com
Medical Research Council	News, research, clinical trials, though not only about cancer	www.mrc.ac.uk
Memorial Sloane-Kettering Cancer Center	Website of the leading cancer-treatment centre in the US	Tel: 001 212 639 2000 www.mskcc.com
National Translational Cancer Research Network (NHS)	Fast-tracking research for patients	www.ntrac.org.uk
Orthomolecular Oncology	Website of a UK-based charity about treating disease with natural substances; not an easy site to navigate, but contains a wealth of useful information on holistic and complementary approaches to cancer	www.canceraction.org.
Patient.co.uk	An extensive general medical site with information on specific diseases, a great deal of information about the	www.patient.co.uk

	workings of the NHS, and many useful features such as a list of the leading experts and consultants for various conditions, and comparative hospital performances; edited by two GPs	
Royal Marsden Hospital	This currently offers 35 titles in the Patient Information series, providing information on different types of cancer, treatments, living with the side-effects and adjusting to changes caused by cancer	www.royalmarsden.org
Steve Dunn's Cancer Guide	A comprehensive guide on how to become your own cancer researcher, and how to work your way through and evaluate the massive amount of information available on cancer	www.cancerguide.org
TENOVUS	UK Cancer Information Centre	Helpline: 0808 808 1010 9 a.m.–4.30 p.m. www.tenovus.com
University of Birmingham, UK	A small but very manageable site	www.cancerhelp.org.uk
University of Pennsylvania Oncolink	Includes disease-orientated and medical speciality-orientated menus; clinical trials; global resources for	www.oncolink.org

	cancer information; symptom management and financial issues; little is offered in the way of education, but has a great deal of information on research and clinical trials; good links to other US sites	
US National Cancer Institute	Largest cancer website in the world, based in Washington, DC	www.cancer.gov
What About Me …	Organization offering parallel cancer care: outlines options when cancer patients need to make decisions; offers the expertise of conventional doctors and surgeons coupled with holistic practitioners; can enhance the effectiveness of both systems, and improve the individual's quality of life and outlook; names team members available for advice	www.bartistic.co.uk/wam
What Is Cancer?	An interesting, unusual approach to cancer using the wisdom of the body to control processes like immunity; for those interested in the mind-body connection and who want to use it to improve health and survival	www.what-is-cancer.com

2. Pioneering Hospitals Offering Integrated Cancer Care

2.1 The Hammersmith Hospital, London

Professor Karol Sikora was the first oncologist to decide that integrated cancer medicine was the way of the future. Impressed by the improved quality of life and health of the people attending the Bristol Cancer Help Centre, and the large number of people with cancer choosing to have complementary therapies, he decided to team up with Bristol in the mid-1980s to create a bespoke supportive-care unit within the Hammersmith Hospital, offering support and gentle therapeutic care to help people through their cancer treatments. In the late 1990s, this centre won the Prince of Wales' Foundation for Integrated Health's Award for Good Practice in Integrated Healthcare as the best example of integrated medicine within the UK.

2.2 The Mount Vernon Hospital and The Lynda Jackson Macmillan Centre, Middlesex

In the 1990s, the Mount Vernon Hospital followed suit and built a unit in a purpose-built setting funded by Cancer Relief Macmillan. The passion to build this unit and the service within it initially came from radiographer Judy Young, supported by forward-looking oncologist Dr Jane Maher. Now, this Centre offers state-of-the-art information, support and complementary therapies for those using the hospital and the surrounding community.

The Drop-in Centre is the hub of the Lynda Jackson Macmillan Centre, and aims to provide information and support to people affected by cancer at any stage of the illness. It provides the opportunity for people to discuss issues with a member of staff face-to-face in a safe and confidential setting. All are welcome. Anyone can drop in at the Centre without referral to discuss anything associated with cancer or its treatments, or to just 'talk things through' on any other concerns they may have related to the illness. The staff always do their best to deal with any questions or concerns, or suggest someone who can.

The Centre is usually open Monday to Friday from 9.30 a.m. – 1 p.m. and 2 – 4.30 p.m., and closed on weekends and Bank Holidays. The helpline (tel: 01923 844 014) is available during opening hours, and an answerphone is used out of hours; messages left are replied to during the next working day.

2.3 Wirral Holistic Care Services, near Liverpool

In the Wirral, an impressive integrated medicine service has been set up by Nurse Dorothy Crowther, who runs one of the deeper-reaching programmes of self-help to be found within the NHS setting. Nurse Crowther has dedicated the Wirral Holistic Care Services to helping people cope with cancer because she recognized that cancer patients want more than the standard NHS fare.

Initial evaluations suggest that the service is going a long way towards meeting the extra needs of people with cancer. Available therapies include aromatherapy, kinesiology, reflexology and meditation. The help is based on a model of care that endorses putting the patient and patient choice first. The helpline (tel: 0151 604 7316) is available Monday to Friday, from 10 a.m. – 4 p.m.

2.4 Rossendale Integrated Medicine Service, Lake District

This superb integrated medicine service at Rossendale in the Lake District in the North of England is one of the few (Complementary and Alternative Medicine) units in the country to have successfully won two lottery grants to set up an integrated medicine service that people with cancer so desperately need. Having survived the test of time, this unit has gone from strength to strength, and offers support and complementary therapies within the local community to those who have a wide range of medical conditions.

2.5 The Royal Surrey Hospital, The Fountain Centre

The Fountain Centre exists solely due to the passion of cancer carer Monica Rowland, whose husband Peter benefited greatly from holistic care, and the small team of local complementary therapists, who fought so hard to win a corner of the St Luke's Cancer Centre in the Royal Surrey Hospital to build a specialized supportive care unit. They then went on to raise the funds to furnish and staff the centre to provide a haven for people with cancer within a hospital setting.

The Centre's primary objective is to offer support to patients and their families at the time of diagnosis and initial treatment, or on relapse. It fosters a holistic approach, providing support, information and therapy to restore health in mind and spirit as well as body.

2.6 The Harley Street Oncology Centre, London

The Harley Street Oncology Centre in London has been the first private hospital to provide a supportive care package to all of its clients routinely alongside radio- or chemotherapy. No one is forced to take up this offer, of course, but each patient who receives treatment is entitled to six counselling sessions and several sessions of relaxing massage, aromatherapy or reflexology.

2.7 The Cromwell Hospital, London

The Cromwell Hospital is the first hospital in the UK to offer the Cancer Lifeline Kit and Mentor Service created by Dr Rosy Daniel routinely to patients in their care. They are currently piloting this as an effective way of providing a complete integrated care package to all patients.

In Summary ...

It is encouraging to see the lead that has been taken by these units, and I am sure that it will not be long until virtually all cancer-treatment centres and hospices will have some form of integrated supportive care routinely available.

3. Alternative Cancer Medicines

3.1 Websites Offering Information on Alternative Cancer Treatments

www.allabouthealth.com
www.alternativemedicine.com
www.anticancerherb.com (Indian carctol site)
www.cancerdecisions.com
www.cancerguide.org
www.cancernet.nci.nih.gov
www.cancure.org
www.carctolhome.com

www.healthy.net
www.howtopreventcancer.com
www.np.edu.sg
www.sph.uth.tmc.edu

3.2 Scientific Information on Alternative Cancer Medicine

Key organizations holding reliable scientific information on alternative cancer medicine are:

- **The Research Council for Complementary Medicine, UK**
- **Department of Alternative Cancer Medicine, University of Houston, Texas**

National Center for Complementary and Alternative Medicines	Comprehensive and up-to-date US site that offers complementary and alternative treatment information, alerts, research, clinical trials, news and more	www.nccam.nih.gov
Orthomolecular Oncology	A UK-based charity all about treating disease with natural substances; not an easy site to navigate, but containing a wealth of useful information on holistic and complementary approaches to cancer	www.canceraction.org
Quality Counts	A great deal of information on various cancers, conventional medical treatments and a wide variety of alternative remedies, all from published articles and news items and, therefore, need to be acted on with caution	www.qualitycounts.com

The Annie Appleseed Project	The Annie Appleseed Project informs, educates, advocates and raises awareness for people with cancer, and family or friends interested in or using CAM; many contributors of the reports are patients; has sections on breast-cancer, ovarian and gynaecological cancer issues	www.annieappleseedproject.org
Alkalyze For Health	Personal and environmental information on cancer cases and holistic approaches to treatment	www.alkalyzeforhealth.net
CanCure	A non-profit organization dedicated to researching and providing information on alternative cancer treatments and therapies; US site with information on alternative cancer therapies and clinics, including some in UK	www.cancure.org

3.3 Alternative Cancer Medicines

Included here are expanded details of the entries mentioned in Chapter 5 on the latest developments in alternative cancer medicine in the fields of:

1. Anti-cancer Nutrients
2. Herbal Medicine
3. Hormone Therapy
4. Metabolic Therapy

5. Immunotherapy
6. Neuroendocrine Therapy
7. Physical Therapies
8. Nutritional Therapies
9. Mind–body Medicine

The rationale for each of these forms of alternative cancer medicine is covered in Part 1, Chapter 5. While the number of options available may make it difficult to choose what is right for you, it will give you a good basis for discussion with any alternative cancer doctors or clinics you may choose to visit.

You will find alternative cancer doctors listed in Section 4, and alternative cancer clinics in Section 5, below.

3.3.1 Anti-cancer Nutrients

See Chapter 5, page 103. These may also be used alongside conventional treatments to increase potency.

3.3.1a Antioxidant vitamins and minerals

Use and Dosage after Medical Treatment

Antioxidant vitamins and minerals are used alongside orthodox medical treatments as well as, in some cases, as a form of alternative medicine. They are used to help the body reduce free-radical damage and strengthen the immune system. Dosage varies according to the patient's condition and weight, but a baseline level of antioxidants for the first year post-diagnosis of cancer is:

Vitamin C
Food state   500 mg three times per day (non-acid form of vitamin C that is more potent than ascorbic acid; equivalent to 1 g of ascorbic acid three times daily)

OR
Calcium ascorbate   1 g three times per day

Beta-carotene
Food State   13.5 mg/day (NOT TO BE TAKEN BY SMOKERS)

OR

Carrot juice   One-and-a-half pints daily

Please note: Reduce your dose of beta-carotene appropriately depending on the amount of juice taken each day.

Vitamin E

Food state   400 iu/day (800 iu/day for men with prostate cancer)

Please note: Stop taking vitamin E two weeks prior to surgery and resume a week afterwards as it is slightly anticoagulant.

Vitamin B Complex

Food state   50 mg/day

Selenium

200 mcg/day

Zinc

As elemental zinc   15 mg/day
As zinc orotate   100 mg/day
As zinc citrate   50 mg/day

Please note: Zinc dosages should be reduced to a third of these levels three months after the end of treatment to prevent excess accumulation of zinc in the tissues. Taken during treatment, zinc helps to promote tissue-healing. Increase to the higher level if treatment is resumed, or during periods of infection or tissue inflammation.

See Part 1, Chapter 7 for Professor Prasad's recommendations for use and dosage during medical treatment. His latest scientific findings have shown that taking higher levels of antioxidants during chemotherapy can potentiate beneficial effects.

How to Use

Antioxidant formulations are usually taken orally in tablet form and may be self-administered. It is desirable to take antioxidants alongside conventional treatments, as they enhance the latter's effectiveness.

Antioxidant vitamins and minerals are also given intravenously in mega-doses in alternative cancer clinics, rather like a form of natural chemotherapy in an effort to destroy tumours. High-dose vitamin C and vitamin B_{17}, or laetrile, which contains cyanide, are used in this way.

Drug Interaction and Special Precautions

- Most controversial has been the potential conflict between antioxidants and chemotherapy or radiotherapy and the fear that the former may make the latter less potent. However, recent research from Professor Prasad in the US has shown the converse to be true. In fact, he says that cancer patients should take higher doses that usual during these treatments as the cancer cells then become more, not less, sensitized to treatment (see Part 1, Chapter 7).
- Smokers should not take beta-carotene as supplements as this has been shown to be associated with an increased risk of lung cancer (while, paradoxically, those with high levels of beta-carotene in the blood from their diet are shown to be protected).
- Doses of selenium should not be exceeded as levels greater than 400 mcg/day may become toxic.
- High-dose vitamin A should not be taken as this is associated with an increased risk of osteoporosis in women.
- Vitamin E should be stopped two weeks before surgical treatment and resumed one week afterwards, as it is slightly anti-coagulant.

Mechanism of Action

A free radical is an unstable molecule with an unpaired electron that steals an electron from another molecule, thereby producing harmful effects. Free radicals are produced in the body by external harmful influences such as radiation, fried or barbecued foods and environmental pollution, and by internal processes as a by-product of metabolism. Free radicals are also produced during radio- and chemotherapy. To protect the body against these free radicals, it is important that the body has sufficient quantities of antioxidants.

An antioxidant is a natural biochemical substance that protects living cells against damage from free radicals. If unblocked or left uncontrolled, oxidation can lead to cellular ageing, degeneration, allergies, arthritis, heart disease, cancer and other illnesses. Antioxidants in the body react readily with free radicals and neutralize them before they can cause damage. Antioxidant nutrients include vitamins A, C and E; beta-carotene; selenium; zinc; co-enzyme Q10, Pycnogenol (grapeseed extract); L-glutathione; superoxide dismutase and bioflavonoids. When antioxidants are taken in combination, the effect is even stronger than when used individually.

The amount of antioxidants in the system can make a critical difference between a normal-functioning immune system and the initiation of a potential cancer process. When free-radical production exceeds the ability of the immune system to neutralize these harmful agents, then progressive cellular damage may begin. When this damage becomes chronic, the next step is chronic or serious degenerative disease, including cancer.

Free radicals are particularly dangerous as they have a tendency to attack and destroy the fragile membranes surrounding cells, thus making the body more vulnerable to various cancer initiators and promoters. In addition, free radicals themselves may interact with cellular DNA, causing mutations that can lead to cancer formation.[1]

Although antioxidants can be found naturally in foods, supplementing with antioxidants may be necessary to offset intense free-radical activity, especially if the diet is or has been nutritionally inadequate for some time. Although many antioxidants, such as vitamin C, can neutralize free radicals, on doing so, the antioxidant become inert and loses its ability to neutralize further free radicals. Newer, 'cascading' antioxidants retain their neutralizing ability and are therefore more potent than the antioxidant vitamins.

Level of Evidence

The importance of antioxidants to the optimal functioning of bodily systems such as the immune system has been studied through a variety of scientific and laboratory studies. There are over 10,000 peer-reviewed reports of the role of antioxidants in cancer prevention and treatment, ranging from epidemiological and pure science to prospective, randomized, controlled trials.

In China, a prospective trial in which 50,000 people were given selenium, vitamin E, beta-carotene and zinc at the above dosages showed a 13.5 per cent decrease in death due to cancer of all types after five years.

Source and Price

High-quality 'food-state' vitamins and minerals that are highly bioavailable to the body are made by Nature's Own.

The cost of a month's supply at the levels above is £58.16, or £1.94/day.

References

- The Nutrition and Cancer Database (Bristol Cancer Help Centre), containing over 7,000 scientific references to the role of antioxidants in preventing and treating cancer
- Goodman, S. and Daniel, R., *Cancer and Nutrition: The Positive Scientific Evidence* (Bristol Cancer Help Centre, 1994)
- Kindles, A. R., Radman, M., 'Tumour promoter induces sister chromatic exchanges', *Proceedings of the National Academy of Sciences* 75 (1978): 6149–53

- Holford, P. *Say No to Cancer* (Piatkus Books, 1999)
- Olivier, S., *The Breast Cancer Prevention and Recovery Diet* (Penguin Books, 2000)
- Plant, J. A. *Your Life in Your Hands* (Virgin Publishing, 2001)

3.3.1b Herbal antioxidant preparations

Neways International have developed a product called Cascading Revenol that contains 23 antioxidants in a regenerative formulation that has a sustained-release delivery system to enhance the body's ability to neutralize damaging free radicals.

Cascading Revenol's formulation regenerates 'spent' antioxidant molecules, enabling them to neutralize multiple free radicals. So, instead of only one free radical being destroyed per antioxidant molecule, each molecule is able to continuously neutralise free radicals.

The formulation combines water-soluble white pine bark (Pycnogenol) and oil-soluble grapeseed extract together with turmeric extract (curcuminoids). Key minerals and trace elements such as zinc, copper and selenium are complexed with amino acids to promote absorption through the intestinal tract. Vitamin C is supplied in an esterfied form that enhances its power and residual retention in the body for up to three days.

Other ingredients in the formulation include decaffeinated green-tea extract, inositol, co-enzyme Q10, vitamin E, carotenoid complex, ellagic acid, astaxanthin, resveratrol, glutathione, *Rosmarinus officinalis* extract, citrus bioflavonoid complex, quercetin, taurine, N-acetylcysteine and potassium sulphate. This combination of potent antioxidants makes Cascading Revenol one of the most effective antioxidant products currently available.

Cascading Revenol is taken orally as capsules and may be self-administered. It costs £65.80 for a month's supply. Intravenous antioxidant therapy is available from the alternative doctors and clinics listed on pages 331–351). The cost is available upon enquiry.

Fruit and vegetable formulations

Juice Plus have created an excellent source of natural antioxidants in their highly concentrated vegetable and fruit capsules (see Part 1, Chapter 5, page 104).

3.3.1c Multi-mineral formulations

Use and Dosage

Multi-minerals are used to help provide the body with the appropriate level of minerals for optimal functioning, and strengthen the immune and tissue systems. Dosage varies according to the patient's condition and the preparation used.

How to Use
Multi-minerals are usually taken orally and may be self-administered. (In alternative cancer clinics, they may be given by physicians as part of an intravenous metabolic therapy with high-dose antioxidant vitamins.)

Drug Interaction and Special Precautions
It is important not to take over the recommended level of selenium (200–400 mg/day) as high doses can be toxic. Zinc at high doses accumulates in the body and it is recommended to drop to a maintenance dose as described after three months. To assess accurately your need for minerals and when you have taken enough, get blood analyses done at Biolab or the Diagnostic Clinic (see Resources Directory).

Mechanism of Action
Selenium has key effects on DNA metabolism, cell-membrane integrity, and optimal functioning of both the liver and pancreas. Thus, it can interfere with both the initiation and promotion of cancer development. Glutathione peroxidase protects tissues against free-radical damage, and its anti-cancer effects are greatly dependent on the availability of selenium.[1]

Like selenium, zinc supports many aspects of the immune system, and its deficiency can potentially make the body more vulnerable to certain cancers. Zinc is necessary for the free-radical-quenching activity of superoxidase dismutase (SOD), a powerful antioxidant that breaks down free-radical superoxide to form hydrogen peroxide. A deficiency of zinc can lead to depressed activity of NK (natural-killer) and other white blood cells.[2]

Copper is also essential for the proper functioning of a wide range of immune cells, including antibody-forming cells, T-helper cells and macrophages, all of which help to defend the body against cancer.[3] It is a cofactor for many important enzymes – called cuproenzymes – which speed up the body's energy-yielding (oxidation) reactions. It is also involved in healing processes, excretion of certain toxins (purines), maintaining connective-tissue integrity and formation of red blood cells. A deficiency of this element can lead to a lowered resistance to infection.

Chromium has been observed to be useful in the treatment of pancreatic cancer.

Level of Evidence
The importance of minerals to the optimal functioning of bodily systems such as the immune system has been studied in a vast number of scientific and laboratory studies.

Source and Price

Neways International has formulated a liquid multi-vitamin/mineral product called Maximol Solution, which contains 67 essential and trace minerals, 17 essential vitamins, 21 amino acids and three enzymes. To provide greater absorption of all of these ingredients into the circulatory system, Maximol has been formulated with organic fulvic acid, identified as playing a key role in the absorption of minerals and nutrients in plants and animals. Providing the minerals in a microcolloidal state makes them much easier to absorb and utilize in the body.

Maximol costs £24.43 for a one-month supply. It should be taken at the level of the recommended daily dose. Most vitamin companies also produce multi-mineral tablets and these too, should be taken at the recommended daily dose.

References

1. Schrauzer, G. N. 'Selenium in nutritional cancer prophylaxis: An update', in Prasad, K .N., (ed) *Vitamins, Nutrition and Cancer* (Basel: Karger, 1984)
2. Boik, J. 'Zinc: Dietary micronutrients and their effects on cancer', in *Cancer and Natural Treatment* (Princeton, MN: Oregon Medical Press, 1995): 147
3. Gershwin, M. E. et al., 'The potential impact of nutritional factors on immunological responsiveness', in *Nutrition and Immunity* (Orlando, FL: Academic Press, 1985): 222

3.3.1d Essential fatty acids and essential sugars

Essential fatty acids are those which cannot be made by the body, but are essential for life and health. A very rich source is found in flaxseed (linseed) and the oil made from it. Linseeds can also be eaten whole or ground up and sprinkled over food.

Flaxseed (Linseed) Oil

Use and Dosage

Flaxseed oil is used to promote immune system and tissue functioning to improve the body's defences against cancer. It is high in the vital omega-3 fatty acids, which are essential to a properly functioning immune system. A typical recommended amount of pure virgin, cold-pressed flaxseed oil is 1–2 tbs/day. Flaxseed tablets are taken at levels of 1.5 g/day.

How to Use

Buy cold-pressed (unrefined) flaxseed oil. It has a short shelf life, so must be purchased as fresh as possible, and kept tightly sealed in the fridge. Since flaxseed oil is highly unsaturated, it readily oxidizes when exposed to air. It should be sold in dark-coloured glass bottles as it also breaks down on exposure to light.

This can be self-administered and taken with food, either as oil in dressings on salads or poured onto hot food after cooking. Never heat flaxseed oil as this will destroy its beneficial properties. It can also be taken in the form of freshly ground linseeds or as capsules/tablets.

Mechanism of Action

The omega-3 fatty acid in flaxseed/linseed oil called alpha-linolenic acid (LNA) helps maintain levels of health-promoting eicosanoids (biological activators that regulate all biological activities) and inhibits the production of tumour-promoting ones. LNA enhances immune function and cellular oxygen use, thereby inhibiting tumour growth.

Level of Evidence

A $20-million study by the National Cancer Institute (NCI) in 1990 found that flaxseed oil, but not fish oil, reduced the growth of breast cancers and metastases in laboratory animals compared with cancerous growths in animals receiving corn oil.[1] Although the NCI study was halted before its completion, it determined that flaxseed oil has a strong anti-cancer effect provided that the particular oil is high in lignans. Flaxseed oil contains up to 100 times more lignans than many other plant foods. Studies showed that test animals receiving flaxseed oil had a significant reduction in tumour size and number (greater than 50 per cent reduction) after one to two months.

Once in the gastrointestinal tract, lignans are converted into enterolactone and enterodiol, believed to be the compounds in flaxseed responsible for the anti-cancer effect. Researchers have found that lignans can bind to oestrogen receptors in the body and obstruct the cancer-enhancing effects of oestrogen on breast tissue.

Source and Price

Flaxseed oil purchased by the bottle typically costs between £6–12/month. It is available in most good healthfood stores.

References

1. Fritsche, K. L. and Johnston, P. V. 'Effect of dietary alpha-linolenic acid on growth, metastasis, fatty acid profile and prostaglandin production of two murine mammary adenocarcinomas', *Journal of Nutrition* 120 (1990): 1601–9

Note: Essential fatty acids (EFAs) are also found in nuts, seeds and oily fish, and must be built into a healthy nutritional programme. Lipoic acid is a useful cofactor that is often taken alone or in conjunction with EFAs. A popular preparation taken as part of an anti-cancer regime is Udo's Oil. BioCare also does a good mixture of EFAs that can be taken in tablet form daily.

A new, more controversial, theory, put forward by the company Mannatech, is that the body also requires essential sugars, which cannot be made by the body.

They are postulating that eight of the 200 monosaccharide sugars that we know about are essential for cell-to-cell communication, and that only two of these are easily obtainable from our diet. They believe that cancer and other diseases occur because of a deficiency in these essential sugars, and sell the product called Ambrotose, which ensures that a healthy supply is maintained.

A number of alternative cancer doctors are now building Ambrotose routinely into their protocols, and some people ascribe their remarkable recovery to the product.

For more information, see www.glycoscience.org.

3.3.1e Co-enzyme Q10

Use and Dosage

For the cancer patient, the primary role of co-enzyme Q10 is to help increase energy levels, reduce free-radical damage and increase white-cell activity. The dose range is 90–400 mg/day, with 90 mg/day as a maintenance dose if the condition is stable and 400 mg/day if there is active cancer in the body.

How to Use

Co-enzyme Q10 can be self-administered.

Drug Interactions and Special Precautions

Patients undergoing Adriamycin (doxorubicin hydrochloride) chemotherapy should not take co-enzyme Q10 at the same time as it may increase tissue levels of a potentially toxic metabolite of this chemotherapy agent. However, if taken before and after Adriamycin, it can reduce the toxicity of the drug on heart tissue.

Mechanism of Action

Co-enzyme Q10 is used by the cells in a process called 'aerobic metabolism'. Through this process, the energy for cell growth and maintenance is created within organelles in each cell called 'mitochondria'.[1] Co-enzyme Q10 as an antioxidant can also protect cells from free-radical damage.

Level of Evidence

In patients with cancer, co-enzyme Q10 can protect the heart from anthracycline-induced cardiotoxicity[2] and stimulate the immune system.[3] It appears that co-enzyme Q10 also has an indirect anti-cancer activity through its stimulatory effect on the immune system, observed in animal studies and in people without cancer. The ability to protect the heart and enhance the immune system make co-enzyme Q10 a valuable part of alternative treatment, particularly if a patient is receiving or has received chemotherapy.

Source and Price

Co-enzyme Q10 or ubiquinone is available from health food shops and many chemists. The price is around £10 per 40 90 mg tablets.

References

1. Ernster, L. and Forsmark-Andree, P., 'Ubiquinol: an endogenous antioxidant in aerobic organisms', *Clinical Investigator* 72 [suppl 8] (1993): S60–5
2. Folkers, K. and Wolaniuk, A., 'Research on coenzyme Q10 in clinical treatment and in immunomodulation', *Drugs Under Experimental and Clinical Research*, XI.8 (1985): 539–45
3. Folkers, K. *et al.*, 'Increase in levels of IgG in serum of patients treated with coenzyme Q10', *Research Communications in Chemical Pathology and Pharmacology* 38.2 (1982): 335–8

3.3.1f Immune stimulants

Inositol/IP-6

Use and Dosage

This is used for the prevention and treatment of cancer. The dose range is 3–6 g/day in three doses. The higher dosage is for active treatment of cancer, and the lower one is for maintenance once remission has been achieved.

How to Use

Inositol can be self-administered, and is excellent for reviving immune function during and after chemotherapy, and as part of a holistic health creation programme.

Mechanism of Action

Inositol has a powerful immune-stimulating action, particularly the production of vital NK cells, while raising white-cell numbers and activity in general.

It is found in virtually all cells of the body and helps the liver remove excess fat from its tissues, preventing liver stagnation from fat and bile accumulation.

Level of Evidence
John Potter, PhD, a researcher at Fred Hutchinson Cancer Research Center in Seattle, Washington, has identified inositol hexaphosphate (IP-6) as one of 15 different classes of phytochemicals with known anti-cancer activity.[1]

It has also been shown to have direct and indirect immune-stimulating properties.

Source and Price
A supply of 120 IP-6 tablets (880 mg) costs £21.95/month while 414 g of IP-6 powder will cost you £69.95.

References
1. Steinmetz, K. A. and Potter, J. D., 'Vegetables, fruit and cancer mechanisms', *Cancer Causes and Control 2* (1991): 427–42

Biobran
Strong claims have been made for the use of BioBran, a polysaccharide complex produced from rice-bran hemicellulose. It is activated by carbohydrase generated by cultivating mushroom mycelia.

Use and Dosage
Biobran is self-administered. It is prescribed at the level of 1–3 g/day for those with cancer.

Drug Interactions and Special Precautions
None known.

Mechanism of Action
BioBran has a strong stimulant effect on the activation of NK (natural-killer) cells. It is said to be an immunopotentiator, immunomodulator, inhibitor of viral growth, inhibitor of tumour-cell growth, a superoxide scavenger, and enhancer of pancreatic and hepatic function; it also improves glucose tolerance and reduces the side-effects of chemotherapy.

Level of Evidence
In studies carried out at the Sano Surgical Clinic by Kihachiro Takhara, MD, the BioBran group had significantly higher NK-cell activation levels and survival rate than the control group.

Source and Price
BioBran costs around £3/g. So, 3 g/day would cost you £9 and a month's supply about £270. This puts BioBran out of the reach of most people with cancer, so the preferred immune stimulant is usually IP-6 or coriolus mushroom (see page 108).

3.3.2 Herbal Medicine

See Chapter 5, page 105.

3.3.2a Aloe vera

Use and Dosage
To treat skin burns, use twice daily on the affected skin and continue for up to six weeks after radiotherapy has ended.

To aim for a direct anti-cancer effect, people take up to 200 ml of juice per day in divided doses.

Taken as aloe vera juice, one tablespoon three times a day will help heal the gut lining during and after chemotherapy. This dosage will also help with radiation cystitis.

How to Use
It is perfectly safe to self-administer aloe vera cream, juice or tablets. Using this herbal medicine during conventional cancer treatment is positively recommended. It can also be applied directly to burned skin from the broken surface of an aloe leaf.

Drug Interactions and Special Precautions
None reported.

Mechanism of Action
Aloe vera contains a variety of vitamins, minerals, amino acids, essential fats and enzymes. However, its most potent constituent appears to be acemannan. This water-soluble compound has been found to enhance immune function in mice by increasing the numbers and activity of T cells and macrophages.[1]

While the therapeutic efficacy of acemannan for human cancer remains to be proven, the compound has demonstrated anti-cancer activity in animals.[2] The antitumour activity seems to be, in part, due to its ability to inhibit cancer cell formation, platelet clumping, and the production of harmful eicosanoids and inflammatory reactions.[3]

Level of Evidence
Aloe vera has a strong anecdotal or folk-medicine tradition that is increasingly being supported by science.

Source and Price
- Aloe vera cream is widely available.
- Aloe vera juice – use Aloe Gold from Nature's Own/Cytoplan as, at this time, it has the highest level of aloe of any proprietary brand.
- High-strength aloe vera tablets cost £3.79 per month from healthfood shops.

References
1. Zhang, L. and Tizard, I. R., 'Activation of mouse macrophage cell line by acemannan: the major carbohydrate fraction from aloe vera gel', *Immunopharmacology* 35.2 (1996): 119–28
2. Harris, C. *et al.*, 'Efficacy of acemannan in treatment of canine and feline spontaneous neoplasms', *Molecular Biology* 3.2 (1991): 207–13
3. Boik, J., 'Conducting research on natural agents', in *Cancer and Natural Medicine: A Textbook of Basic Science and Clinical Research* (Princeton, MN: Oregon Medical Press, 1995): 177

3.3.2b Amygdalin or laetrile

Use and Dosage
Dr Michael B. Schachter, of the Schachter Center for Complementary Medicine in Suffern, New York, has used amygdalin for more than 20 years with cancer patients. He has found that 500 mg, one to three times daily, can be taken safely as an oral supplement. It can also be safely administered intravenously. By eating amygdalin-rich foods, patients may also obtain substantial amounts through diet. One source is bitter apricot kernels, which appear to be safe at the rate of three to five apricot kernels three times a day.

The injectable form is more concentrated, enabling the delivery of higher doses in a shorter period of time. After several weeks and if the patient responds well to treatment, the physician may reduce the dosage and prescribe tablets to replace injections. This therapy is usually used in conjunction with proteolytic enzymes, and a diet of fresh fruit and vegetables, and whole-grains, with the elimination of meat and dairy products for the duration of the treatment.

How to Use
Initially, intravenous injections need to be administered by a qualified medical practitioner. Subsequent treatments or initial treatment using amygdalin tablets and apricot kernels for nutritional support may be done at home.

Drug Interactions and Special Precautions
It is essential not to take too much amygdalin as cyanide is a poison. Always take it under medical guidance. However, a review of laboratory and clinical studies observed no toxic effects from consistent amygdalin use in either mice or humans.[1]

Mechanism of Action
Amygdalin consists of two sugar molecules – a benzaldehyde ring and a cyanide radical. These two molecules are split off by the enzyme beta-glucosidase (found in high quantities in cancer cells) and replaced by glucuronic acid. This results in a selective toxicity only to cancer cells and relative non-toxicity to normal cells as the enzyme glucuronidase, which splits off the glucuronic acid, is found in low quantities in normal cells. The glucuronic acid and the remaining benzaldehyde are then split off from the cyanide molecule, which is then toxic to the cancer cell.

An additional mechanism that protects normal cells from cyanide is their content of the enzyme rhodanase. This enzyme adds a sulphur atom to any free cyanide to form thiocyanate, a relatively harmless substance. Cancer cells lack significant amounts of this enzyme and so, it is believed, are more susceptible to cyanide poisoning.

Level of Evidence
Unfortunately, amygdalin/laetrile has been the subject of much controversy over the years. According to Dr Ralph Moss, positive research findings on the compound have been consistently suppressed by the pharmaceutical industry, allegedly because it is non-patentable.

Amygdalin has been found to have direct anti-cancer potential, particularly against secondary cancers, where a 60 per cent reduction in lung metastases – albeit in animals – has been reported.[2]

Source and Price
The compound can be purchased from World Without Cancer Inc., No. 303, 111 Kane

Concourse, Bay Harbor Island, Florida 33154, in the US; order by calling +(305) 861 0685 or order it via the Internet from www.worldwithoutcancer.com.

Prices for treatment at alternative medicine clinics vary and are available upon enquiry. Typically, though:

- initial 21 days of intravenous injections costs around £480
- initial 21 days of oral tablets costs about £300
- subsequent treatment for the next three months is approximately £800.

References

1. Brown, W. E., Wood, C. D. and Smith, A. N., 'Sodium cyanide as a cancer chemotherapeutic agent. Laboratory and clinical studies', *American Journal of Obstetrics and Gynecology* 80 (1960): 907
2. Moss, R. W., *The Cancer Industry: Unravelling the Politics* (New York: Paragon House, 1989)

3.3.2c Astragalus

Use and Dosage

Astragalus membranaceus can be taken orally as a tincture, tablet, capsule or powdered herb. The usual dosage is 3–6 g/day of the dried root or 250 mg twice daily of the concentrated root extract. This is used by UK doctor Robert Jacobs to raise energy levels prior to starting other Chinese herbs as part of an integrated cancer-treatment protocol.

How to Use

Astragalus may be self-administered and is safe to use alongside conventional cancer treatment.

Drug Interactions and Special Precautions

None reported.

Mechanism of Action

Clinical studies in China have shown *Astragalus* to be effective when used as a preventive measure against the common cold. Research in animals indicates that the herb seems to work by stimulating and boosting several aspects of the immune system – namely, phagocytic (cell-destroying) activity of monocytes and macrophages, interferon production, NK (natural-killer)-cell activity, T-cell activity and other antiviral mechanisms.[1–3]

The active constituents of *Astragalus* are complex polysaccharides known as saponin glycosides, astraglycosides, flavinoid glycosides and aglycones. These polysaccharides stimulate the immune system.

The herb has also been found to help reverse the chemotherapy-induced immunosuppression with the drug cyclophosphamide.[4]

Level of Evidence

Most of the data relating to clinical efficacy is derived from Chinese studies. There have been several clinical studies providing evidence to support the use of *Astragalus* for stimulating the immune system.

Source and Price

A bottle of 100 capsules (470 mg) costs approximately £11 per month from healthfood shops.

References

1. Chang, H. M. and But, P. P. H. (eds), *Pharmacology and Applications of Chinese Materia Medica* (Singapore: World Scientific, 1987): 1041–6
2. Zhao, K. S. *et al.*, 'Enhancement of the immune response in mice by *Astragalus membranaceus*', *Immunopharmacology* 20 (1988): 225–33
3. Boik, J., 'Antitumour and anticancer effects of botanical agents', in *Cancer & Natural Medicine: A Textbook of Basic Science and Clinical Research* (Princeton, MN: Oregon Medical Press, 1996): 120–8
4. Chu, D. T., Wong, W., Mavligit, G., 'Immunotherapy with Chinese medicinal herbs. 11. Reversal of cyclophosphamide-induced immune suppression by administration of fractionated *Astragalus membranaceus in vivo*', *Journal of Clinical and Laboratory Immunology* 25 (1998): 125–9

3.3.2d Carctol

Use and Dosage

Carctol is used by Dr Nandlal Tiwari on its own, taken orally as capsules – two capsules, four times a day, for a 70-kg person, after meals and before bedtime. While taking these supplements, Dr Tiwari advises a vegetarian diet and dietary restrictions prohibiting the consumption of sour, acidic food and drink. Patients must also consume large quantities of boiled refrigerated (or filtered) water (3 to 5 litres daily), avoid constipation and take a digestive enzyme with each dose of the medication.

How to Use

Some of the herbs in Carctol are classed in the UK as medicines, which means that the product can be obtained by prescription only. However, because it has not gone through the process of licensing as a medicine (which costs millions of pounds), it is therefore an unlicensed medicine. A doctor is allowed to prescribe an unlicensed medicine if he believes that it will be of benefit. A list of doctors who will prescribe Carctol is to be found on page 335.

Dr Tiwari recommends that the medicine be taken for at least two months before assessing its effectiveness. If there is no improvement of general condition or stabilization of the cancer within this time, he advises stopping the treatment. Carctol can also be taken to help offset the side-effects of chemotherapy, and is safe and beneficial when taken alongside orthodox treatment.

Drug Interactions and Special Precautions

No drug interactions have been reported. However, Carctol must not be taken if there is severe constipation or any obstruction to the passage of food through the bowel.

Mechanism of Action

None of the herbs used in Carctol have a direct anti-cancer effect but, in combination, they appear to produce unexpected remarkable recoveries. It is believed that its effect is in part due to changing the pH of the body from being more acid to more alkaline. The Carctol formulation has been developed to strengthen the immune system, neutralize the toxicity of chemotherapy agents, support liver and kidney function, improve digestion and weight gain, and calm the nervous system. The precise anti-cancer mechanism of action is not known.

Level of Evidence

Dr Tiwari has done a case study of 1,900 patients who have used Carctol (see www.anticancerherb.com), most of whom had been pronounced beyond medical help by their conventional medical team. Over 25 per cent of those studied reported a 75–100 per cent improvement in their condition with Carctol, while a further 30 per cent reported a 50–75 per cent improvement. The best results have been seen with those who had gastrointestinal and haematological cancers. I have been working with this medicine in the UK since February 2000, and have myself witnessed some remarkable recoveries. There have also been other reported benefits such as increased energy, recovery of appetite, weight gain and a general improvement in feelings of well-being.

Source and Price
Cankut Herbs in Bristol is currently the sole source of Carctol in the UK, and only with a doctor's prescription. Their helpline number is 0117 973 6052. It has been Cankut founder Mrs Amlani's charitable mission to bring the possible benefits of Carctol to the awareness of those with cancer throughout the world. The cost of Carctol is around £90 a month, plus the cost of the digestive enzymes, around £10 per month, from healthfood shops.

3.2.2e Cat's Claw (Uncaria Tomentosa)

Use and Dosage
In relation to cancer, cat's claw is useful because of its immune-boosting properties. It may be taken as a tea, powder or capsules. The dosage is 20 mg/day of the root extract, increasing up to 60 mg/day in more serious cases.

How to Use
Cat's claw may be self-administered.

Drug Interactions and Special Precautions
Cat's claw must not be taken during chemotherapy as it may worsen the drop in levels of red blood cells.

Mechanism of Action
Recent studies indicate that the particular species of cat's claw, *Uncaria tomentosa*, contains substances that have immune- and digestion-enhancing properties.[1] The beneficial constituents of the herb include several types of antioxidant compounds (polyphones, triterpenes and the plant steroids beta-sitosterol, stigmasterol and campesterol). The presence of these compounds is thought to account for the antioxidant and antitumour properties of cat's claw.

Level of Evidence
There have been scientific studies of the plant's constituent elements and their properties.

Source and Price
The cost of 90 capsules is about £6.50 a month from healthfood stores.

References
1. 'Oxindole alkaloids, from una de gato (cat's claw), have immune-stimulating properties', *US Patent No. 4,844,901*

3.3.2f Echinacea

Use and Dosage

Echinacea root extract can be taken orally as a tincture in water, or as tablets or capsules at the level of 225 mg twice daily.

How to Use

It may be self-administered.

Drug Interactions and Special Precautions

No interactions are reported. Long-term use of E *Echinacea* is not recommended. Use for approximately six weeks only as an immune-boosting tonic.

Mechanism of Action

In recent years, *Echinacea* has been shown to act as a potent immune-booster. It stimulates the production of white blood cells to protect against bacteria, and helps the body to produce more interferon for greater protection against viruses.

The plant's main active constituents are polysaccharides, betaine, alkalides and echinolone, all of which appear to be key to its immune-boosting ability by increasing macrophage production, the white cells that help to destroy cancer cells.[1]

Level of Evidence

A study in healthy men found that, after five days of taking 30 drops of *Echinacea* extract three times a day, their white blood cells had doubled their activity (cell-destroying, phagocytic capacity).[2]

There is no doubt that this herb has well-known immunostimulant properties, and studies of patients with inoperable metastatic oesophageal or colorectal cancer have found the herb to increase NK-cell activity by 221 per cent. In addition, one of its phytochemicals – arabinogalactan – stimulates the tumour-killing activity of macrophages.

In addition to immune support, *Echinacea* exerts a direct antiviral activity, and helps prevent the spread of bacteria by inhibiting a bacterial enzyme called 'hyaluronidase'. This bacterial enzyme can break through the body's first line of defence, protective membranes such as the skin or mucous membranes, thereby allowing disease-causing organisms to enter the body.

Source and Price
The cost of 100 capsules (250 mg) is £6 a month, available from healthfood shops.

References
1. Melchart, D. *et al.*, 'Immunomodulation with *Echinacea:* a systematic review of controlled clinical trials', *Phytomedicine* 1 (1994): 245–54
2. Erhard, M. *et al.*, 'Effects of *Echinacea, Aconium, Lachesis* and *Apis* extracts and their combinations on phagocytosis of human granulocytes', *Phytother Res* 8 (1994): 14–7

3.3.2g Essiac or Rene Caisse herbs

Use and Dosage
Essiac herbal medicine is usually taken orally at the level of 15 ml in 30 ml of water, before breakfast and again at night, two hours after food.

How to Use
Essiac can be self-administered and used alongside orthodox cancer treatment. Although now purchased as tablets and as drops, Essiac was originally prepared by Rene Caisse as a herbal drink requiring careful preparation. Once the drink has been prepared from its constituent herbs, it can be stored in sterilized bottles and refrigerated. Before use, the bottle must be shaken well.

Drug Interactions and Special Precautions
No drug interactions reported. Some doctors advise against taking the herbal formula during pregnancy.

Mechanism of Action
Essiac is formulated from four herbs – sheep sorrel (*Rumen acetosella*), burdock root (*Arctium lappa*), slippery elm (*Ulmus fulva*) and Indian rhubarb (*Rheum palmatum*). Studies of each of these components have demonstrated significant anti-cancer activity.[1]

Emodin, one of the main constituents in rhubarb, can inhibit various cancer-cell lines,[2] and reduce tumour-cell numbers and increase survival time in leukaemic mice.[3] Indian rhubarb has also been shown to exhibit immune-boosting properties, and can help cleanse the liver of toxic wastes and improve the supply of oxygen to tissues.

Japanese researchers have identified a potent factor in burdock that can block cell mutation.[4]

Sheep sorrel possesses strong antitumour activity and other immune-boosting properties.[5]
Slippery elm is rich in vitamins and minerals, and helps support the healing of mucous membranes.

Level of Evidence

Although Essiac has never been tested in randomized clinical trials, Caisse and her associates recorded many impressive case histories and anecdotal success-stories. Nevertheless, the evidence relating to its constituent elements and their likely actions are based on hard scientific evidence.

Source and Price

Essiac is available as a liquid medicine from Argyll Herbs, and from many healthfood shops as a liquid, powder and tablets.

References

1. Moss, R., *Essiac Cancer Therapy: The Independent Consumer's Guide* (New York: Equinox Press, 1992): 146–7. (In this book, Moss reviews the technical cancer-related research on Essiac, and the many substances isolated from herbs in Essiac showing specific kinds of anti-cancer activity.)
2. Chen, Q. H. *et al.*, 'Studies on Chinese rhubarb XII. Effect of anthraquinone derivatives on the respiration and glycolysis of Ehrlich ascites carcinoma cells', *Acta Pharmaceutica Sinica* 15 (1980): 65–70
3. Lu, M. and Chen, Q. H. 'Biochemical study of Chinese rhubarb XXIX. Inhibitory effects of anthraquinone derivatives on P338 leukaemia in mice', *Journal of China Pharmacology University* 20 (1989): 155–7
4. Morita, K. *et al.*, 'A desmutagenic factor isolated from burdock', *Mutation Research* 129 (1984): 25–31
5. Cyong, J. C. *et al.*, *Journal of Ethnopharmacology* 19 (1987): 279–83

3.3.2h Garlic

Use and Dosage

The dose of garlic is one clove or 2 g/day of fresh raw garlic, equivalent to 650 mg of garlic powder or 6 mg of allicin and other active constituents. Fresh raw garlic is good on buttered toast with tahini, or in olive oil as a dressing for pasta and salads.

How to Use
Garlic can be self-administered and is beneficial used alongside orthodox cancer treatment. Cooking the garlic will lessen the therapeutic benefits.

Drug Interactions and Special Precautions
Garlic has a mild anticoagulant (blood-thinning) effect and may affect the dose requirement of anticoagulant medications.

Mechanism of Action
Garlic contains an abundance of sulphur-containing compounds, especially allylic sulphides. Sulphide compounds enhance the action of cellular enzymes capable of neutralising carcinogens.

Allicin, one of garlic's main biologically active components, is released when garlic is crushed. It has been shown to decrease breast and prostate cancer cell proliferation in laboratory studies.[1, 2] Research into cancer at universities in Pennsylvania and Texas in the US has identified two other compounds – diallyl sulphide and S-allyl cysteine – that are active against cancer in crushed garlic.

In addition to containing substances that appear to inhibit the initiation and promotion of cancer development, garlic also seems to strengthen the immune system response to tumours.[3]

Garlic extract seems able to enhance NK-cell activity, improve the therapeutic ratio between T helper/suppressor cells, stimulate macrophages to greater activity and enable lymphocytes to become even more cytotoxic (able to kill cells) against tumours. Garlic may also block cancer cells from sticking to blood vessels, thereby helping to prevent metastases (spreading).[4]

Level of Evidence
Pure scientific research supports garlic's ability to work as a cancer inhibitor and, thus, as a valuable addition to alternative cancer therapy. Epidemiological studies have also shown garlic to help in the prevention of cancer.

Source and Price
The cost of 60 high-strength (600 mg) enteric-coated garlic tablets is £15 per month from healthfood stores, or you can take raw garlic in salad dressings and pâtés.

References

1. Pinto, J. T. *et al.*, 'Effects of garlic thioallylic derivatives on growth, glutathione concentration, and polyamine formation of human prostate carcinoma cells in culture', *American Journal of Clinical Nutrition* 66 (1997): 398–405

2. Li, G. *et al.*, 'Antiproliferative effects of garlic constituents in cultured human breast cancer cells', *Oncology Reports 2* (1995): 787–91

3. Lau, B. H. S. *et al.*, '*Allium sativum* (garlic) and cancer prevention', *Nutrition Research* 10 (1990): 937–48

4. Lin, R. S., *Garlic and Health: Recent Advances in Research* (Irvine, CA: International Academy of Health and Fitness, 1994): 23

3.3.2i Green tea (catechins)

Use and Dosage

When brewing green tea, pour hot – but not boiling – water over the leaves. Brewing time is just a minute or two. Boiling water is too harsh for green tea, and will damage the flavour and its vital ingredients. It is taken without milk and sugar. The tea can be drunk throughout the day in place of ordinary tea as a cancer preventative or treatment: 4–7 cups/day is recommended.

Alternatively, take catechins as polyphenols in capsule form called Tegreen 97, made by Pharmanex, two 250-mg capsules three times a day. For prevention, one capsule of Tegreen per day is recommended.

How to Use

Green tea and catechin capsules can be self-administered. Green tea should be kept in a cool, dry place, avoiding heat and light.

Drug Interactions and Special Precautions

There are reports of allergic reactions to green tea. Use of catechins while breastfeeding is not advised. It is also mildly anticoagulant, so should be taken with caution by those on anticoagulant drugs. It is high in potassium and should be avoided by those on a low-potassium diet.

Mechanism of Action

Green tea (*Camellia sinensis*) contains a substance called 'epigallocatechin gallate', shown to inhibit the growth of cancer and to lower cholesterol.[1] This is one of a number of chemical compounds known as 'polyphenolic catechins', which are many times stronger than vitamin E in defending the body against cancer-producing free radicals.[2]

The catechins found in green tea support immune system responsiveness and have powerful anti-cancer effects.[3] Studies indicate that green tea can reduce the risk of cancers of the liver and throat.[4,5] Green tea flavonols (the active bioflavonoids in the tea) and catechin supplements may offer substantial protection if consumed on a regular basis.

Level of Evidence

Pure scientific research has established the findings concerning green tea's constituents and their mechanism of action. There have also been epidemiological studies to establish the cancer-preventing properties of green tea.

Source and Price

Green teabags cost £3–10 per month, and can be found in most healthfood stores and some supermarkets.

The amount of polyphenol activity in green tealeaves varies depending on the climate, season, horticultural practices and the position of the leaf on the harvested shoot. A green-tea concentrate can be made by lightly steaming and drying the leaves of the tea plant. This steaming process preserves polyphenol activity.

References

1. Chisaka, T. *et al.*, 'The effect of crude drugs on experimental hypercholesterolemia: Mode of action of (-)epigallocatechin gallate in tea leaves', *Chemical and Pharmacology Bulletin* 36.1 (1988): 227–33
2. Bu-Abbas, A. *et al.*, 'Marked antimutagenic potential of aqueous green tea extracts: Mechanism of action', *Mutagenesis* 9 (1994): 325–31
3. Mukhtar, H. et al., 'Green tea and skin: Anticarcinogenic effects', *Journal of Investigative Dermatology* 102 (1994): 3–7
4. Klaunig, J. E., 'Chemopreventative effects of green tea components on hepatic carcinogenesis', *Preventative Medicine* 21 (1992): 510–19
5. Gao, Y. T. *et al.*, 'Reduced risk of esophageal cancer associated with green tea consumption', *Journal of the National Cancer Institute* 86 (1994): 855–8

3.3.2j Iscador (mistletoe)

Use and Dosage

Iscador is usually injected. The dose is individually determined.

How to Use

Iscador has to be prescribed by a doctor, and it is best to see an anthroposophical or homoeopathic doctor for this purpose. Once prescribed at the correct dosage and type for the given individual, the Iscador can be collected for home use. This requires that you either learn how to inject yourself, as a diabetic does, or having your local practice nurse or GP do it for you. Occasionally, it is prescribed as drops, most commonly for a brain tumour or secondary cancer. There is often an initial flu-like illness when treatment begins, evidence that a strong immune reaction is being provoked in the body.

Usually, Iscador is not used at the same time as orthodox cancer medicine.

Drug Interactions and Special Precautions

Iscador is safe when given at the right dosage, but it can cause adverse reactions if taken in excess. It is, therefore, important to use it only with the supervision of a properly trained anthroposophical or homoeopathic doctor.

Mechanism of Action

The therapeutic success of Iscador has been reported in nearly 5,000 cases studied so far. In animal experiments, it has been found to kill cancer cells, stimulate the immune system and significantly inhibit tumour formation.[1]

The activity of various immune cells increases significantly within 24 hours of injecting Iscador.[2,3] These effects are likely to explain the findings that Iscador selectively inhibits the growth of different types of tumour cells.[4]

Level of Evidence

The evidence for the effectiveness of Iscador is of a high quality. Studies using RCT (randomized clinical trial) methodology have judged the effects of Iscador to be clinically significant. There is also compelling laboratory as well as anecdotal evidence to support its use.

Source and Price

Iscador can be obtained on NHS prescription if prescribed by a GP, consultant or specialist anthroposophical or homoeopathic doctor. The main distributor of Iscador in the UK is Weleda (Heanor Road, Ilkeston, Derbyshire, tel: 0115 944 8200), the major anthroposophical supplier in the UK. It does an 'Iscador Patient Pack', containing all the relevant information about taking the treatment plus a countrywide list of UK anthroposophical physicians, most of whom prescribe Iscador on an outpatient basis. It is also prescribed by doctors at homoeo-pathic hospitals in London, Bristol and Glasgow.

The main anthroposophical clinic in the UK is Park Attwood (tel: 01299 861 444) in Worcestershire, where you can go to be put on Iscador during a two-week inpatient stay under doctor-and-nurse supervision. This costs £204 per day, including doctor appointments, and massage sessions, movement and art therapy, treatments with herbal compresses and aromatherapy. On leaving, you will be given a month's supply of Iscador. Park Attwood is keen that no one be denied access to their services for financial reasons, and will help those who cannot afford the fees to obtain help to meet the costs. Iscador injections bought privately cost approximately £6 each, and around three are required per week during treatment. If obtained on NHS prescription, the cost is the prescription charge alone.

References

1. Kiene, H., 'Clinical studies on mistletoe therapy for cancerous diseases: A review', *Therapeutikon* 3.6 (1989): 347–50
2. Hajito, T. and Lanzrein, C., 'Natural killer and antibody-dependent cell-mediated cytotox-ity and large granular lymphocyte frequencies in *Viscum album*-treated breast cancer patients', *Oncology* 43 [suppl] (1986): 93–7
3. Hajito, T., 'Immunomodulatory effects of Iscador: A *Viscum album* preparation', *Oncology* 43 [suppl] (1986): 51–65
4. Nienhaus, J., 'Tumour inhibition and thymus stimulation with mistletoe preparations', *Elemente Naturowissenschaft* 13 (1970): 45–54

3.3.2k Mushrooms and their extracts

Use and Dosage

The mushrooms *maitake*, *shiitake*, *Coriolus versicolor* and *reishi* are available as powders, with a therapeutic dose of around 500 mg three times a day.

Maitake mushroom extract is also available as MGM3, and has a dose range of 3–6 g/day in three divided doses. The 6-g dose is for those who have been recently diagnosed or who have cancer present in the body whereas the 3-g level is for those whose condition is stable.

The dose of *Coriolus* is usually one capsule three times daily before food, but this can be as much as four capsules three times a day in those who are immunocompromised.

How to Use

The mushrooms can be eaten fresh, or taken medicinally as a liquid extract or powder. They are self-administered and can be used alongside conventional cancer treatment.

Drug Interactions and Special Precautions

There are occasionally allergic reactions to these mushrooms, but no reported drug interactions.

Mechanism of Action

The *maitake* mushroom has demonstrated potent activity against cancer, inhibiting both its development and spread, according to Hiroaki Nanba, PhD, of the Department of Immunology at Kobe Women's College of Pharmacy in Japan. Animal research suggests the these supplements increase the body's ability to destroy tumours.[1]

Research has shown the *shiitake* mushroom contains an antitumour polysaccharide called 'lentinan', which appears to activate T lymphocytes, macrophages and other immune cells that mediate the release of cytokines. Lentinan has also shown potential antitumour activity in humans, whether given orally or by injection. It is currently being studied as an additional treatment to protect cells from the damaging effects of chemotherapy agents.[2]

Compounds in these mushrooms increase the tumour-fighting activity of NK cells and improve antibody responses, although *maitake* mushrooms seem to have the strongest and most consistent effects.

Coriolus is the mushroom most favoured by alternative cancer doctor Julian Kenyon and is available from his Dove Clinics. He believes it to be the strongest immunostimulant mushroom.

Reishi has been well investigated by Pharmanex, and its product ReishiMax GLP is available from its UK distributor Nu Skin.

Level of Evidence

The evidence supporting the positive effects of these mushrooms comes from studies both in the laboratory and in people, and from case studies.

Source and Price

These mushrooms may be bought from East Asian food suppliers, or even from good greengrocers. *Maitake* and *shiitake* mushroom extracts are available fresh or dried, or in capsules or as tinctures, and are available in specialist healthfood stores. The liquid extract is available from The Nutri Centre in London, where it costs £39.95 for 30 ml, or £29.95 for 120 capsules of the powdered extract. *Coriolus* is also available from The Nutri Centre. The cost of MGM3 is £64.95 for 50 250-mg capsules.

References

1. Adachi, K. *et al.*, 'Potentiation of host-mediated antitumour activity in mice by beta-glucan obtained from *Grifola frondosa* (maitake)', *Chemical and Pharmacology Bulletin* 35.1 (1987): 262–70

2. Matsuoka, H. *et al.*, 'Usefulness of lymphocyte subset change as an indicator for predicting survival time and effectiveness of treatment with the immunopotentiator lentinan', *Anticancer Research* 15 (1995): 2291–6

3.3.2l Noni juice

Use and Dosage

Noni (*Morinda citrifolia*) may be taken as fruit juice, tea or tablets. The dosage depends on the condition of the patient.

How to Use

Noni juice is self-administered and can be used alongside conventional treatment.

Ideally, noni extracts should be taken on an empty stomach about half an hour before meals, twice daily. The process of digesting food is thought to interfere with the medicinal value of the alkaloid compounds in the juice.

Drug Interactions and Special Precautions

There are no reported drug interactions.

If the dose is too high, then the side-effects of burping and loose stools can occur. This can be avoided by lowering the dose.

Mechanism of Action

Over 140 active constituents have been identified in different parts of the noni plant. The juice contains a wide variety of substances, including vitamin C, selenium, sodium, potassium, polysaccharides and many useful phytochemicals.

Scientific studies investigating noni as an anti-cancer agent are encouraging.[1,2] A study by a team of scientists from the University of Hawaii used laboratory mice to test the medicinal properties of noni fruit against Lewis lung cancer (artificially implanted into the lungs of the mice).[3] The mice left untreated died within 9–12 days while the mice given noni juice in consistent daily dosages lived significantly longer, with almost half of them living for more than 50 days. The study was repeated several times with similar results. The average survival time was 123 per cent longer with noni.

The scientists discovered that noni juice contained a polysaccharide compound called 6-D-glucopyranose pentaacetate. It is this that stimulates the activity of macrophages and T lymphocytes, thus enabling the immune system to attack the cancerous cells.[4]

Scientific research on the medicinal uses of noni was presented at the 83rd, 84th and 85th Annual Meetings of the American Association for Cancer Research. These conferences concluded that the chemical constituents of noni juice acted indirectly by enhancing the ability of the immune system to deal with the invading malignancy by boosting macrophage/lymphocyte activity.

Damnacanthal, an anthraquinone compound in the fruit, has also been shown to block or inhibit the activation of *ras* oncogenes that, when activated, can initiate many types of cancers.

Level of Evidence

The evidence of noni effectiveness is based on animal and laboratory studies together with anecdotal evidence in humans.

Source and Price

One litre of Hawaiian Noni Juice costs £24.68 per month from Healthy Solutions.

References

1. Hirazumi, A. and Furusawa, E., 'Immunomodulation contributes to the anticancer activity of *Morinda citrifolia* (noni) fruit juice', *Proceedings of the Western Pharmacology Society* 39 (1996): 7–9
2. Hirazumi, A. and Furusawa, E., 'An immunomodulatory polysaccharide-rich substance from the fruit juice of *Morinda citrifolia* (noni) with antitumour activity', *Phytotherapy Research* 13.5 (1999): 380–7
3. Hirazumi, A. and Furusawa, E., 'Anticancer activity of *Morinda citrifolia* (noni) on intraperitoneally implanted Lewis lung carcinoma in syngeneic mice', *Proceedings of the Western Pharmacology Society* 37 (1994): 145–6
4. Ibid.

3.3.2m Pau D'arco

Use and Dosage
This is taken orally as capsules or as powdered dry bark. The dosage may vary according to the condition of the patient, but it is usual to take one 250-mg tablet three times per day with meals.

How to Use
Pau d'arco is self-administered and is safe to use alongside conventional cancer treatment.

Drug Interactions and Special Precautions
There are none reported.

Mechanism of Action
The main active ingredient is a substance called 'lapachol', which has a molecular composition uniquely suited to inducing strong biological activity against cancer.[1]

Level of Evidence
In one study of nine patients with various cancers (liver, kidney, breast and prostate) given pure lapachol in 250-mg capsules with meals, all nine showed tumour shrinkage and a reduction in tumour-related pain; three patients experienced complete remission – and all with no side-effects.[2]

In studies of mice injected with leukaemia cells, the lifespan of animals given lapachol was 80 per cent greater than that of the control group.[3]

Source and Price
Pau d'arco is available from The Nutri Centre, in London, at £8.95 for 60 100-mg capsules. It is also available in tincture form at £6.99 for 30 ml.

References
1. Rao, K. V., 'Quinone natural products. Streptonigrin (NSC-45383) and lapachol (NSC-11905) structure-activity relationships', *Cancer Chemotherapy Reports (Part 2)* 4.4 (1974): 11–17
2. Santana, C. F. *et al.*, 'Preliminary observations with the use of lapachol in human patients bearing malignant neoplasms', *Revista de Instituto de Antibioticos* 20 (1980/81): 61–68
3. Linardi, M. D. C. *et al.*, 'A lapachol derivative active against mouse lymphocyte leukemia P-388', *Journal of Medicinal Chemistry* 18.11 (1975): 1159–62

3.3.2n PC-SPES

Use and Dosage

Taken as tablets, the active treatment for prostate cancer is initially four tablets three times a day. This should reduce prostate-specific antigen (PSA) levels. Once a new, lower level is stable and maintained, the dose can be halved to six tablets per day taken as two tablets three times a day.

How to Use

PC-SPES can be self-administered.

Drug Interactions and Special Precautions

PC-SPES has been reported to have 'an acceptable toxicity profile'. It does raise the risk of venous thrombosis by 8 per cent, so individuals who are at high risk of blood-clotting due to vascular disease must use this treatment with caution. It is also inadvisable to take it together with stilboestrol treatment for prostate cancer, as that by itself can carry up to a 35 per cent clotting risk.

Mechanism of Action

This combination of herbs contains flavonoids that are antioxidant, anti-inflammatory and anti-carcinogenic. PC-SPES also contains compounds that may enhance immune function. It also has components that interfere with testosterone metabolism and prevent it from binding to prostate cells. Individual components of PC-SPES can work together to block prostate cancer progression by blocking androgen-supported prostate cell growth and by causing cell death.

A recent phase II study assessed the efficacy and toxicity of PC-SPES in patients with advanced prostate cancer. The study concluded that this herbal combination may be active against prostate cancer.[1]

Level of Evidence

The findings from pure science and randomized controlled trials, and anecdotal evidence for the use of PC-SPES is compelling.

Source and Price

The supply of PC-SPES has been interrupted at this time due to controversy following the discovery of some medicinal contaminants in some samples of commercially available PC-SPES.

These contaminants included a warfarin-like compound, used to prevent blood-clotting, and a compound similar to stilboestrol, used in mainstream treatment of prostate cancer. Efforts are currently being made to reestablish a reliable supply of PC-SPES.

When available, 60 capsules will usually cost £89.95 from The Nutri Centre. This was also available at a lower price from the American supplier Botanics (tel: +(516) 432 1758).

References
1. Small, E. J. *et al.*, 'Prospective trial of the herbal supplement PC-SPES in patients with progressive prostate cancer', *Journal of Clinical Oncology* 18.21 (2000): 3595–603

3.3.2o Turmeric (curcumin)

Use and Dosage
Curcumin is taken orally as a powder or capsule at levels of 400 mg three times a day.

How to Use
Curcumin can be self-administered and taken alongside conventional cancer treatment.

Drug Interactions and Special Precautions
Turmeric is safe. It has been used in food for centuries with no adverse reactions. However, people with gallstones and who are pregnant should avoid turmeric due to its mildly stimulant effect on smooth muscle.

Mechanism of Action
The main active component of turmeric is a yellow pigment called curcumin, which possesses both anti-inflammatory and antioxidant properties. Part of the therapeutic effect may be that curcumin helps reduce the production of prostaglandin E2 (PGE2) and other 'bad' eicosanoids that promote tumour growth.[1] Curcumin also plays a role in the production of the cancer-detox enzyme glutathione-S-transferase.

Level of Evidence
Research indicates that turmeric can inhibit cancer at various stages of its development.[2] After one month, smokers who took two 750-mg tablets of turmeric daily had a significant reduction in the level of urinary mutagens (from cigarette-smoking) compared with no change in that of the controls.[3] Dietary curcumin can suppress colon tumour size significantly (by more than 57 per cent) and may also inhibit the progression of the cancer.

Source and Price
The cost of 100 capsules (400 mg) is £6.50 per month from healthfood shops.

References
1. Rao, C. V. *et al.*, 'Chemoprevention of colon carcinogenesis by dietary curcumin, a naturally occurring plant phenolic compound', *Cancer Research* 5.2 (1995): 259–66
2. Nagabhushan, M. and Bhide, S. V., 'Curcumin as an inhibitor of cancer', *Journal of the American College of Nutrition* 11.2 (1992): 192–98
3. Polasa, K. *et al.*, 'Effect of turmeric on urinary mutagens in smokers', *Mutagen* 7.2 (1992): 107–9

3.3.2p Other important herbal and food extracts

For information on graviola, lycopene, saw palmetto, mangosteen, wormwood, Chinese herbs and ukrain, please see Chapter 5, pages 109–11.

3.3.3 Hormone Therapy

Many cancers of the breast are hormone-sensitive, and can be helped by the use of progesterone cream and indole-3-carbinol to reduce the impact of oestrogen on the tumour.

3.3.3a Natural progesterone

Use and Dosage
Natural progesterone is used to control hot flushes and menopausal symptoms in women and men who have been put onto hormonal therapy to control breast or prostate cancer. It is also used to help prevent osteoporosis in women who are on oestrogen-blocking drugs. It is a prescription-only medication and the dose is decided by the prescribing doctor.

How to Use
Natural progesterone is taken either orally or applied as a skin cream, rubbed into the fine-skinned areas of the body such as the inner arm or inner thigh at the prescribed level. Any patient receiving hormonal therapy should do so only under medical supervision. Natural progesterone needs to be prescribed by a doctor. It is safe to use while undergoing conventional cancer treatment. Progesterone is safe to take with other drugs. Some women do have unacceptable side-effects while taking progesterone, and the dosage has to be tailored carefully to the individual.

Mechanism of Action

Studies have shown that low levels of natural progesterone in the body can increase the risk of breast cancer. A study by the Johns Hopkins Medical School, published in the *American Journal of Epidemiology* in 1981, tested the hypothesis that progesterone deficiency plays a major role in breast cancer. The study took 20 years to complete, and followed two groups of women: one with normal progesterone levels and another with low progesterone levels. It was found that the occurrence of breast cancer was 5.4 times greater in the women in the low-progesterone group.

In one double-blind randomized study,[1] researchers examined the use of topical progesterone (cream) and/or topical oestrogen and breast duct cell growth. Forty premenopausal women scheduled to have breast surgery to remove a presumably benign lump were divided into four groups and asked to apply a gel to their breasts daily for 10–13 days before surgery. One group used a placebo, one group used progesterone, one group used oestrogen (oestradiol) and one group used a combination of progesterone and oestrogen. Blood tests were taken on the day of surgery, and breast tissue was taken during surgery and tested for hormone levels and rate of cell growth. The women using progesterone had more dramatically reduced cell growth rates than any of the other groups, whereas those using a combination of progesterone and oestrogen had rates similar to that of the placebo group.

This study provides some of the first direct evidence that both oestradiol and progesterone are well absorbed through the skin, that 10–13 days of topical (skin) application significantly increases the concentration of hormone levels in breast cells, that oestradiol significantly increases breast cell hyperplasia (abnormally increased cell growth) and that progesterone decreases cell-proliferation rates even when oestrogen is being supplemented.

Proponents of the benefits of natural progesterone believe that the very high levels of breast cancer in the West are due to women being in a state of oestrogen dominance due to excess body weight, a diet high in animal fat and a lack of exercise. They prescribe progesterone to help overcome this risky condition of oestrogen dominance.

Level of Evidence

The evidence cited above is from high-quality randomized controlled trials, which suggests that these arguments for the benefits of natural progesterone should be seriously considered.

Source and Price

Progesterone cream is available by prescription from Higher Nature (tel: 01435 884 668) at a cost of £19 (1.5 per cent strength) and £24 (3 per cent strength) per tube, and from Healthy

Solutions at a cost of £18.82 for a 60-ml jar. Progesterone is also available from conventional doctors, but this tends to be the synthetic variety, which is reported to produce more side-effects such as water retention, weight gain and mood disturbances, which are rarely reported with the natural progesterone cream.

References

1. Chang, K. J., Lee, T. T. Y. and Linares-Cruz, G., 'Influences of percutaneous administration of estradiol on human breast epithelial cell cycle in vivo', *Fertility and Sterility* 63 (1995): 7865–91

3.3.3b Indole-3-Carbinol (I3C)

Use and Dosage

Taken orally as tablets, the effective dose established in human studies is 6–7 mg/kg/day. This amounts to an average dose of around 500 mg/day.

How to Use

Indole-3-carbinol can be self-administered and used safely alongside orthodox cancer treatment.

Mechanism of Action

Indole-3-carbinol has been shown to boost the production of enzymes that reduce the formation of malignant tissue, promote hormonal balance, work with antioxidants to prevent free-radical damage and detoxify body tissues.

In 1991, researchers at the Institute for Hormone Research in New York found that, by using I3C, they were able to convert up to 50 per cent of the more potent form of oestrogen (known as oestradiol) into the weaker 2-hydroxyoestrone form. In women, 2-hydroxyoestrone is considered to be a more protective form of oestrogen as it effectively blocks the strong signals for growth sent by oestradiol to cancer cells.[1]

Researchers at the Strang Cancer Research Laboratory in New York, in 1997, found that, when I3C changes oestradiol into the weaker form of oestrogen, it stops breast-cancer cells from growing by up to 60 per cent and provokes the cancer cells to self-destruct.

Subsequent studies at the University of California at Berkeley have shown that indole-3-carbinol inhibits a certain type of human breast-cancer cell from growing by as much as 90 per cent in laboratory experiments.[2]

Professor Gary Firestone is co-author of a report in the 13 February 1998 issue of the *Journal of Biological Chemistry* that indicates that I3C appears to interfere with the cell cycle by turning off a gene for an enzyme that is important in the growth cycle and, thus, stops the growth of cancer cells without killing normal cells.

Level of Evidence

Although the findings above are from laboratory studies, the argument for the potential use of this treatment especially for women with breast cancer is a strong one.

Source and Price

The cost of 60 capsules (250 mg) is £39.95 per month.

References

1. Michnoviez, J. J., Bradlow, H. L. 'Altered estrogen metabolism and excretion in humans following consumption of indole-3-carbinol', *Nutrition and Cancer* 16.1 (1991): 59–66
2. Cover, C. M. et al., 'Indole-3-carbinol and tamoxifen cooperate to arrest the cell cycle of MCF7 human breast cancer cells', *Cancer Research* 59 (1999): 1244–51

3.3.4 Metabolic Therapy

See Chapter 5, page 112.

Intravenous metabolic therapy

This is given by alternative medicine doctors in their own practices or as part of an integrated medicine regime in an alternative cancer clinic.

The most regularly used substances are:

a. High-dose vitamin C (see page 269)
b. Vitamin B_{17} (laetrile or amygdalin) (see page 281)
c. Ukrain (see page 111).

Anti-cancer substances

3.3.4d Shark and Bovine Cartilage

Use and Dosage

Cartilage is taken orally as capsules or powder or, occasionally, as an oil extract. For more pronounced effects, Dr William Lane, a pioneer of the use of shark cartilage, recommends 1 g/kg body weight/day of the powder. Bovine cartilage is usually given at lower dosages than this.

How to Use

Cartilage can be self-administered, but it has an unpleasant taste. Ideally, it should be used under medical supervision.

Drug Interactions and Special Precautions

No drug interactions have been reported, but there is a serious contraindication.

IT IS VITAL NOT TO TAKE SHARK CARTILAGE WHILE PREGNANT AS IT CAN INHIBIT THE PROPER DEVELOPMENT OF THE PLACENTAL BLOOD SUPPLY TO THE BABY.

Mechanism of Action

To grow, all tumours require the development of new blood vessels, a process known as 'angiogenesis'. Significant interest in shark cartilage was generated in 1992 with the book *Sharks Don't Get Cancer* by Dr Lane. He highlighted that shark cartilage contains no blood vessels and its protein component has strong angiogenesis-inhibiting properties. But before the book, there was already compelling research as to the possible role of bovine cartilage as an inhibitor of blood-vessel development, which can cut off the supply of nutrients to a tumour and, thus, hamper its ability to grow. The cartilage approach, when combined with other immune-enhancing agents, has proved a useful addition in helping to reduce tumour growth and induce remission. In mainstream medicine, trials are underway with the drug thalidomide as an angiogenesis-inhibitor.

Level of Evidence

Dr Lane reports that shark cartilage appears to be effective against solid tumours and has seen tumour reduction rates of 15–67 per cent in advanced prostate tumours.

In 1990, Japanese researcher T. Oikawa further confirmed the clinical benefits of shark cartilage by finding a 'significant inhibition of angiogenesis' with the substance.[1] Shark cartilage is currently undergoing tests by the US Food and Drug Administration (FDA) for its clinical efficacy.

Source and Price
The cost of 45 capsules is £15.09 per month, or £44.25 for 250 g of powder from The Nutri Centre.

References
1. Oikawa, T. *et al.*, 'A novel angiogenic inhibitor derived from Japanese shark cartilage. Extraction and estimation of inhibitory activities toward tumour and embryonic angiogenesis', *Cancer Lettes* 52 (1990): 181–86

3.3.4e Hydrazine sulphate

Use and Dosage
Dosage is typically a 60-mg capsule, taken three to four times a day after meals.

How to Use
Hydrazine sulphate can be self-administered, but medical supervision is recommended.

Drug Interactions and Special Precautions
Please note: HYDRAZINE SULPHATE MUST NOT BE USED IN CONJUNCTION WITH ALCOHOL, ANTIDEPRESSANTS, SLEEPING PILLS OR TRANQUILLIZERS.

Pain medications may be safely used without interaction with hydrazine sulphate, but dosages of more than 25 mg/day of vitamin B_6 and more than 3 g/day of vitamin C may interfere with hydrazine sulphate activity.

Mechanism of Action
Dr Joseph Gold points out that the weight loss caused by the cancer process can often be more life-threatening than the invasiveness of the tumour itself. The weight loss seen in cancer – called 'cachexia' – is due to loss of lean tissue and muscle as well as fat. Advanced cancerous tumours appear to grow at the expense of the body's healthy tissue. The constant high metabolic demand of the growing tumours uses up first the body's fat and sugar reserves, followed by the muscle and protein reserves.

By blocking a particular enzyme in the liver that is involved in the generation of glucose from other substances, hydrazine sulphate can inhibit this weight-loss process. Hydrazine sulphate also improves the appetite, increases the sense of well-being and often results in weight gain in those who have lost weight. It may also contribute directly to tumour shrinkage by helping to deprive it of its glucose supply.

Level of Evidence

Research on hydrazine sulphate indicates that it can lead to significant subjective improvements (notably by controlling pain and nausea) as well as to favourable clinical outcomes for many types of cancer.[1]

A study of 740 cancer patients (200 with lung cancer, 138 with stomach cancer, 66 with breast cancer, 31 with melanoma and others) reported tumour stabilization or regression in 51 per cent of patients, while 46.6 per cent of the patients reported symptomatic improvements such as fewer respiratory problems and a decrease in fever.[2, 3]

For more clinical information about hydrazine sulphate, healthcare professionals may contact Syracuse Research Institute, Joseph Gold, MD, 600 East Genesee Street, Syracuse, New York 13202; tel: +(315) 472 6616.

Source and Price

The cost of 100 capsules (60 mg) is £52.50 per month from The Nutri Centre.

References

1. Gold, J., 'Hydrazine sulphate: A current perspective', *Nutrition and Cancer* 9.2-3 (1987): 59–66
2. Filov, V. A. *et al.*, 'Results of clinical evaluation of hydrazine sulphate', *Voprosy Onkologii* 36.6 (1990): 721–76
3. Gershanovich, M. L. *et al.*, 'Results of clinical study of antitumour action of hydrazine sulphate', *Nutrition and Cancer* 3 (1981): 7–12

3.3.4f Urea

Use and Dosage

Urea treatment is occasionally used in an attempt to control the growth of liver secondaries. The dose should be prescribed by a doctor.

How to Use

Urea can be taken orally as tablets or powder and self-administered. Urea is also injected, which requires medical administration. It is recommended that urea therapy be taken under medical supervision.

Mechanism of Action

The theory behind urea therapy is that it alters the chemical properties of the cellular surfaces around malignant tumour cells, thereby disrupting the processes necessary for uncontrolled cellular growth.[1]

Level of Evidence

Professor E. F. Demopoulas of the Medical School of Athens University has used this substance to treat cancer patients. He has found that a 50 per cent urea solution injected directly into a mass of large fast-growing tumours was effective. Injections around the tumour site were even more effective.[2] Significant healing responses were reported in 15 of 22 patients diagnosed with cancer that had metastasized to the liver. (However, this evidence is from a case study, rather than randomized controlled trials.)

Source and Price

Urea is available in a powder form (in a formula with creatine monohydrate) from Innovative Therapeutics, PO Box 512, 200 Franklin Street, Carlyle, IL 62231; tel: +(888) 688 9922, Mon-Fri 9 a.m. – 5 p.m., Email: orders@innovativetherapeutics.com, info@innovativethera-peuics.com

References

1. Pelton, R., Overholser, L., *Alternatives in Cancer Therapy* (New York: Fireside/Simon & Schuster, 1994): Chapter 20, Footnote 5. Tumour cell surfaces contain large amounts of surfactants (glycoproteins and other large molecular surface-active agents), which have hydrophobic and hydrophilic properties at nonpolar sites, respectively, producing a structured water matrix surrounding cancer cells that is markedly different from that surrounding normal cells.
2. Ibid.
3. Demopoulas, E. D. *et al.*, 'Eleven years of oral urea treatment in liver malignancies', *Clinical Oncology* 7 (1981): 281–89

3.3.4g Enzyme Therapy

The most commonly used enzyme preparation for enzyme therapy is Wobenzyme, which can be obtained in Germany.

3.3.4h Cesium

This can be obtained from the US and must be used under medical supervision.

3.3.4i The Rath Vitamin C Protocol

See Chapter 5, page 114.

3.3.4j Amitriptyline

This antidepressant is being promoted by the Samantha Dixon Trust as an adjuvant treatment for some brain tumours.

3.3.4k Aspirin

Aspirin and other anti-inflammatory drugs can be used to prevent cancer of the colon and pancreas.

3.3.5 Immunotherapy

See Chapter 5, page 115 for details of the Issels Theory.

Vaccine therapy

3.3.5a Coley's Toxins

Source and Price
For more information, contact Innovative Therapeutics in the US on +(888) 688 9922.

3.3.5b BCG and Melanoma Vaccine

Professor Gus Dalgleish of St George's Hospital, London.

Another source is the Japanese Maruyama vaccine, made from polysaccharides extracted from the tubercle bacillus, available from the Research Institute of Vaccine Therapy for Tumours and Infectious Disease, Nippon Medical School, 1-5, Sendagi, Bunkyo-Ku, Tokyo 113-8706, Japan.

3.3.5c T/Tn antigen breast cancer vaccine

Source
For more information on the T/Tn vaccine, contact the Heather Bligh Clinic in the US on +(847) 578 3435.

Please note: VACCINE TREATMENT CANNOT BE USED AT THE SAME TIME AS CHEMOTHERAPY.

References
- Springer, G. F., 'T and Tn general carcinoma autoantigens', *Science*, 224 (1984): 1198–206
- Springer, G. F., 'T/Tn antigen: Two decades of experience in early immuno-detection and therapy of human carcinoma', *Jung Foundation Proceedings* (Stuttgart, Germany: G. Thieme, in press)

3.3.5d VG-1000 vaccine

Use and Availability
This new treatment is now available at the Immuno-Augmentative Clinic in Freeport, Grand Bahamas, and also from the CHIPSA Center for Integrative Medicine in Tijuana, Mexico. Both these facilities were selected for their long and varied expertise in the treatment of difficult cancer cases.

Research Evidence
The University of Texas Center for Alternative Medicine (UT-CAM) is one of 10 research centres established by the Office of Alternative Medicine (OAM) at the US National Institutes of Health (NIH) to evaluate alternative therapies. UT-CAM's review of VG-1000 therapy is available on its website at www.mdanderson.org/cimer.

3.3.5e Hansi

Use and Availability
The Homoeopathic Natural Activator of the Immunologic System (HANSI) product is available from Juan Jose Hirschmann, who can be contacted through his website at http://hansiargentina.cjb.net/. You can also fax your medical history for review. Contact hansiargentina@hotmail.com for more details, tel: +54 (011) 4612 4641.

It is also available from World Health Advanced Technologies at http://www.worldhealthadvancedtec.com/, which has a list of doctors who use it. In addition, Hospital de Diagnostico in San Salvador is now offering this therapy.

Dr Shaw in California also makes a form of HANSI available (see www.drshawlac.tothe.net/hansiwo1.html).

There has been some confusion as to who has the correct formula for HANSI, and the rights to sell it and where the formulas are manufactured. I would recommend researching the authenticity of the product before using it.

3.3.5f Dendritic cell therapy

Source

Dendritic cell therapy is available in the UK from Dr Julian Kenyon at the Dove Clinic for Integrated Medicine in Winchester and Harley Street, London. The cost is available on enquiry. Dr Kenyon collects tumour antigen from urine after treating the individual with high dose vitamin C treatment given intravenously.

Dendritic cell therapy is also available from Dr Thomas Nesselhut in Germany who collects the necessary antigen and cells from blood samples – a technique favoured by some immunologists (tel: 00 49 5 527 2056). Again, the cost is available on enquiry. Professor Dalgleish is available to help with an appropriate medical referral.

3.3.5g Immuno-Augmentative Therapy (IAT)

Source

Although Dr Burton died in 1993, IAT is still offered today at the clinic he founded in Freeport on Grand Bahama Island.[1] For more information on IAT, contact IAT Centre in Grand Bahama, tel: 001 (242) 352-4755.

Reference

1. Clement, R. J. *et al.*, 'Peritoneal Mesothelioma' *Quantum Treatment* 1 (1988), 68-73.

3.3.5h TVZ-7 lymphocyte treatment

While Coley's Toxins and Burton's Immuno-Augmentative Therapy are examples of non-specific immunotherapy, TVZ-7 is an example of specific immunotherapy. In TVZ-7, particular components of the immune system are targeted and activated for a more precise response. Dr Ravi Devgan of Toronto, Canada has used TVZ-7 with his patients and has seen positive results. He indicates it is one of the most potent immune modulators he is aware of.

Source

For more information on TV-7, contact Integrated Biologics in the US, tel: 001 (617) 938-9088.

3.3.6 Neuroendocrine Therapy

See Chapter 5, page 120.

3.3.6a Adrenaline therapy

Use and Dosage

Adrenaline therapy is used to combat adrenal exhaustion. The dosage is prescribed individually for each person dependent on their constitution and response.

How to use

Adrenaline therapy involves self-administration of injections and supplements.

Mechanism of Action

A detailed explanation of Dr Fryda's theory is available in *Adrenaline Deficiency as the Cause of Cancer* (translated into English by Dr Robert Jacobs, 2000).

Level of Evidence

The authors are not aware of any scientific evidence for this approach at present. However, there is anecdotal evidence for the use of this therapy.

Source and Price

In the UK, adrenaline therapy is performed by Dr Fritz Schellander and Dr Julian Kenyon. Dr Fryda is virtually retired, but does conduct the therapy personally with small numbers of clients, by referral from the UK's holistic and alternative cancer doctors.

3.3.6b Insulin Potentation Therapy (IPT)

See Chapter 5, page 120.

3.3.7 Physical Therapies

3.3.7a Heat therapy

Use

Hyperthermia is used for the treatment of cancer and may involve either increasing the temperature of the whole body or just tissue locally at the site of a cancer tumour. Heat can be localized with the use of microwave diathermy or ultrasound. Diathermy raises the body temperature by applying radio-frequency electromagnetic energy. Ultrasound causes an increase in body temperature as a result of friction produced at the molecular level as the high-energy sound waves strike the different body tissues. These procedures are particularly effective in controlling superficial tumours located on or near the skin. In whole body hyperthermia, the temperature of the whole body is taken up gradually, whilst the individual is sedated. This is done under extremely vigilant medical supervision. This type of treatment is often used in conjunction with low-dose chemotherapy or radiotherapy whose effect can be greatly potentiated by the heat treatment. This can therefore be a useful option for those who do not feel able or well enough to embark upon full dose chemotherapy.

Special Precautions
Patients must be strong to tolerate this therapy as enduring the high body temperatures which are induced in whole-body hyperthermia is fairly unpleasant. Caution is advised with patients who have cardiovascular disease due to the extra stress which high body temperatures place upon the heart and microwave diathermy should never be used by people with pacemakers. This therapy must always be done under expert medical supervision.

Mechanism of Action
Studies have shown that hyperthermia treatment modifies cell membranes, helping to weaken them, which makes the tumour cells more susceptible to chemotherapy, radiation and immune attack.

Level of Evidence
Several laboratory and human studies have shown that hyperthermia can play an important role in the treatment of some cancers. At the Duke Hyperthermia Program of the Duke University Medical Centre in Durham, North Carolina, considerable success has been reported using hyperthermia to treat soft-tissue sarcomas and recurrences of breast cancer.

Source and Price
Hyperthermia is available in Britain at the Liongate Clinic in Tunbridge Wells, under Dr Fritz Schellander (cost available on enquiry), tel: 01892 543535. Hyperthermia is available in Germany under its pioneer, Professor Douwes on 0049 8061 494217 (cost available on enquiry).

Reference
- Dewhirst, M., Professor of Radiation Oncology and Director of the Duke Hyperthermia Program at the Duke University Medical Centre, Durham, North Carolina (personal communication, 1996)

3.3.7b Light Therapy

It is used most commonly in tumours that are close to the surface of the body either under the skin or accessible via scopes, (as the light will only penetrate properly up to a few millimetres).

The light sensitive substances include photofrin, and aminolevulinic acid, foscan and naturally occurring substances like *Spirulina platensis*, a blue green algae used by pioneer Dr Bill Porter for 'cytoluminescent therapy' (CLT) in Ireland. Dr Porter's therapy is being researched by himself and American Ralph Moss.

Cancers successfully treated include oesophageal, lung cancers close to the bronchus (windpipe) and skin cancers. For deeper tumours, light can be administered by laser needles.

Light therapy is also practised by Dr Julian Kenyon at the Dove Clinic in Winchester.

A good source of information is Professor Stanley Brown, Director of Leeds Centre for Photobiology and Photodynamic Therapy.

3.3.7c Detoxification

Dietary Detoxification

Dietary detoxification involves taking a very clean light diet for 2-6 weeks, to allow the body to shed excessive toxins naturally. This can be done by following the Clean Machine regime in the *Cancer Lifeline Recipes* by Jane Sen, within the Cancer Lifeline Kit. This process is ideally supported with liver herbs (see below). When this detox is finished, a healthy eating pattern should be established by following the 'Eat Right' recipes.

Liver Detoxification

This is required whenever overall detoxification of the body is being undertaken either as part of an anti-cancer treatment or after heavy cancer treatment. It is achieved through either coffee enemas or by taking Liver Herbs.

Coffee Enemas

These have been shown to increase the liver's enzyme activity by up to seven times which speeds up the process of elimination of toxins from the body greatly. It is very noticeable that those using coffee enemas quickly find their skin and even the whites of their eyes becoming visibly clearer within days. Coffee enemas are performed at home by the individual. The best way of doing this is by getting a gravity feed enema kit from a chemist. About a pint of coffee is made from ground fresh coffee that is made half as strong as coffee that would be drunk. The other big difference from making coffee to drink is that the coffee is simmered for ten minutes. It is then left to cool to blood temperature and filtered before putting into the enema kit. Thereafter it is run into the rectum via the nozzle provided. It is best to lie comfortably supported by pillows on one side, in bed or on a sofa covered with towels as it necessary to attempt to hold the coffee in the rectum for around 20 minutes. Whilst in the rectum much of the coffee is absorbed straight into the portal vein which runs directly to the liver. Once the coffee hits the liver it has a direct stimulant effect with a great enhancement on the cleansing of the blood. After the 20 minutes is up, the remaining coffee is then released into a lavatory, commode, bowl or bucket as convenient, and disposed of with a good cleaning and sterilization procedure observed of the container used to catch the residue.

For many, the prospect of having an enema is repugnant and similar results can be observed by taking Liver Detox Herbs. A good 'Liver Herbs' preparation is available from Argyll Herbs at £20.45 for 450 ml.

Chest Detoxification

This is required if the lungs have become very congested with mucus or fluid or if there is a cough that persists. Chest Herbs are also available from Argyll Herbs at £20.45 for 450ml.

Lymph Detoxification

Lymph detoxification is necessary if the lymph flow has become sluggish and the tissues appear congested or 'water-logged'. Lymph herbs are available from Argyll Herbs at £20.45 for 450 ml.

Skin Detoxification

This is performed with lymph drainage massage or skin brushing techniques.

Chemotherapy Detox Herbs

These herbs are usually made from Chinese herbs and particularly good ones are available from Anna-Maria Lavin at Kailash, in St Johns Wood, London. Tel: 0207 722 3939.

Radiation Detox Remedies

These are available both from homoeopathy and flower remedy ranges. The homoeopathic radiation remedy is called *Rad Brom*. This can be taken at the 200X strength on a daily basis both during and for a week after radiotherapy to help antidote the effects. It can also be taken at the 30X strength in which case it will be needed about 6-hourly. The weaker 6X strength may be needed hourly. *Rad Brom* is available from homoeopathic chemists and health food shops. The radiation flower remedy is made by Galen and is available from the Bristol Cancer

Help Centre shop on 0117 980 9504. Excellent radiation cream made by Louise Brackenbury is also available from the Bristol shop.

Colonic Irrigation

Another fairly radical form of detox is achieved by colonic irrigation. In this treatment the colon is filled with a large quantity of warm saline solution administered through the rectum. The fluid is then released and with it any debris which has adhered over time to the wall of the colon. Often surprisingly large amounts of accumulated matter are shed and it is believed that this helps the bowel to work more efficiently in its eliminatory function thereafter.

Reducing Your Exposure to Toxins

It is advisable where possible to limit your exposure to toxins in your home where you may be exposed to toxic chemicals in many household products, cosmetics and personal care products. Although none of these products alone may present a critical toxic exposure, when many little exposures are added together they can present a cumulative toxic load that stresses the body's immune system and damages cells.[1]

Many chemicals used in cosmetics and personal care products do not require full safety testing before they are allowed to be marketed and used by millions of consumers. Dr Samuel Epstein has long highlighted the potential danger of certain chemical substances in many of the personal care products that we commonly use. A useful summary can be found in *The Safe Shopper's Bible* by Epstein and Steinman. It is therefore good to attempt to use products that are known to be free of chemical carcinogens wherever possible.

Source and Price

Neways International offers an extensive range of personal care, skin, hair care and household products that contain effective and safe ingredients.

The catalogue and price list, detailing an extensive range of personal care, cosmetics and household products that are free from ingredients that may harm you, is available from Healthy Solutions on 01454 418972.

References
1. Steinman, D. and Epstein, S. S., *The Safe Shopper's Bible* (New York: Macmillan, 1994)

Viral, Bacterial and Parasite Elimination

At least 15 per cent of all cancers are currently known to be caused by viruses. For example most cancer of the cervix, many lymphomas and leukaemias and primary liver cancer are caused by viruses. These are just the cancers we know about with viral origins. We also know that stomach and oesophageal cancers can be associated with the bacteria *Helicobacter pylori*. In addition to this there are cancers that are linked with the presence of parasites in the body, which also create a source of irritation. It is strongly suspected that many more cancers will be found to have infective origins in the future. This is probably the reason why there are such high cancer rates associated with the eating of meats and animal fats as these infective agents are often passed through the animal food chain.

These infective causes of cancer must be eliminated from the body in order to stabilize your health. This will occur in part by the overall raising of immune function through healthy eating, exercise and improved mental state. However it can also be wise to take anti-viral medicine such as *Echinacea* (mentioned earlier). Pre-cancerous cervical problems can be treated locally with a mixture of the herb Golden Seal with Tea Tree Oil in an almond oil carrier given as a douche on a daily basis, although laser and cone biopsy are strongly recommended for CIN2 and 3 lesions. The presence of *Helicobacter* in the gut can be assessed by your doctor and, if present, be treated with antibiotics.

Parasites in the gut are traditionally treated with the herb wormwood and strong claims are being made for the use of wormwood with an anti-candida diet by Dr Gerald Green for the effective treatment of cancer. Wormwood tablets are available from the Nutri-Centre at £7.49 for 100 tablets. Wormwood and Clove tablets that are also used for this purpose are available for £12.89 for 100.

However, more recently there has been a fascinating advance in complementary medicine known as complex homoeopathy. In this speciality the practitioner is able to pinpoint the presence of infective agents in the system, often long after the acute illness they created, which can be continuing to cause problems. The agents discovered are then treated with homoeopathic drops and the overall effect is to lift this infective burden from the body. This form of medicine has been pioneered by Dr Adrian Lindeman, in Devon, who has now trained a number of practitioners. Being first checked and then treated by a complex homoeopath can be a very useful part of the overall jigsaw puzzle for the recovery of your health and well-being.

Three good practitioners in the UK are Janice Seeley, in Devon (tel: 01884 425 8143); Tim Part, in Bath (tel: 01225 329355); and Mark Salmon, in London (tel: 0207 221 3899).

Electro-magnetic Radiation and Geopathic Stress

Help is available from Jennifer and Robin Clark who provide Charges Card to lessen the impact of electro-magnetic fields. They are to be found at 30 Manor Drive, Merriot, Somerset,

UK, tel: 01460 789914, email: card@rclark.com

Further reading on this subject is:

Earth Radiation by Kathe Bachler (Wordmasters Ltd, 1989)
The Body Electric by Robert Becker and Gary Seldon (NY: Quill, 1985)
Terminal Shock by Bob De Matteo (Toronto: NC Press Ltd, 1986)

3.3.7d Oxygen therapy

Hyperbaric oxygen chambers are to be found in some centres for those with MS.

3.3.7e Electro-magnetic therapies

These include:

- the Kosmed or Scenar bio-energy device from Russia
- the Bio-ionic system offered by the Bio-Physical Therapy Centre in London, tel: 0207 487 3777
- the Zapper – a tool devised by Hulda Clarke which is said to eliminate parasites from the system
- negative ion therapy proposed by the late John Knopp.

3.3.8 Nutritional Therapies

See Chapter 5, page 122.

Jane Sen – Health Creation Nutrition Mentor Service

I recommend Jane Sen for personal nutritional and healthy cooking advice. To get individual help from Jane, contact her via her website www.janesen.com, email her on info@janesen.com, write to her at Jane Sen, PO Box 4, Tetbury, Glos GL9 1BE, UK, or fax her on 01454 299810.

Jane's recipe books and teaching materials include:

The Cancer Lifeline Recipe Cards, Health Creation
More Healing Foods (Thorsons)
Eat to Beat Cancer (Thorsons, with Dr Rosy Daniel)

Videos:

Delicious and Dairy Free
Juicing and Raw Power
Sweet and Unrefined

These are all available from www.healthcreation.co.uk, tel: 0845 009 3366
The books and recipe cards are also available from Waterstones bookshops.

Organizations offering nutritional therapies

British Association of Nutritional Therapists	Professional body providing lists of individual nutritional therapists and telephone numbers	Tel: 08706 061284 www.bant.org.uk
The Gerson Support Group UK	The Gerson Support Group has been established in the UK to advise, assist, inform and educate those wanting to undertake the Gerson nutritional therapy for cancer and other degenerative diseases	Tel: 01372 817 652 www.gersonsupportgroup.org.uk Gerson Support Group (UK) PO Box 74, Leatherhead, Surrey, KT22 7YD
Gerson Mexico	Dr Melendez Dr Bravo	See international clinics, Mexico
The Nutritional Cancer Therapy Trust	The Nutritional Cancer Therapy Trust provides nutritional therapy including prescribed individual diets and supplements aimed at achieving long-term remission. Director Chris Ashton says, 'We are naturopathic and	Tel: 01636 612707 www.defeatingcancer.co.uk

	holistic in our application of bio-medical therapies based on the ongoing university level research into nutritional science.'	
Nutrition Society	Nutritional therapists	Tel: 0207 602 0228 www.nutritionsociety.org
Orthomolecular Oncology	A UK-based charity to do with treating disease with natural substances. The site contains a wealth of useful information on holistic and complementary approaches to cancer	www.canceraction.org
Soil Association	Provides information on sources of organic fruit and vegetables	Tel: 0117 929 0661 www.soilassociation.org
Vegan Society	Information, recipes, advice, publications and merchandise	Tel: 01424 427393 www.vegansociety.com
Vegetarian Society	Information, advice, recipes, cookery courses	Tel: 0161 925 2000 www.vegsoc.org

Nutritional and metabolic testing organizations

Biolab	Blood, sweat, hair analysis	Tel: 0207 636 5959 www.biolab.co.uk
Biomed	Blood, sweat, hair analysis	Tel: 01342 322854

The Diagnostic Clinic	State-of-the-art diagnostic service in London run by Dr Rajendra Sharma	Tel: 0207 009 4650 www.thediagnosticclinic.com
The Institute for Allergy and Environmental Therapy	Maintains a Register of Practitioners specialising in allergy diagnosis and treatment; information and local lists of therapists	Ffynnonwen, Llangwyrfon, Aberystwyth SY23 4EY Tel/Fax: 01974 241376 www.allergy.org.uk
Neurotech International Ltd	This firm performs highly technical immune, genetic and neuro-endocrine testing for alternative cancer doctors	Lansdowne House, Christchurch Road, Bournemouth BH1 3JT Tel: 01202 510 910

Protective anti-cancer phyto-chemicals in food

For a full explanation of the scientifically researched properties of these phyto-chemicals, see Suzannah Olivier's book – *The Breast Cancer Prevention and Recovery Book*.

Alfalfa	Saponins, sterols, flavonoids, coumarines and alkaloids, vitamins and minerals
Allium vegetables: Onions, Spring Onions, Garlic, Leeks, Chives	Allium compounds – diallyl sulphide and allyl methyl trisulphide
Almonds	Protease inhibitors, phytate, genistein, lignans and benzaldehyde
Apples	Chlorogenic acid and caffeic acid

Broccoli, Cabbage, Brussels Sprouts, Collards, Kale, Bok Choy, Kohl Rabi, Arugula, Horseradish, Radish, Swede and Turnip	Dithiolthiones, isothyocyanates, glucosinolates, indole-3- carbinol and sulphurophanes (in broccoli)
Broccoli, sprouted and Cauliflower seeds	10-100 x higher levels of sulphurophane than the plant
Burdock Root (Gobo – a component of the herbal cancer remedy Essiac or Rene Caisse Herbs)	Benzaldehyde, phytosterols, glycosides, mokko lactone and arctic acid
Citrus Fruits	Coumarines and D-Limonene, hesperatin, narangenin, glutathione and bioflavonoids
Flax Oil	Omega-3 fats and antioxidants
Garlic	Selenium, germanium, nntioxidants, isoflavones and allyl sulphide
Ginger	Antioxidants, gingerol and carotenes
Grapes	Antioxidants and ellagic acid (raisins also contain tannins and caffeic acid)
Licorice	Triterpenoids
Linseeds	Lignans, omega-3 essential fatty acids and alpha linolenic acid
Mushrooms: *Maitake, Reishi* and *Shiitake*	Polysaccharide immune stimulants (which boost interferon and interleukin levels), selenium, antioxidants, lignans and adaptagenic compounds

Nettles   Carotenes, chlorophyll, folic acid and selenium

Nuts and Seeds (Fresh):   Protease inhibitors, essential fats and antioxidants
particularly Almonds,
Walnuts, Black Walnuts,
Pecans, Sunflower, Sesame
and Linseed (Flax Seed)

Olive Oil   Specific antioxidants

Orange-, Red- and   Beta-carotene and proanthocyanidins (among the most
Purple-coloured foods   powerful antioxidants known)
such as: Apricots,
Cantaloupe, Melons,
Carrots, Yellow and Red
Peppers, Beetroot,
Squashes, Sweet
Potatoes, Red and
Black Berries

Parsley   Phytosterols, carotenes, folic acid, chlorophyll, vitamin C,
                           essential oils terpenes and pinenes, and polyacetylene

Pineapple   Bromelain; protease inhibitors; citric, folic, malic and clorogenic
                           acids

Potatoes   Protease inhibitors, chlorogenic acid and vitamin C

Pulses and Beans   Protease inhibitors, lignans, genistein and phytosterols

Rice, brown   Rice bran saccharide

Seaweeds: Kombu, Kelp,   Antioxidants, carotenes, selenium, iodine, alginic acid, the full
Nori, Arame, Laver   range of minerals and trace elements, and vitamin B_{12}
Bread, Dulse, Wakame,

Soy Products	Isoflavones genistein and diadzein, phytic acid, saponins, phytosterols, protease inhibitors, omega-3 fats and lecithin
Tea, Black	Polyphenols theaflavin and thearubigin which interfere with initiation, promotion and growth stages of cancer
Tea, Green	Epicatechin which is the strongest anti-mutagen of any plant yet examined and also contains epigallocatechin-3-gallate
Teas, All Leaf	Anti-mutagenic tannins, antioxidants and polyphenols
Tomatoes	Antioxidants, flavonoids, lycopene, chlorogenic acid, coumarines, carotenes and carotenoids
Turmeric	Curcumin

3.3.9 Mind–Body Medicine

Mind–body centres and therapies

Bristol Cancer Help Centre, England, UK

Bristol Cancer Help Centre is the leading UK charity that has pioneered and specializes in the holistic Bristol Approach to cancer care. Founded by Penny Brohn, who had breast cancer, and her great friend Pat Pilkington, MBE, the Bristol Approach is for people living with cancer and those close to them. The Bristol Approach combines the full range of physical, emotional and spiritual support. The Centre runs residential two- and five-day courses for people with cancer and their close family and friends. For those who live in the Avon, Somerset and Wiltshire area, Cancerpoint is a bookable individual appointment service.

Tel: 0117 980 9500; Helpline: 0117 980 9505; Website: www.bristolcancerhelp.org

Cancer Treatment Centers of America

Excellent mind–body approach to transform the experience of cancer.

Tel: 001 (847) 872-6067; Contact: Timothy Birdsall; E-mail: Tim.Birdsall@mrmc-ctca.com

Block Center for Integrated Cancer Care, Illinois

Excellent mind–body approach to transform the experience of cancer. Recommended by the Center for Mind–Body Medicine, Washington DC.

Tel: 001 (847) 492-3040; Contact: Keith Block, MD; Website: www.blockmd.com

Commonweal Center, California

The Commonweal Cancer Help Program (CCHP) is a week-long retreat for people with cancer. Their goal is to help participants live better and, where possible, longer lives. The Cancer Help Program addresses the unmet needs of people with cancer. These include finding balanced information on choices in healing, mainstream and complementary therapies; exploring emotional and spiritual dimensions of cancer; discovering that illness can sometimes lead to a richer and fuller life; and experiencing genuine community with others facing a cancer diagnosis.

The Cancer Help Program offers an integrated program of healing that includes daily group support sessions led by a psychotherapist, massage, yoga, meditation, deep relaxation, imagery work, symbolic learning through sandtray, poetry, exploration of sacred space, and a gourmet vegetarian diet. Evening sessions, led by Commonweal co-founder Michael Lerner, explore choices in healing, mainstream therapies, integrative therapies, pain and suffering, and death and dying.

Widely considered the premier programme of its kind in the United States, the CCHP draws participants from across the United States, Canada, and Europe.

Tel: 001 (415) 868 0870; Website: www.commonweal.org

Center for Integrated Healing in Vancouver, BC

Has an introductory programme that consists of 12 hours of seminars and workshops over a two-day period, including an introduction to complementary cancer care and healing, meditation, healthful nutrition, visualization, group sharing, decision making, vitamins, supplements and an opportunity to discuss a wide variety of complementary cancer care modalities with the Center's practitioners. They help put together an integrated cancer care program, that might also include Floressence, MRV vaccine, 714X, and hydrazine sulphate.

Tel: 001 (604) 734 7125; Website: www.healing.bc.ca

Simonton Cancer Center, California

The Simonton Cancer Center now offers a wide variety of on-line resources and aids for those who wish to learn more about the Simonton method. Affirmations for getting well and on-line movies for relaxation and guided imagery.

Website: www.simontoncenter.com

Gawler Foundation, Yarra Valley Living Centre, Melbourne, Australia

Life and living programme – a 10-day residential programme for people affected by cancer. In this programme they focus on what people affected by cancer can do to help themselves – how to develop peace of mind, how to provide active support, how to get the best from any treatment received and how to get the best from the immune system and self-healing techniques. This is based on the fact that there are many things that people experiencing cancer and their support people can do to meet and overcome the challenges cancer presents.

Tel: + (613) 5967-1730; Fax: 03-5967-1715; E-mail: info@gawler.org or programs@gawler.org; Website: www.gawler.org,

Slánú Cancer Help Centre, Galway, Ireland

Slánú is a Cancer Help Centre specializing in emotional and psychological support for people with a cancer diagnosis or life-threatening illness. They run a drop-in centre, helpline, counselling service, courses and a residential programme. Slánú is unique in Ireland. It is the only centre that runs a fully residential programme for people with a life-threatening illness. The programme offers time and space to explore illness in a caring and supportive environment. Individuals are encouraged to learn from their disease, to look on it as a turning point. The aim is to provide a programme of support, education and complementary therapies through which people with any life-threatening illness can begin the process of enhancing the quality of their lives.

Tel: 00353 91 550050; Website: www.slanu.ie

Cancer Bridge, Hexham, England

The team at Cancer Bridge run four residential weekends a year for specific groups. These are open to approximately 10 people. Cancer Bridge also runs day courses and a one-to-one therapy programme for those with cancer. The programmes help individuals to live positively and develop and strengthen their skills in coping with cancer.

This programme will empower and increase self-awareness, introducing participants to complementary therapies and help to identify the connection between mind, body and spirit.

It also enables people to prioritize and begin to work towards things important in their life. The team includes doctors, complementary therapists, counsellors, art therapists, healers, a vegetarian cook and staff involved in meditation, movement and relaxation.

Tel: 01454-605551; Website: www.cancerbridge.org.uk

Breast Cancer Care, Scotland

Information, support, advice.

Tel: 0141 221 2244; Helpline: 0808 800 6000

Breast Cancer Haven, London and Hereford, England

Breast Cancer Haven is committed to creating a national network of Havens recognized as centres of excellence in breast-cancer support. They aim to lead the way in complementary and alternative medicine in helping to heal the mind, body and spirit through group support and individual therapy programmes. They are committed to working together with healthcare professionals to promote integrated breast-cancer care.

London Haven: Tel: 0207 384 0000; Hereford Haven: Tel: 01432 361061; Website: www.thehaventrust.org.uk

Health Creation Programme and Cancer Lifeline Kit (available nationally and internationally as it is a portable self-help kit)

The Health Creation Programme is part of the Cancer Lifeline Kit by Dr Rosy Daniel (author of this book). It is a six-month structured, interactive self-help programme to enable those with cancer to make a full health and lifestyle review independently or with the support of a Health Creation Mentor. This has been designed to meet the needs of those wishing to heal or prevent cancer who are not able to get to a residential mind–body cancer centre.

Helpline: 0845 009 3366; Website: www.healthcreation.co.uk

HeartMath

HeartMath was created by Doc Childre, an author, researcher and consultant to leaders in business, science, medicine and education. HeartMath is a system for unlocking the heart's innate intelligence. Recognized and highly respected in the fields of psychology, mind–body medicine, new science, business and personal development, HeartMath offers a new psychology and physiology based on the power of the heart providing an innovative approach to healthy and fulfilling living.

www.heartmath.com; E-mail: inquiry@heartmath.com

The Journey

Brandon Bays' 'Journey' is a gentle yet powerful guided process for permanent freedom from any emotional, physical or life issue. The results are profound and the Journey has released people from every kind of life issue, including relationship, career and money problems; creative blocks; ME, allergies, chronic pain and many other physical conditions; long-held patterns of anger, fear, depression and stress; sexual blocks and addictions; abuse and loss traumas. It is a great tool for those with cancer who wish to heal their emotional past. Highly recommended.

Website: www.thejourney.com; www.brandonbays.com

The Order of Love

The Order of Love was created by Bert Hellinger. It was in his systemic therapy work that Bert discovered that the family system, just like any other system, has its own natural order and when that order is disrupted, the effects are felt by subsequent generations as the system tries to right itself. There appear to be certain natural laws operating to maintain that order and permit the free flow of love between family members.

According to Bert Hellinger's systemic therapy, the solution to life in a family occurs when each of its members takes his/her appropriate and actual place, takes upon his/her roles in life, taking care of himself/herself and avoiding intervening in others' destinies. This system is highly recommended for healing family dysfunction.

Website: www.hellinger.com

Counselling and psychotherapy and group work

See pages 362–5 to find therapists.

Hypnotherapy

See page 360 to find therapists.

Emotional Freedom Therapy

Based on impressive new discoveries involving the body's subtle energies, EFT has been clinically effective in thousands of cases. Read the actual clinical cases and testimonials regarding dramatic relief for trauma and abuse, panic and anxiety, fears and phobias, depression, addictive cravings, children's issues and hundreds of physical symptoms including pain relief, headaches, body pains and breathing difficulties. Properly applied, over 80 per cent achieve either noticeable improvement or complete cessation of the problem. It is the missing piece to the healing puzzle. It often works where nothing else will. It is usually rapid, long lasting and gentle. There are no drugs or equipment involved. It is easily learned by anyone and can be self applied.

Website: www.emofree.com

NLP (Neuro-linguistic Programming) (Professional Guild)

NLP is a set of insights and skills with which you actively use your mind and your emotions and your body to run your own life more successfully and to communicate with other people with extraordinary effectiveness.

NLP is an ever-growing collection of information, insights and mental techniques that can enable you to improve how you think, behave and feel – and assist others to do the same.

Website: www.professionalguildofnlp.com

Art therapy

See pages 365–9.

Music therapy

See pages 365–9.

Drumming

US-based dynamic training programmes, research and the latest insights into health and well-being.

Website: www.ubdrumcircles.com; also check the Health Rhythms section of: www.remo.com

Voice Workshops

Chloë Goodchild invites all to work through sacred chant, spoken and sung poetry, movement, improvisation and song. She is an exceptional woman who creates a singing community where people discover exciting new ways of expressing themselves with others while creating great warmth and feeling.

Tel: 0117 927 7020; E-mail: now@thenakedvoice.com; Website: www.thenakedvoice.com

Tantra training

See page 368.

Laughter training
Dhyan Sutorius is a teacher of laughing meditation in Duivendrecht, The Netherlands.
  Tel: 0031-20-690-0289; Centre in Favour of Laughter

Happiness training
The Happiness Project is a remarkable success story that continues to unfold day by day. The cast of The Happiness Project includes top psychologists, life coaches, business leaders, spiritual ministers, leading physicians, great musicians, actors and poets – all of whom are fired with a passion to serve and inspire. Formed in 1996 by Robert Holden, they are rapidly approaching their tenth year in existence and offer seminars and training for health and business.
  Tel: 01865 244414; Website: www.happiness.co.uk

Clown Medicine with Patch Adams
Patch Adams graduated as a medical doctor in 1971, convinced of the powerful connection between environment and wellness. He holds the belief that the health of an individual cannot be separated from the health of the family, community and the world. In consequence, Patch and some friends founded the Gesundheit Institute, which ran as a free community hospital for 12 years.
  Website: www.patchadams.org

Relaxation
See page 367.

Meditation
See pages 366–7.

Visualization
See page 368.

Hatha Yoga and Pranayama
See page 369.

Five Rhythms Dance
See page 366.

4. Alternative Cancer Doctors

4.1 By Speciality

4.1a Immunotherapy

Dr Julian Kenyon	Dove Clinic for Integrated Medicine, Winchester	Tel: 01962 718000 www.doveclinic.com
Professor Gus Dalgleish	St George's Medical School, London	Tel: 020 8672 9944
Dr Thomas Nesselhut	Dendritic Cell Therapy, Duderstadt, Germany	Tel: 0049 5527 2056 www.tumor-therapy.de/

4.1b Hyperthermia

Dr Fritz Schellander	Liongate Clinic, Tunbridge Wells	Tel: 01892 543535
Professor Douwes	Klinik St Georg, Germany	Tel: +011 49 8061 435 www.klinik.st.georg.de

4.1c Metabolic Therapy

Dr Simmi Khanna	Chiltern Clinic of Natural Therapeutics. Oxygen and other therapies	Tel: 07000 567876 Tel: 01494 472110
Dr Fritz Schellander	Liongate Clinic, Tunbridge Wells	Tel: 01892 543535
Dr Nicola Hembry	IV metabolic therapy, Bristol	Tel: 0117 949 3366
Dr Michael Wetzler	IV metabolic therapy, London and Baldock, Hertfordshire	Tel: 0207 935 5251 Tel: 01462 893586

Dr Patrick Kingsley	Leicester	Tel: 01530 223622
Dr Rodney Adeniyi-Jones	The Regent Clinic, London	Tel: 020 7486 6354
Dr Julian Kenyon	The Dove Clinic, Winchester, Hampshire	Tel: 01962 718000 Tel: 01962 717800 www.doveclinic.com

The Dove Clinic tailors tests and treatments to the individual. They offer a wide spectrum of complementary treatments and therapies under the direction of one of the leading experts in the field, Dr Julian Kenyon. They may use laetrile and dendritic cell therapy to reduce tumour size, C-statin from bindweed for angiogenesis inhibition, homoeopathy, diet and nutrition, autohaemotherapy or intravenous ozone, acupuncture, wholebody negative ionization, and lifestyle changes/mind–body approaches. They treat late-stage cancers and many chronic diseases.

Dr Wendy Denning	Integrated Medicine Centre, London, offers IV metabolic therapy	Tel: 0207 224 5111
Dr Avril Crolick	Integrated Medicine Centre, London, offers IV metabolic therapy	Tel: 0207 224 5111
Etienne Callebout, MD	London	Tel: 0207 255 2232 Mobile: 07930 336348 Fax: 01582 769832

Etienne Callebout uses numerous herbs, nutritional supplements, enzymes and substances uniquely tailored to fight cancer, along with a detoxification regime, an overhaul of the patient's diet and psychological healing strategies. He alternates protocols so that the malignancy gets hit from different angles at different times.

He may use 714X, aloe vera, amygdalin (laetrile), bovine cartilage, DMSO, Wobe-Mugos and other enzymes, glandulars, green tea, iscador, flaxseed oil, *Maitake*, vaccines, shark cartilage and other homoeopathic and herbal remedies.

4.1d Iscador therapy, homoeopathy and complex homoeopathy

Dr Peter Fisher and Dr Sosie Cassab	NHS treatment at the Royal Homoeopathic Hospital, London	Tel: 01547 550331
Dr Elizabeth Thompson	NHS treatment at the Bristol Homoeopathic Hospital	Tel: 0117 973 1231
Dr David Reilly	NHS treatment at the Glasgow Homoeopathic Hospital	Tel: 0141 211 1600
Dr A. U. Ramakrishnan	Madras, Boston, London and Singapore. Offers strongly potentized anti-cancer remedies with high levels of success	www.drramakrishnan.com
Dr Roger Lichy	Homoeopath who also specializes in homoeopathy for cancer and mental difficulties	Tel: 0207 267 8487
Dr Rajendra Sharma,	Diagnostic Clinic, London. Homoeopath and diagnostician	Tel: 0207 009 4650
Dr George Lewith	Homoeopath in Southampton and London	Tel: 023 8033 4752
Dr Peter Grundweld	Anthroposophical doctor prescribing iscador at the Helios Centre, Bristol	Tel: 0117 949 9668
Dr Maurice Orange	Anthroposophical Clinic, Park Attwood, Worcestershire	Tel: 01299 861444 Fax: 01299 861375 www.parkattwood.org

The Anthrosophical Clinic uses anthroposophical medicine and integrates complementary and orthodox medicine. The Clinic is designed, staffed and licensed to care for 14 in-patients and to conduct outpatient appointments. Care is offered for a range of illnesses including cancer. It uses a combination of treatments, including anthroposophical approaches, in conjunction with conventional medication when needed. They treat a wide range of illnesses including cardiovascular diseases, musculo-skeletal disorders, neurological problems, immunological disorders and cancer.

Dr Robert Jacobs	Naturopath and complex homoeopath	Tel: 01202 829189

Dr Jacobs is a specialist in complex homoeopathy, Chinese herbalism, and electromagnetic therapies. He also has a special interest in geopathic stress.

Weleda UK	Heanor Rd, Ilkeston, Derbyshire For a full list of UK anthroposophical doctors prescribing iscador.	www.weleda.co.uk

4.1e Nutritional Medicine

Dr Charles Innes	Gerson Doctor Gerson Therapy support group, UK	Tel: 0207 221 2266 Contact Lesley Pearce Tel: 01372 817 652
Dr Jan de Vries (Naturopath)	Jan de Vries Healthcare, Auchenkyle Clinic, Troon, Scotland Chorley, Lancashire Barnet, Herts	Info@jandevries health.co.uk Helpline: 01292 318846 (Mon-Fri 9a.m.–4.30p.m.) Troon, tel: 01292 311414 Lancs, tel: 01254 830122 Herts, tel: 0208 441 8352
The Nutritional Cancer Therapy Trust	Naturopathic and holistic application of biomedical therapies. Be aware that the Trust is against all forms of medical treatment.	Tel: 01636 612707

| Dr Mark Draper | Mark runs his patient service from Malvern Integrated Health Centre. He also runs a cancer nutrition training programme for healthcare professionals called Nutrition Matters | Tel: 01684 560124 |

4.1f Herbal Medicine

Ayurvedic Medicine

| Dr Mosaraf Ali | Integrated Medical Centre, London | Tel: 0207 224 5111 |

Carctol Therapy (Doctors known to Dr Daniel)

Dr Rosy Daniel	Bath	Tel: 01225 423333
Dr Pippa Harrold	Bath	Tel: 01225 423333
Dr Roger Lichy	London	Tel: 0207 267 8487
Dr Michael Wetzler	London,	Tel: 0207 935 5251
	Baldock, Herts	Tel: 01462 893586
Dr Nicola Hembry	Bristol	Tel: 07720 062109
Dr Rodney Adeniyi-Jones	London	Tel: 0207 486 6354
Dr Milind Jani	Brighton & Hove	Tel: 01273 777448/748600
Dr Fritz Schellander	Tunbridge Wells	Tel: 01892 543535
Dr Robert Jacobs	Bournemouth	Tel: 01202 829189
Dr Andre Young-Snell	Hove	Tel: 01273 778123
Dr Rajendra Sharma	London	Tel: 0207 009 4650
Dr Max Mackay-James	Dorset	Tel: 01305 262626
Dr P. C. Tatham	Durham	Tel: 0191 384 6242
Dr Anne Curtis	Jersey	Tel: 07797 717897

Chinese Herbs

| Dr Robert Jacobs (Naturopath and complex homoeopath), England | Specialist in complex homoeopathy, Chinese herbalism, and electromagnetic therapies, he also has a special interest in geopathic stress | Tel: 01202 829189 |

| Anna Maria Lavin, London | Chinese herbs and acupuncture | Tel: 0207 722 3939 |

4.1g Women's Medicine

| Dr Sarah Miller | Woman-to-Woman service for holistic gynaecological help | Tel: 01275 464149 |

4.1h Mind–Body Integrated Medicine Doctors

Dr Rosy Daniel	Bath	Tel: 01225 423333
Dr Pippa Harrold	Bath	Tel: 01225 423333
Dr Roger Lichy	London	Tel: 0207 267 8487
Dr Michael Wetzler	London	Tel: 0207 935 5251
	Baldock, Herts	Tel: 01462 893586
Dr Mark Atkinson	10 Harley Street, London	Tel: 020 7467 8301
Dr Sarah Miller	Near Bristol (and at the Bristol Cancer Help Centre)	Tel: 01275 464149
Dr Nimrod Sheinman	Israel	nimush@internet-zahav.net
Dr Michael Lerner	Commonwheal in California	www.commonweal.org

5. Alternative Cancer Clinics (International)

Austria

The Kroiss-Cancer-Center for Alternative Cancer Therapy

Run by Dr Thomas Kroiss in Vienna, especially known for treating cancer of the breast, lung, colon/rectum, prostate, brain, ovary and leukaemia, liver metastases and bone metastases. Their speciality is Electromagnetic Wave Therapy and they also use hyperthermia, 'LT' Chinese herb speciality, cryosurgery, carnivora, Ukrain, vaccines, PC-SPES and megamin.

Tel: 0043-1-982 57 67; Fax: 0043-1-982 69 92; Website: www.kroisscancercenter.com

Bahamas

Immuno-Augmentative Therapy

The clinic, run by Dr John Clement, uses IAT or Immuno-Augmentative Therapy, a nontoxic method to help control many forms of cancer. IAT doesn't always shrink tumours, but it does help stabilize the patient's immune system and increase the quality of life. Best results have been obtained with mesothelioma, bladder, kidney, colon, lung, myelomas, ovarian and prostate cancer. Inflammatory cancers and skin metastases, as well as some forms of other cancers have had variable results. Even some non-Hodgkin's and Hodgkin's lymphoma cases have been successfully treated here. IAT treats the immune system, not cancer, by bringing the body's natural defence system back into balance through building systemic levels of tumour-killing immune complexes to the levels that would be found naturally in a balanced immune system. IAT involves injecting the patient with various products that have been extracted from the patient's own blood, then refined and processed into an immune-boosting 'serum'. They also use the vaccine VG1000. Patients may need to stay for 4–8 weeks on the first visit and then return periodically for additional diagnosis and treatment.

Tel: 001 (242) 7455 352; Fax: 001 (242) 3201 352, Website: http://www.iatclinic.com, E-mail:burtonh101@aol.com

Canada

Centre for Integrated Healing, Vancouver

This mainly mind–body cancer centre puts together an integrated cancer care programme that might also include medicines such as Floressence, MRV vaccine, 714X, cimetidine, indomethacin and hydrazine sulfate.

Tel: 001 (604) 734-7125; Website: www.healing.bc.ca

Jim Chan, ND, Vancouver

Jim is an acupuncturist and doctor of Chinese Medicine. He works with cancer patients using alternative therapies and nutrition. He has a very good reputation.

Tel: 001 (604) 435-3786

Cose, Inc., Rock Forest, Quebec

This centre is primarily run by Gaston Naessens, Françoise Naessens, Stephane Sdicu and Daniel Sdicu. They treat cancer and multiple sclerosis, rheumatoid arthritis and degenerative diseases. Their main therapy is 714X. **Note:** The clinic is currently closed, but it may be reopening.

For info on 714X and Gaston Naessens, go to www.cerbe.com

Highline Oxyzone, Oxygen Therapies, Vernon, BC

Provides adjunctive therapies for cancer, HIV/AIDS, post-stroke, chronic brain-trauma neurological conditions such as MS, cerebral palsy and auto-immune disorders. They use ozone, hyperbaric oxygen therapy, detoxification, lymphatic drainage and intravenous vitamin therapies.

Tel: 001 (250) 503-2111; Fax: 001 (250) 542-1574

HOC Centre for Progressive Medicine – Dr Thao Nguyen in Coquitlam, BC

A hyperbaric oxygen centre with a naturopathic physician on staff. It uses hyperbaric oxygen, hydrogen peroxide, ozone, Bio-Oxidative Medicine, Balneotherapy and IV/Chelation. The focus is on neurological conditions as well as adjunctive care for cancer and HIV/AIDS.

Tel: 001 (604) 520-3941; Fax: 001 (604) 520-9869

Abram Hoffer, MD, PhD, British Columbia

Dr Hoffer is considered a pioneer in the use of nutritional substances for healing. He uses high doses of vitamin C along with other supplements; and a low-fat, low-sugar, dairy-free diet.

Tel: 001 (250) 386-8756; Website: http://www.islandnet.com/~hoffer

Kelowna Naturopathic Clinic, Kelowna, BC

Run by Dr Garrett Swetlikoff, ND, he is a naturopathic physician who has a family practice and utilizes biological medicine. He uses a wide variety of modalities, including but not limited to clinical nutrition, botanical medicine, homoeopathy, intravenous high-dose vitamin/minerals, Ukrain, B_{17} oral and IV, neural therapy, ozone, IV hydrogen peroxide, photo oxidation, thymus injections, IV DMSO, Heckel whole-body hyperthermia, Insulin Potentiation Therapy, potassium and insulin IV, *Helixor* mistletoe therapy, photocell, clodronate, heparin, pulsed electromagnetic field therapy, ionized O_2, blood and urine vaccines, sanum pleomorphic remedies, IV garlic, PC-SPES, chelation therapy IV and oral enzymes, various diets and a lot of 'care and love' – his words.

Tel: 001 (250) 868-2205; E-mail: gswetlikoff@home.com

The Nasri Chelation Clinic

Dr Durenfeld and Dr Nasri use a variety of approaches including vitamin C, hyaluronan, HA, hyperthermia, Intravenous Poly MVA with hyaluronic acid, iscador, laetrile, tumorin, hydrogen peroxide, neural therapy, Wobe-Mugos, dendritic vaccine, infra-red sauna. They also use low-dose chemotherapy, non-steroidal anti-inflammatory drugs and high doses of vitamin C, all of which are combined with hyaluronic acid, which is a targeting carrier molecule. The use of hyaluronic acid allows for better penetration of the drug to the tumour, and also better targeting, so the severe side-effects of drugs are not felt. In operation since 1986.

Tel (Barrie): 001 (705) 735-2354 (Toronto): 001 (647) 293-5363; Website: www.nasrichelation.com

Pacific Center, Vancouver

Run by Rachelle Herdman, ND, MD. They treat chronic problems including cancer; autoimmune, neurological, cardiovascular and digestive disorders and chronic fatigue. Treatments include: nutrition, diet, Ayurvedic medicine, homoeopathy, botanical medicine and teas, herbal tincture, plant extracts, supplements, mind–body medicine and in-depth counselling.

 Tel: 001 (604) 734-0244

Richmond Alternative Medical Clinic, Richmond, BC

Dr Martin Kowk, ND, MSAOM, RAC, uses Traditional Chinese Medicine (TCM), herbal medicine, acupuncture, acupoint injections, clinical nutrition, homoeopathic medicine, chelation therapy, ozone, IV therapy and more. They also treat autoimmune disorders and do amalgam and heavy metal detoxification.

 Tel: 001 (604) 207-0167

Schafer's Health Centre, Saskatchewan

Is run by Dr Sir Leo J. Schafer, MH, RHC, LCSP, also treats AIDS and degenerative diseases. He uses herbology, magnets, diet, nutrition, Rife, and over 220 herbal formulas. They also sell Rife machines. In operation over 20 years.

 Tel: 001 (306) 228-2512

Vital Path Health Centre, British Columbia

Treats cancer, fibromyalgia, liver disease and stroke using hyperbaric oxygen, homoeopathy, oxygen, Chinese herbs, Essiac and Hoxsey in some cases, diet, and acupuncture. Psychological therapies are also used, such as guided imagery and positive affirmations.

 Tel: 001 (250) 549-1400; Website: http://www.vitalpathhealthcentre.com

Cuba

Ozone Research Center, Havana

Carlos Hernandez Castro, PhD, treats senile dementia, Parkinson's, arthritis, diabetic neuroangiopathy and glaucoma. Primary therapy is ozone therapy.

 Tel: 0053-721-0588

Denmark

Humlegaarden

An international cancer clinic, situated north of Copenhagen, using innovative and holistic methods in the treatment of cancer. In some cases, chemotherapy may be used. They treat most cancers, even late-stage cancers, brain, prostate, pancreas, kidney, cervical, lung and liver.

The alternative therapies they use include: mistletoe, ReVia, sensitivity testing of cancer tissue, anti-angiogenesis by tetrathiomolybdate, diet, hyperthermia, light therapy, galvanotherapy, electroporation, echinacea, anthroposophical and homoeopathic remedies, magnet field therapy, ozone treatment, vitamins and minerals, herbal teas and psychotherapy.

The typical treatment stay is three weeks.

Tel: 0045 491 32 465; Fax: 0045 491 34 498

Ecuador

Robert B. Wickman DO ND, Quito

Wickman is an osteopathic doctor, specializing in diseases of the nervous system and spinal column. He has treated many cancers, even advanced ones. He uses IPT therapy, diet and supplements.

Tel: 00593-2-241-274; E-mail: Rbw66_2000@yahoo.com

Germany

Professor Douwes, Klinik St Georg

Specializes in hyperthermia for all (and especially advanced) cancers. He is a trained oncologist who has sought to improve his outcomes by working with a combination of alternative and orthodox medicines. He has a very positive attitude and will often take you on when others have given up!

Tel: 0049-8061-494215; Fax: 0049-8061-494217

Dr Waldraut Fryda

Neuro-endocrine adrenaline therapy. Dr Fryda worked for many years with the pioneers of immuno-therapy like Dr Josef Issels. Nearly retired, she carries many of the pearls of wisdom discovered in these early days and will take on a few private patients for her own amazing adrenaline regeneration therapy. This is particularly relevant if cancer has followed a period of severe stress and emotional burnout.

By referral from Dr Bob Jacobs, Dr Fritz Schellander.

Dr Thomas Nesselhut
Specializes in dendritic cell therapy. A trained oncologist, he has decided to improve his results by working to re-activate the immune system. Highly recommended pioneer in his field.
   Tel: 00 49 5527 2056.

Issels therapy
The pioneer centre for immunotherapy, which has led the way for most of the new alternative cancer therapies.
   Website: www.issels.com

Bio Med Klinik, Bad Borgzabern
Run by E. Dieter Hager, MD, PhD, since 1989. They treat cancer as well as other immuno-deficiencies, including chronic fatigue syndrome. They use many therapies including hormone therapy, hyperthermia, immunotherapy (ASI/tumour vaccination), thymus peptides and electrotherapy (galvanotherapy), complementary oncology, immunology and hyperthermia.
   Tel: 00 49 6343 7050; Website: www.biomed-klinik.de/bmgruwolen.htm

Hartmut Baltin, MD, located between Salzburg and Munich
Treats cancer, multiple sclerosis, HIV and autoimmune diseases. He uses diet, plant extracts, hyperthermia, ozone, vaccinations, minerals, vitamins, psychotherapy, surgery, and acupuncture.
   Tel: 00 49 08052 4176

Hufeland Clinic for Holistic Immunotherapy, Bad Mergentheim
Uses a treatment based on a well-established concept developed by Dr Josef Issels, which is a holistic approach using fever therapy, hyperthermia and immuno-biological medicine. They treat most cancers including breast, melanoma, prostate, colon, kidney, brain and sarcomas, as well as arteriosclerosis. They also use colonics, eumetabolics, homoeopathy, vitamins, minerals, enzymes, ozone, oxygen, hydrogen peroxide, chelation, hydrotherapy, acupuncture and nutrition.
   Tel: 0049 7931 5360; Website: www.hufeland-klinik.de/Englisch/hufeland_clinic.htm

Institute for Immunology and Thymus Research, Bad Harzburg (outside Hanover)
Is run by Milan C. Pesic, MD. They have had the best response with treating the cancers of the lung, bladder, colon, pancreas, breast, Hodgkin's and non-Hodgkin's lymphomas, and Kaposi's sarcoma. They use THX/Thymex-L, a thymus extract, for immune stimulation.
Tel: 0049 5322-960541

Hong Kong

Optimum Health Centre, Causeway Bay
Is run by Alexander Yuan, BA, DC, ND, DHt. It was established in 1987 and is one of the oldest and largest health centres in Hong Kong. They treat a full range of health problems, including AIDS and cancer. They use gastrointestinal tract cleansing; colon hydrotherapy; herbal, nutritional and constitutional hydrotherapy; ionic therapy; enzymes; supplements and diet.
Tel: 00 852 2577 3798; Website: www.naturalhealing.com.hk

Hungary

United Cancer Research Institute, Budapest
Run by Dr Laszlo K. Csatary and Eva Csatary. This clinic uses a Virus Therapy that they have been researching and developing for over 30 years. They have cancer patients that are in remission since their clinic opened.
They can be reached via a Fort Lauderdale phone/fax number: 001 954 525 3120.

Israel

Joseph Brenner, M.D., Tel-Aviv
Dr Brenner mainly treats cancer using nutrition, megadoses of vitamins and minerals, laetrile, iscador, non-steroidal anti-inflammatory drugs, shark cartilage, neytumorin, carcinomium copmostium (HEEL), herbs and acupuncture.
Tel: 00972-3-5467733 or 00972-3-5467739

Italy

Giancarlo Pizza, MD, Sant'Orsola-Malpighi Hospital, Bologna
Treatment is out-patient at the clinic. Additional follow-up, both at home and visiting the clinic may be required. Best results are in renal cancer, but they treat most cancers. They use specific and non-specific transfer factor, low-dose IL-2 injected intralymphatically, interferon, LAK cells (lymphokine activated killer cells), interferon-alpha and hormone therapy. Currently they have a proposed research study on transfer factor as a form of immunothera-

py for advanced metastatic prostate cancer stage D3. NFAM has a write up on this clinic at http://www.med.unibo.it

Tel: 0039 051 636 2478; Fax: 0039 051 636 2476

Japan

Holistic Keihoku Hospital, Tokyo, run by Tsuneo Kobayashi, MD

They treat many cancers including cancers of the bone, breast and liver; ovarian and colon cancers; as well as cirrhosis of the liver; and chronic hepatitis. They use lymphocyte therapy, LAK therapy, plasma exchange, herbal therapy, refreshment therapy (enhancement of natural healing), psycho-immunomodulation and immuno-thermo-chemotherapy.

Tel: 0081 0339 467 271

Obitsu Sankei Clinic and Hospital

The excellent holistic clinic and hospital are known to Dr Daniel. Acupuncture, Chinese Herbal Medicine and Chi Gong are practised in an ideal residential setting for true integrated medicine. The clinic is in Ikeeukuro, Tokyo. The hospital is in the Saitama prefecture: Obitsu Sankei Hospital, in the Kayagae, Saitama prefecture, Japan.

Tel (Clinic, Tokyo): 0081 6359 851 080

Kenya

Spring of Life Therapeutic Center

Uses Polyatomic Oxygen Therapy and Apheresis in treating cancer. Detoxification and boosting the immune system are major parts of their approach. They use intravenous treatments, colonic enemas, diet and supplementation.

Tel: 00254 733 708 041

Mexico

American Metabolic Institute and St. Joseph Hospital, La Mesa, Mexico, Geronimo Rubio, MD

American Metabolic uses up to 150 different nontoxic medications and therapies to re-train the immune system to eliminate cancer. For ten years they have been treating degenerative diseases, particularly cancer, with a wide variety of alternative protocols. A metabolic therapy programme is aimed to stimulate the patient's immune system to eliminate cancer. A variety of approaches are used including chelation therapy, supplements, enzymes, lymphatic therapy, acupuncture, oxygen therapies, immunotherapy, colon therapy, Rife frequency-generator technology, botanicals, specialized herbal medicines, shark liver oil, intravenously delivered laetrile (amygdalin), cranial electro-stimulation, reflexology, nutritional therapy, detoxification and counselling. In some cases they may also use low-dose radiation or chemotherapy. There is an optional 7- to 21-day tissue cleanse and complete mercury amalgam removal programme. American Metabolics uses vaccines that are cultured from the patient's blood and tumour antigen. Although all forms of cancer are treated, they appear to have had the most success with lymphomas and cancers of the liver, brain, breast, pancreas and lung.

Tel: 0052-1-800-388-1083; Mexico: 0052 6621 7602; Website: www.ami-health.com

Baja Nutri Care, in the Playas area of Tijuana, Mexico

The Gerson Institute has initiated a license agreement with Baja Nutri Care, a new treatment centre co-owned and operated by the two most knowledgeable and devoted Gerson physicians in the world: Dr Alicia Melendez and Dr Luz Maria Bravo.

Tel: 0052 619-685-5353; Tel: (within US) 888-4-GERSON

CHIPSA, Center for Integrative Medicine, Playas de Tijuana, Tijuana, BC, Mexico

CHIPSA, the home of the Center for Integrative Medicine, is a full-service hospital where 24-hour care is provided by fully licensed physicians and nurses and a full range of on-call medical specialists. CHIPSA treats all forms of cancer. The Center is one of the few places in the world where patients can receive Coley's Toxins. They use a modified Gerson Diet. They also use the VG-1000 vaccine, CoQ10, ozone therapy, hyperthermia, laetrile, DMSO, Wobe enzymes, chelation, biological dentistry, diet, supplements and a variety of other approaches.

Tel:1-877-424-4772 or 1-877-4-CHIPSA; Tel 00 52 66 80-2903; Fax: 00 52 66 80-29-08; Website: www.chipsa.com

Gerson Healing Center of America, The Gerson Institute and the Oasis of Hope

The Gerson Healing Center of America has an office in Bonita, California, but the main clinic is in the Oasis of Hope in Mexico (see below). The Gerson Institute does not own, operate or control any treatment facility. They maintain a licensing programme with clinics to ensure that patients are receiving true, 100 per cent Gerson care. They advise you to ensure any clinic offering Gerson therapy is Gerson Institute Licensed to provide the genuine Gerson Therapy. They will also advise on how the Gerson Therapy can help you.

Tel: 001 (619) 685-5353; Tel: 1-888-4GERSON (within US)

New Hope Clinic, Tijuana, Mexico

Founded by Dr Stephen Linsteadt, ND, and directed by Dr Jorge Llamas, MD. It is best known for the use of BioElectric Cancer Therapy (ECT) based on the groundbreaking research of Dr Nordenstrom and Dr Pekar. Immune system modulators, innate immune enhancement vaccines, selective cytokines, therapeutic enzymes and mycoplasma vaccines, as well as natural and potent biological remedies from Germany are utilized in conjunction with bio-energetic therapies, which are tested for compatibility and effectiveness before being administered to the client. Quantum Medicine protocols and the use of bio-energetic technologies identify and eliminate the real cause of disease. Cancer is seen as the result of extreme dysregulation in the body's cellular respiration, communication and genetic systems. Therapies are aimed at removing the obstacles to self-regulation by cancelling out the electromagnetic hold of toxins and other pathological elements using bio-photon, bio-resonance and low level laser technologies. These technologies and natural substances, along with BioElectric Therapy, are used to re-establish optimal cellular and bio-electrical function thereby gently destroying cancerous cells or transforming them into healthy productive cells.

Emotional traumas and inner conflicts contributing to blockages in the body's energetic pathways are also assessed and effective self-healing modalities are employed.

Tel: 619-778-4454; Toll Free: 1-888-532-0897; E-mail: newhope@newhopeclinic.com; Website: www.newhopeclinic.com

Oasis of Hope Hospital (Contreras Clinic), Tijuana, Mexico

Also known as The Contreras Clinic, The Oasis of Hope Hospital has been treating cancer since 1963. It is run by Dr Ernesto Contreras, MD and his son, Dr Francisco Contreras, MD. They have treated over 100,000 patients over 35 years with a good success rate. The hospital is very clean and modern. The staff speak English. It is particularly famous for its long and successful use of laetrile and enzyme therapy, but they also have a cancer-prevention programme and offer a large variety of therapies including Managed Nutrition and the Body-Mind-and-Spirit approach. They are currently the only facility authorized by The Issel's Foundation to use the name of Issels and the Issels Treatment. The Issels Treatment Center is a separate entity within the Oasis hospital.

Oasis uses mostly alternative therapies, but in certain situations they may use a combination of both conventional and alternative therapies. For example, for liver cancer they use a combination of 5FU (chemotherapy) with laetrile and inject it directly into the liver. They are having good success with this approach. There are several programmes including a 4-day programme for people undergoing chemotherapy who want to complement it with alternative approaches.

Tel: 011 52 664 631 61 00 or 888 500-4673 (within US) to arrange a free phone consultation with one of their doctors; Website: www.oasisofhope.com

Stella Maris Clinic, Dr Alvarez, Tijuana, Mexico

Stella Maris Clinic offers help for the cancer patient and those with other degenerative diseases through natural methods, metabolic therapy and nutritional support. Their basic 21-day therapy includes detoxification, lymphatic massage, an IV cocktail of laetrile, DMSO and ascorbic acid, enzyme therapy, vaccine therapy, European mistletoe, nutritional guidance and individualized protocols to rebuild the immune system. This is a well-run, impressive clinic.

Tel: 011-52-66-46-343444; Tel: 800-662-1319 or 619-662-1319 (within US); Website: www.stellamarisclinic.com

New Zealand

Bay of Plenty Environmental Health Clinic, Tauranga

Run by Mike Godfrey, MBBS. In addition to cancer they treat Alzheimer's, cardiovascular disorders and other chronic diseases using nutrition, immuno-supportive therapies, detoxification, chelation, acupuncture and homoeopathy. They also do mercury amalgam investigations.

Tel: 0064 07 578 5899

Philippines

Bio Medical Health Center, Pasay City, Metro Manila

Treats chronic degenerative, vascular and heart diseases using homoeopathy, chelation and Chinese Medicine.

Tel: 0063-702-827-1444

Portugal

Health Center, Lisbon

Run by Serge Jurasunas, MD. It was established over 15 years ago. They treat most cancers, especially breast, stomach, prostate, colon, pancreas and brain; as well as multiple sclerosis, and Parkinson's. The therapies they use include: Geoxy 132, chitin, Ukrain therapy, bamboo leaf extract, SGE, SOD, LEM, aloe vera injections, xian tian, propermyl, DMSO, enzymatic, hematoxilan, live cell, tributyrrate, nucleic acid, and peptides.

Tel: 00351-1-347-1117

South America

Centro De Rejuvenecimiento Cellular Por Oxigenoterapia Hiperbarica, Palmira, Colombia

Uses adjuvant hyperbaric oxygen treatment, especially for those receiving radiation or chemotherapy, mostly breast and prostate cancers. They also use nutritional and vitamin therapy.

Tel: 0057 (02) 272 45 44; Fax: 0057 (02) 273 32 28

Medicina Bio Energetica, Dr Elias Bechara Simancas, Cali

Uses allopathic and alternative, including hyperbaric oxygen, Bio Energetic Medicine, homoeopathic medicine, acupuncture, chelation, vitamin and nutritional medicine.

Tel: 0057 (02) 661 78 36; E-mail: ebechasim@hotmail.com

Clinica de Medicina Biologica del Dr Arturo, Cali

Uses allopathic and alternative, including hyperbaric oxygen, Bio Energetic Medicine, homoeopathic medicine, acupuncture, chelation, vitamin and nutritional medicine.

Tel: 0057 (02) 554 12 87

Spain

J. Buxalleu Font, Barcelona

Treats solid tumours using self-vaccination with gamma globulin. Has used this therapy since 1965.

Tel: 0034 93 792 0489

Las Mariposas Clinic, Malaga, Spain and Barcelona

Treats any problem with chronic diseases and degeneration, especially cancer. Their clinic, as far as we know, is the only clinic in the world that offers a full refund of all clinical consultation fees to any cancer patient treated by them who does not see any noticeable improvements within 90 days after following their therapy. Their programme uses HLB – high blood resolution – analysis to allow them to tailor their approach to your specific endogenic (immune) status and hormonal needs, EAP (Electro-Acupuncture) treatment and Dr Budwig's protocol. They have recently opened a second clinic in Barcelona called the Centro de Medicinas Alternativas.

Tel: 0034 95 205 7171

Switzerland

Aeskulup, Brunnen

Has approaches similar to Klinik St Georg in Germany and they are a well-known clinic in Switzerland. They use classic homoeopathy, neural therapy, Traditional Chinese Medicine, acupuncture, anthroposophic medicine (mistletoe), fever therapy (hyperthermia), blood-oxygen therapy, ozone therapy, hyperthermia – whole-body and local – galvanotherapy and more.

Tel: 0041 41 825 48 61; E-mail: info@aeskulap.com; Website: www.aeskulap.com/e/index.htm

Lukas Klinik, Arlesheim

They use mistletoe in their treatment programmes. They aim to give special consideration not only to the physical situation of the sick individual but also to his or her soul and spirit. The work is based on the insights gained in anthroposophical medicine which was developed by Rudolf Steiner and Ita Wegman.

Tel: 0041 61 706 7171; Website: www.lukasklinik.ch/English/Default1.htm

Paracelsus Klinik Center for Holistic Medicine and Dentistry

Combines holistic medicine, naturopathic treatments and biological dentistry. They work with some clinics in the US.

Tel: 0041 (0)71 335 7171 or 7177

Serafin Naturheilpraxis AG, Wolfhalden

Uses electro-acupuncture, chiropractic, darkfield microscopy, laser therapy, pain management, immune system modulations and most natural healing methods for treating chronic diseases including cancer. This includes enzymes, mistletoe, thymus therapy, hyperthermia and vaccines.

Tel: 0041 (0)71 891 32 40; Fax: 0041 (0)71 891 32 47; E-mail: cheitz@searfin.ch; Website: www.serafin.ch/coco.htm

US

Please note that legislation in the US is much tighter than in Mexico and Central/South America, which is why many of the alternative cancer clinics are set up over the Mexican border.

American Biologics has an office in Chula Vista, but the clinic is in Mexico.

American Metabolic Institute has an office in San Diego, but the clinic is in Mexico.

Bio-Medical Center (Hoxsey Clinic) has an office in in San Ysidro, but the clinic is in Mexico.

Europa Institute of Integrated Medicine: contact a consultant for the clinic, Dr Carolyn Bormann, who has an office in Twin Peaks, but the clinic is in Mexico.

Genesis West Research Institute for Biological Medicine has an office in Irvine, but the Clinic is in Tijuana, Mexico

Gerson Healing Centers of America has an office in San Diego, but the main clinic is in Mexico at Oasis of Hope.

Institute of Chronic Disease has an office in San Ysidro, with a clinic in Mexico.

International BioCare Hospital and Medical Center is in Mexico – they use the Alivizatos Treatment.

Oasis Hospital has offices in San Ysidro and Chula Vista, but the clinic is in Mexico. It is also called the Contreras Clinic.

Arizona

Aidan Inc., Tempe

A research-based facility that provides complementary and unique approaches to treating cancer. Their treatment approach is designed to help stimulate a person's own immune system to recognize and attack tumour cells. They believe defective or inadequate antigen (cell surface information) presentation and inadequate T-cell recognition of tumour cells are the root cause of the development of most malignancies. They also believe that people with malignancies can have a much higher requirement of vitamin C and that vitamin C, given in adequate intravenous doses, can exert potent anti-tumour effects. They also use C-Statin as an antiangiogenesis inhibitor to enhance the effectiveness of immune-based therapies and a homoeopathic form of dendritic cell therapy.

Tel: 800-529-0269 (from inside the US only); Website: www.aidan-az.com

Integrative Health Care, PC, Scottsdale

Run by Alan Christianson, ND. Treats almost any type of cancer, even later-stage cancers. They use metabolic therapies for those not undergoing conventional care. For those doing conventional treatments, they use intravenous nutrition and botanical medicines to prevent side-effects and help efficacy of chemo/radiation.

Tel: 001 (480) 657-0003; Website: www.integrativehealthcare.com

Immune Therapies International (ITI)

Operate two clinics for people with cancer. One is in Dunwoody, Georgia (Atlanta area – see below) and the other is in Tucson, Arizona.

Their approach uses state-of the art medicine and diagnostic testing which will mobilize the body, mind, spirit and emotions towards ongoing health. Each participant's individualized treatment plan is developed by Dr Jesse A. Stoff MD (H), Director of Integrative Medicine, and his team of health professionals. ITI's model is integrative medicine at its best.

Tel: 001 (866) 471-4743; Website: www.immunerecovery.com/facilities.htm

Georgia

Atlanta Integrative Medical

The Atlanta clinic is located within the Progressive Medical Group. They work with cancer and many immune disorders. Their approach uses state-of-the-art medicine and diagnostic testing which will mobilize the body, mind, spirit and emotions towards ongoing health. Each participant's individualized treatment plan is developed by Dr Jesse A. Stoff MD (H), Director of Integrative Medicine and his team of health professionals. ITI's medical model is integrative medicine at its best.

Tel: 001 (866) 471-4743; Website: www.immunerecovery.com/atlanta.htm

Kentucky

The Foxhollow Clinic of Integrated Biological Medicine, Crestwood

Offers an individualized programme that may include intravenous therapies, metal detox, neuromuscular restructuring, neural therapy, cupping, juicing, immune-strengthening therapies, hormone balancing, stress management, mind–body approaches, nutrition, supplements, energy balancing – rebalancing the energy 'meridians' in your body through homoeopathy, TCM, European biological remedies and anthroposophical medicine. They are a partner clinic with Paracelsus Clinic in Switzerland.

Tel: 001 (502) 241-4304; Tel: (within US) (800) 624-7080; Fax: 001 (502) 241-3935; Website: www.Foxhollow.com

Michigan

Community Supported Anthroposophical Medicine (CSAM), Ann Arbor

Treats many chronic conditions. They have a waiting list for cancer patients. CSAM is a not-for-profit organization dedicated to providing patient care, education and research in healthcare through anthroposophical medicine. Approaches used include diet, iscador, homoeopathy, and adjunct approaches to conventional treatments, or stand alone.

Tel: 001 (734) 677-7990; Website: www.csamwebsite.org

New York

Michael B. Schachter, MD, The Schachter Center, Suffren

Michael is a very warm-hearted doctor for whom nothing seems to be too much trouble. He has had good responses with breast, lung and colon cancers; lymphoma and Hodgkin's. He also treats AIDS, neurological problems and candida. He uses detoxification, EDTA and DMPS chelation, laetrile, DMSO, co-enzyme Q10, hydrogen peroxide, shark cartilage, hydrazine sulfate, biomagnetic therapy and homoeopathy. Highly recommended.

Tel: 001 (845) 368-4700; Website: www.mbschachter.com

Washington

The Leo J. Bolles Clinic, Bellevue

Offers the following services: chelation therapy, IV vitamin therapies, homoeopathy, neural therapy, hydrogen peroxide, detoxification, heavy metal removal, antiviral IV therapy, electro-acupuncture, herbal medicine, oral vitamin therapy, dark field blood evaluation, thermographic analysis, EKG analysis, anti-cancer protocols, chronic fatigue therapies, fibromyalgia treatments, NAET and all phases of preventive medicine.

Tel: 001 (425) 881-2224; Website: www.bollesclinic.com

6. Integrated Medicine Doctors and Services

6.1 UK Integrated Medicine Doctors

These are doctors who offer guidance on the best use of complementary, alternative and orthodox medicine:

| Dr Rosy Daniel and Dr Pippa Harrold | Integrated Cancer Medicine Consultants at the author's centre in Bath | Tel: 01225 423333 |

Dr Roger Lichy	Homoeopath in Bristol and London	Tel: 0207 267 8487
Dr Sarah Miller	Integrated Cancer Medicine Consultant and Women's Medicine in Bristol	Tel: 01275 464149
Dr Michael Wetzler	Integrated Cancer Medicine Consultant in London and Baldock, Herts	Tel: 0207 935 5251 Tel: 01462 893586
Dr George Lewith	Integrated Cancer Medicine Consultant and Homoeopath in Southampton and London	Tel: 023 8033 4752
Dr Rajendra Sharma	Integrated Medicine Consultant and Homoeopath who also runs the Diagnostic Centre in London	Tel: 01425 461740 Tel: 0207 009 4650

6.2 US Integrated or Holistic Cancer Doctors

These are doctors who offer guidance on the best use of complementary, alternative and orthodox medicine:

| James Gordon MD | Integrated Medicine Physician and Director of the Center for Mind–Body Medicine which trains healthcare professionals to be CancerGuides to offer integrated care to those with cancer. | Tel: 001 (202) 966-7338 centre@cmbm.org |
| Dr Michael Lerner | Medical Director of Commonweal in California | Tel: 001 (415) 868 0970 www.commonweal.org |

| Joel Evans MD | Obstetrician, gynaecologist and expert in nutritional and functional medicine | Tel: 001 (203) 656-6635 JEvansMD@aol.com |
| Stephen Sagar MD | Radiation oncologist and acupuncture and reiki practitioner | Tel: 001 (905) 387 9495 Stephen.Sagar@hrcc.on.ca |

6.3 UK Integrated Medicine Services Offering Mind–Body Approaches, Self-help and Complementary Therapies

(For holistic support groups see page 372.)

Bristol Cancer Help Centre	Residential centre offering healing and positive healthcare to people affected by cancer and their supporters	Tel: 0117 980 9500 www.bristolcancerhelp.org
Cancer Bridge, Hexham	Residential centre offering healing and positive healthcare to people affected by cancer and their supporters	Tel: 01434 605551
Rainbow Centre, Bristol	Day centre providing holistic help for children and their carers	Tel: 0117 985 53343

6.4 International Holistic/Integrated Medicine Centres Offering Mind–Body Medicine and Complementary Health Care

| Ian Gawler Foundation, Australia | Yarra Valley Living Centre | Tel: 00 61 359 671730 www.gawler.org |
| Darinkja Zupan, Slovenia | National support service for those seeking to heal cancer | Tel: 00 386 652 5338 |

Tara McInty, Australia	The Sanctuary	Tel: 0061 352 584 562
Dr Michael Lerner, US	Commonweal, California	Tel: 001 (415) 868-0970 www.commonweal.org
Bernie Siegel website, ECap – Exceptional Cancer Patients	Bernie Siegel's site provides tools, information and resources based on the science of mind–body–spirit medicine for the challenges of all chronic illnesses.	www.ecap-online.org

7. Complementary Medicine Organizations for Finding Therapists

Find a practitioner by contacting one of these lead bodies:

7.1 General UK Complementary Umbrella Organizations

British Complementary Medical Association	The British Complementary Medical Association supports the integrity of its therapists and the quality standards with which complementary medicine is delivered to the public	Tel: 0845 345 5977 www.bcma.co.uk
British Dietetic Association	The association promotes training and education with the aim of advancing the science and practice of dietetics	5th Floor, Charles House 148/9 Great Charles Street Birmingham, B3 3HT Tel: 0121 200 8080 www.bda.uk.com
British Holistic Medical Association	An open membership association of professionals and members of	Tel: 01273 725951 www.bhma.org

the public who want to adopt a more holistic approach in their own life and work. Details of the *Journal of Holistic Healthcare*, links to other sites, self-help tapes. Referral possible

Complementary Medical Association	Comprehensive complementary referral service to help find a good practitioner	Tel: 08451 298434 www.the-cma.org.uk
Health Practitioners Association	A multi-disciplinary organization founded in 1935 to represent professional interests and to set standards of training and education for the benefit of patient and practitioner	3 Stoneleigh Drive, Carterton, Oxford, OX18 lEE. Tel: 01993 845805 or 01993 842422
Institute of Complementary Medicine	Directory of practitioners of all disciplines	Tel: 0207 237 5165 www.i-c-m.org.uk
Register of Holistic Health Practitioners (UK)	Register of alternative ayurvedic medicine practitioners, health visitors, nurses, physiotherapists	121 Coral Street, Leicestershire LE4 5BG (SAE please).
UK Therapists	Psychotherapists, counsellors and complementary practitioners	www.uktherapists.com

7.2 Therapeutic Umbrella Organizations for Finding Therapists

ACUPUNCTURE

British Acupuncture Council	Directory of acupuncturists	Tel: 0208 735 0400 www.acupuncture.org.uk

| The British Medical Acupuncture Society | Only fully accredited members of the British Medical Acupuncture Society, holding the Diploma of Medical Acupuncture, may be listed on this site. Individual members of the BMAS are UK-registered medical practitioners (doctors, dentists or vets) | Tel: 01606 786782 www.medical-acupuncture.co.uk |

ALEXANDER TECHNIQUE

| The Professional Association of Alexander Teachers | Practices throughout Britain, private lessons, introductory courses, etc. | Tel: 0121-449 0903 www.paat.org.uk |
| Society of Teachers of Alexander Technique | Physical therapy technique: directory of practitioners | 1st Floor, Linton House, 39-51 Highgate Road, London NW5 1RS Tel: 0845 230 7828 www.stat.org.uk |

ALLERGY THERAPISTS

| The British Institute for Allergy and Environmental Therapy | Maintains a Register of Practitioners specializing in allergy diagnosis and treatment. Information and local lists of therapists | Ffynnonwen, Llangwyrfon, Aberystwyth SY23 4EY Tel: 01974 241376 www.allergy.org.uk |

AROMATHERAPISTS

| The Aromatherapy Organisations Council | This is the UK governing body for aromatherapy, representing 13 professional associations and 85 training establishments | PO BOX 6522, Desborough, Kettering, NN14 2YX Tel/Fax: 0870 7743477 www.aocuk.net |

CHINESE MEDICINE

College of Integrated
Chinese Medicine — Information, clinic, training clinic, register of practitioners. Low-cost treatment available — Tel: 0118 950 8880
www.cicm.org.uk

International College of
Oriental Medicine — Information and training clinic — Tel: 01342 313106/7
www.orientalmed.ac.uk

Register of Chinese
Herbal Medicine — Register of practitioners and information — RCHM, Office 5,
Ferndale Business Centre,
1 Exeter Street, Norwich
NR2 4QB
Tel: 01603 623994
www.rchm.co.uk

CHIROPRACTORS

The British
Chiropractic Association — Members registered with the BCA have completed a minimum of four years' full-time training, graduating with the following qualifications: D.C. B.App.Sc. (Chiro), BSc (Chiro) — Blagrave House,
17 Blagrave Street,
Reading, Berkshire
RG1 1QB
Tel: 0118 950 5950
www.chiropractic-uk.co.uk

CRANIOSACRAL THERAPY

Craniosacral Therapy
Association — Monomark House,
27 Old Gloucester Street,
London, WC1N 3XX
Tel: 07000 784 735
www.craniosacral.co.uk

DOWSING

British Society of Dowsers — Sycamore Barn,
Hastingleigh, Ashford,
Kent TN25 5HU
Tel: 01233 750253
www.britishdowsers.org

FELDENKRAIS

The Feldenkrais Guild UK	Help with mobility through sophisticated and sensitive physical therapy to re-educate new muscle and nerve reflexes when movement may has been disturbed by brain or nerve damage	Leila Malcolm, East Holcombe, Shillingford, Tiverton, Devon EX10 9BR Tel: 07000 785506 www.feldenkrais.co.uk

HEALERS

The British Alliance of Healing Associations	Directory of Healing Organizations (Member of the Confederation of Healing Associations)	For healers in your area contact Mr Wallace Tel: 01502 742224 www.bahahealing.co.uk
Healing Research	For validation of healing see The International Journal of Healing and Caring – online	www.ijhc.org
National Federation of Spiritual Healers	Healer referral service worldwide	Tel: 0845 123 2767 www.nfsh.org.uk
The White Eagle Lodge	Worldwide association of registered healers	Tel: 01730 893300 www.whiteagle.org

HERBALISTS AND FLOWER ESSENCES

Dr Edward Bach Centre	Advisory Centre for Bach Flower Remedies. Professional register of fully qualified therapists trained at the Bach Centre. Details of local practitioners on request	Mount Vernon, Sotwell, Wallingford, Oxon OX1O OPZ Tel: 01491 834678 www.bachcentre.com
Healing Herbs	Help with herbs	PO Box 65, Hereford, HR2 0UW Tel: 01873 890218 www.healing-herbs.co.uk

| National Institute of Medical Herbalists | Directory of qualified herbalists | 56 Longbrook Street, Exeter, EX4 6AH Tel: 01392 426 022 www.nimh.org.uk |

| Register of Chinese Herbal Medicine | Register of practitioners and information | RCHM, Office 5, Ferndale Business Centre, 1 Exeter Street, Norwich NR2 4QB Tel: 01603 623994 www.rchm.co.uk |

HOMOEOPATHS

| The British Homoeopathic Association | Accurate and helpful information about homoeopathy. Directory of homoeopaths | Hahnemann House, 29 Park Street West, Luton LU1 3BE Tel: 0870 444 3950 www.trusthomeopathy.org |

| Glasgow Homoeopathic Hospital | Homoeopathic and iscador treatment | Tel: 0141 211 600 |

| Homoeopathic Medical Association | Represents professional homoeopaths and promotes homoeopathy | www.homeopathy.org |

| Royal London Homeopathic Hospital NHS Trust | Information about homoeopathy and iscador and homoeopathic treatment with Dr Sosie Cassab | Tel: 0207 833 8897 |

| The United Kingdom Homeopathic Medical Association | Qualified homoeopaths (NHNA) bound by a code of ethics, covered by professional indemnity insurance, register on request | 6 Livingstone Road, Gravesend, Kent, DA12 5DZ Tel/Fax: 01474 560336 www.homoeopathy.org |

HYPNOTHERAPISTS

British Society of Clinical Hypnotherapists	A nationwide list of ethical practitioners	The Organising Secretary, 125 Queensgate, Bridlington, East Yorkshire YO16 7JQ Tel: 01262 403103 E-mail: sec@bsch.org.uk www.bsch.org.uk

MASSAGE

British Federation of Massage Practitioners	A professional organization offering membership and insurance to professionally qualified therapists	78 Medow Street, Preston PR1 7BH. Tel/Fax: 01772 881 063 www.jolanta.co.uk
The Massage Training Institute	High quality professional training in Holistic Massage – National Register of M.T.I Practitioners (ethical and insured)	PO Box 44603, London N16 0XQ Tel: 020 7254 7227 www.massagetraining.co.uk

NUTRITIONAL THERAPY

British Association of Nutritional Therapists	Professional body providing lists of nutritional therapists and telephone numbers	Tel: 0870 6061284 www.bant.org.uk
Nutrition Society		www.nutritionsociety.org

OSTEOPATHY

The General Council & Register of Osteopaths	Directory of Osteopaths	Goswell House, 2 Goswell Road, STREET, BA16 0JG Tel: 08707 456984 www.naturopathy.org.uk

REFLEXOLOGY

Association of Reflexologists	For reliable information about registered professional practitioners; accredited training courses; membership – including quarterly journals, seminars and support groups; speakers and presenters. Please send 9" x 7" SAE	27 Old Gloucester Street, London WC1 3XX. Tel: 0870 5673320 or 01273 771061
International Institute of Reflexology (UK) membership	For a fully trained, insured, professional practitioner in reflexology in your area, with the use of the IIR Dip. or MIIR regd	Head Office, 255 Turleigh, Bradford on Avon, Wiltshire, BA15 2HG Tel/Fax: 01225 865899
Reflexology Society	Initials: MRXS or FRXS, Insurance and Code of Ethics, member of BCMA and ICM. Send an SAE for your local practitioner and membership details. Talks and demonstrations can be arranged	127 Bullbrook Drive, Bracknell, Berkshire, RG12 2QR. Tel: 01344 429770
The Scottish Institute of Reflexology	For details of the membership list of qualified reflexologists, contact the Secretary	Flat 1/2, 110 Easterhouse Road, Glasgow, G34 9RG Tel: 0141 773 0018 www.scottish reflexology.org

REIKI

The Reiki Association		Cornbrook Bridge House Clee Hill, Ludlow, Shropshire SY8 3QQ Tel: 01584 891197 www.reikiassociation.org.uk

The United Kingdom Reiki Alliance		PO Box 114, Stowmarket, Suffolk, IP14 4WA Tel: 01449 673449 www.reikialliance.co.uk

SHIATSU

The European Shiatsu Network	Co-ordinates comprehensive training courses throughout Europe leading to professional shiatsu qualifications	Highbanks, Lockeridge, Marlborough, Wiltshire, SN8 4EQ Tel: 01672 861362
The Shiatsu Society	The umbrella organization for shiatsu in the UK, providing a quarterly newsletter and overseeing the professional register of shiatsu Therapists. Registered Practitioners use Initial MRSS and have trained at an approved school	Suite B, Barber House, Storey's Bar Road, Fengate, Peterborough PE1 5YN Tel: 0845 1304560 or 01788 555051 www.shiatsu.org

8. Counselling Organizations for Finding Therapists

Association of Humanistic Psychology Practitioners	Psychology information and directory of practitioners	Tel: 08457 660326 or 0845 707 8506 www.ahpp.org
Association of Professional Therapists	Register of Hypnotherapists, with high standards of training and ethics	Katepwa House, Ashfield Park Avenue, Ross-on-Wye, Herefordshire HR9 5AX Tel: 01989 566 676 www.hypnotherapists.org

British Association for Counselling and Psychotherapy	Information, ethical framework, training, publications, online directory for therapists in your area	Tel: 0870 443 5252 www.bacp.co.uk
British Association of Psychotherapists	Directory of practitioners	37 Mapesbury Road, London NW2 4HJ Tel: 0208 4529823 www.bap-psychotherapy.org
The British Psychoanalytical Society	Directory of practitioners	112a Shirland Road, Maida Vale, London, W9 2EQ Tel: 0207 563 5000 www.psychoanalysis.org.uk
The Cancer Counselling Trust	A charity offering holistic counselling for those with cancer and their supporters	Tel: 0207 704 1137 www.cctrust.org.uk
Centre for Transpersonal Psychology	Courses and Directory of Transpersonal Therapists with a good website to find therapists in your area. Highly recommended for holistic counselling	Tel: 0208 203 6671 www.transpersonal centre.co.uk
Family Therapy	Family Centre	Tel: 0207 854 5880
Institute of Family Therapy	Counselling for recently bereaved families and those with seriously-ill family members	Tel: 0207 391 9150 www.instituteoffamily therapy.org.uk

Institute for Group Analysis	Directory of practitioners	Tel: 0207 431 2693 www.igalondon.org.uk
London Centre for Psychotherapy	Counselling and psychotherapy	32 Leighton Road, Kentish Town, London NW5 2QE Tel: 020 7482 2002/2282 www.lcp-psychotherapy.org.uk
National Association of Holistic Hypnotherapists	Send SAE for list	19 St George's Avenue, Northampton, NN2 6JA www.nahh.skynet.co.uk
Neuro-Linguistic Programming (NLP)	A modern method of re-programming the thought processes to effect transformation; Directory of Practitioners	Tel: 0870 870 4970 (Monday–Thursday, 9.00am to 12.00pm, answerphone at most other times) www.anlp.org
Psychosynthesis Counselling and Psychotherapy Service at the Psychosynthesis and Education Trust	Excellent holistic counselling – highly recommended for those with cancer	92–94 Tooley Street, London Bridge, London, SE1 2TH Tel: 020 7403 2100 www.psychosynthesis.edu/counselling
The Psychotherapy Centre	Counselling and psychotherapy	67 Upper Berkeley Street, London, W1H 7QX Tel: 020 7723 6173 www.the-psychotherapy-centre.org.uk

United Kingdom Council for Psychotherapy (UKCP)	Overseeing accrediting body	167–169 Great Portland Street, London W1W 5PF Tel: 020 7436 3002 www.psychotherapy. org.uk

COUPLES COUNSELLING

British Association for Sexual and Relationship Therapy	Couple counselling	PO Box 13686 London, SW20 9ZH Tel: 020 8543 2707 www.basrt.org.uk
Couple Counselling, Scotland	Couple counselling	Tel: 01382 640340 www.couplecounselling. org
RELATE	Couple counselling	Herbert Gray College, Little Church Street, Rugby, Warwickshire CV21 3AP Tel: 0845 456 1310 Helpline: 0845 130 4010 www.relate.org.uk

9. Self-help Organizations for Finding Classes or Teachers

9.1 General Umbrella Group

UK Self Help	Guide to self-help organizations and internet groups for medical conditions, many for cancer	www.ukselfhelp.info

9.2 Specific Therapies

AUTOGENIC TRAINING

British Association for Autogenic Training	For relaxation and stress management	The Royal London Homoeopathic Hospital, Greenwell Street, London W1W 5BP Tel/Fax: 020 7383 5108

BIOFEEDBACK

Aleph One Ltd., Laurie van Someren at Aleph One Ltd	Provide instruments that feed back signals that indicate muscle activity and relaxation levels	The Old Courthouse, Bottisham, Cambridge CB5 9BA Tel: 01223 811 679 info@aleph1.co.uk

CHI GONG

Qigong Southwest	Qigong (Chi Gong) classes	www.qigong-southwest.co.uk

DANCE

Biodanza – The Dance of Life	System of human integration and growth stimulated by music, movement, rhythm and emotions	Tel: 0208 392 1433 www.biodanza.co.uk
5 Rhythms Moving Centre	Gabrielle Roth's 5 Rhythms Movement Practice facilitates the human need to dance, express, create, let go and find a purpose and connection	www.5rhythmsuk.com

MEDITATION

Friends of the Western Buddhist Order	Classes and courses in meditation and in Buddhism	Tel: 020 8981 8000 www.fwbo.org

Rigpa	Buddhist Meditation Centre	Tel: 0207 700 0185
Transcendental Meditation	Regular classes with ongoing support and refresher classes. Great quality but very expensive	Tel: 08705 143733 www.transcendental-meditation.org.uk
Vipassana Meditation	Theraveda Buddhist Meditation	Tel: 01380 850238 www.ubakhin.com
West London Buddhist Centre	Meditation classes	Tel: 0845 458 5461

RELAXATION

Relaxation for Living Trust	Relaxation Classes	12 New Street, Chipping Norton, Oxon. 0X7 5LF Tel: 01608 646100

STRESS MANAGEMENT

International Stress Management Association	ISMA (UK) is the professional association for people whose work centres on stress management. It exists for the spread of sound knowledge, the maintenance of quality and to resource its members. For general information, send a large stamped, self-addressed envelope	PO Box 348, Waltham Cross EN8 8ZL Tel: 07000 780430 Email: stress@isma.org.uk www.isma.org.uk

TAI CHI

Rising Dragon	Tai Chi teachers' register	Tel: 01432 840860 www.risingdragontaichi.com

TANTRA

Diamond Light Tantra	Tantra training for individuals and couples. Tantra holidays	Tel: 08700 780 584 www.diamondlight tantra.co.uk
School of Awakening	Yogic-bases and tantra training	Tel: 01769 581232 E-mail: info@schoolof awakening.com
Shakti Tantra	Tantra for women	Tel: 01453 752256 www.shaktitantra.co.uk
Sky Dancing Tantra	Tantra training for individuals and couples	Tel: 01865 428374 www.tantralaboratory.com
Tantra Studio	Tantra workshops for individuals and couples	Tel: 01736 788304 www.tantrastudio.co.uk
Transcendence	Tantra training course and information	Tel: 0845 345 8593 www.tantra.uk.com

TRANSFORMATIONAL RITUALS

Spirit Horse Nomadic Circle	Ceremonial transformational workshops held amid 2,000 acres in the Welsh countryside	Tel: 0208 346 3660 www.spirithorse.co.uk

VISUALIZATION

Image Work Association	Dina Glouberman specializes in the use of imagery for personal, professional and management development. She runs the Imagework training courses	Tel: 0870 7875183 www.imagework.co.uk

VOICE

Chloë Goodchild	The Naked Voice workshops	Tel: 0117 927 7020 www.thenakedvoice.com
Jill Purce's Healing Voice Workshops	Sacred chant, breathing and sonorous meditation, ceremonial healing workshops	Tel: 0207 435 2467 www.healingvoice.com

YOGA

British Wheel of Yoga	Information on all aspects of yoga and its practice, network of local branches	Tel: 01529 306 851 www.bwy.org.uk
Yoga Biomedical Trust	Yoga therapy for low back pain, asthma, ME and other stress related conditions	Yoga Therapy Centre, 90–92 Pentonville Street, London, N1 9HS Tel: 020 7689 3040
Yoga For Health Foundation	Yoga therapy and courses	Ickwellbury, Ickwell Green, Near Biggleswade, Bedfordshire SG18 9EF Tel: 01767 627271 www.yogaforhealth foundation.co.uk

10. Support Services

10.1 General Information about Support

BBC Website for cancer	Very good site – lots of information on cancer, treatment, helplines, organizations, support, prevention	www.bbc.co.uk/health/cancer

Cancer Advice	An informative and up-to-date resource for people with cancer – support groups, cancer links, advice centre, ask for opinion, current issues, advice leaflets, etc. Managed by Dr Nick Plowman, leading oncologist, London	www.canceradvice.co.uk
CancerBACUP Scotland	Face-to-face counselling	Tel: 0141 553 2686 www.cancerbacup.org.uk
Cancer Information and Support Centre	For emotional support, information on all aspects of cancer, information on self-help groups local and nationwide	Tel: 0117 928 3369
CancerLink	UK information network and support. Can help bring patients, carers and professionals together in various ways, e.g. Cancer Voice. Has joined forces with Macmillan – same helpline, etc. On-line search engine to find a support group	Tel: 0800 132 905 or 0800 808 0000 www.cancerlink.org
CLAN (Cancer Link Aberdeen and North)	Support and self-help. Centre in Aberdeen offers a wide range of services	Tel: 01224 647000 Freephone: 0800 783 7922 www.clanhouse.org
Cancer Support UK	NHS site for information and support. Information is excellent, but site can be difficult to navigate. Includes sections on obtaining community and emotional support, practical help,	www.cancersupportuk. nhs.uk

	complementary therapies, etc. Also available in Gujerati and Punjabi	
Irish Cancer Society	Information, home-care funding, support groups, nursing	Tel: 00 353 1 800 200 700
Macmillan CancerLine	Publishes directory of cancer support and care organizations in the UK, with telephone numbers, addresses and website addresses; Macmillan CancerLine; can provide financial help and special nurses in hospital and in homes	Freephone: 0808 808 2020, Monday to Friday, 9 a.m. to 6 p.m. for information and emotional support for people living with cancer www.macmillan.org.uk
Macmillan Cancer Relief, Northern Ireland		Tel: 028 9066 1166
Macmillan Cancer Relief, Scotland		Tel: 0131 229 3276
Macmillan Cancer Relief, Wales		Tel: 01446 775679
National Cancer Alliance	Patient and healthcare professionals, co-ordinating services, care and treatment available for people affected by cancer	Tel: 0870 770 2646 www.nationalcancer alliance.co.uk
Northern Cancer Network	Information about cancer services in the northern areas of the UK	www.cancernorth.nhs.uk

| PAC Project – Positive Action on Cancer | Free professional counselling service | Tel: 01373 455255 www.pacproject.org |
| Women's Health | Can put you in touch with self-help support networks | Helpline: 0845 125 5254 www.womenshealthlondon. org.uk |

10.2 Holistic Support Groups

ABACUS The Cancer Self Help Support Group, Bromley	Holistic support	Tel: 0208 467 2565
ABC Support Group, Jersey	Holistic support	Tel: 01534 498980
Bearstead Holistic Cancer and Stress Self Help and Support Centre, Maidstone	Holistic support	Tel: 01622 730133
Breast Cancer Care	Support and information for women and their families	Helpline: 0808 800 6000 www.breastcancercare. org.uk
Breast Cancer Haven	Holistic support and free therapies	Tel (London): 020 7384 0000 Tel (Hereford): 01432 361 061 www.breastcancerhaven. org.uk
Breast Care Campaign	Information on benign breast disorders; campaigns to raise awareness of breast health	www.breastcare.co.uk

Bridport Healing and Cancer Care Centre	Holistic support	Tel: 01308 422459
Camborne/Redruth Cancer Support	Holistic support	Tel: 01726 843576
Cambridge Cancer Help Centre	Holistic support	Tel: 01223 566151
The Cancer Resource Centre	Holistic support	Tel: 0207 924 3924
CancerVIVE Gentle Approach to Cancer Association, Cleveleys	Holistic support	Tel: 01772 682051
Cavendish Cancer Care	Holistic support	27 Wilkinson Street, Sheffield Tel: 0114 278 4600 www.cavcare.org Helpline: 0208 202 4567 General Info: 0208 202 2211
Cherry Lodge Cancer Care, London	Holistic support	Tel: 0208 216 4486
Crawley Cancer Contact Mike Vincent Sue Evans	Holistic support	Tel: 01342 325538 Tel: 01403 823850
Emsworth Cancer Support Group, Hants	Holistic support	Tel: 01243 377913

Gentle Approach to Cancer Association, Blackpool, July Gaywood	Holistic support	Tel: 01772 682051
Gentle Approach to Cancer Association, Cumbria	Holistic support	Tel: 01539 621307
Gentle Approach to Cancer Association, Lancs, Colin Sunderland	Holistic support	Tel: 01772 705465
Macclesfield & District Cancer Support Group	Holistic support	Tel: 01625 828961
Mansfield Self Help Cancer Group	Holistic support	Tel: 01623 624632
Manx Cancer Help Association, Isle of Man	Holistic support	Tel: 01624 852825
The Melangell Centre, Oswestry	Holistic support	Tel: 01691 860408 www.st-melangell.org.uk
Natural Healing Group, Leeds	Holistic support	Tel: 0113 268 5724
New Approaches to Cancer	This is a charity that promotes complementary therapies and holistic treatment for cancer patients and carers. Information and referral service, network of support groups and practitioners	Tel: 0800 389 2662 www.anac.org.uk

Newark Cancer Help Group	Holistic support	Tel: 01636 525655
North East London Cancer Help Centre	Holistic support	Tel: 0208 597 0024
Northumberland Cancer Support Group	Holistic support	Tel: 0191 410 2679 / Tel: 0191 251 0935
Primrose Self Help Centre, Bromsgrove	Holistic support	Tel: 01527 878 780
SASH Support & Self Help, Bristol	Holistic support	Tel: 0117 935 8880
Slánú, Galway Cancer Help Centre	Holistic support	Tel: 00 353 9175 5023 or 00 353 9158 0050
South East Cancer Help Centre	Holistic support	Tel: 0208 668 0974
Stevenage Cancer Support Group	Holistic support	Tel: 01438 352793
Swansea Cancer Self Help Group	Holistic support	Tel: 01792 794233
Tak Tent Cancer Support, Scotland	Information, support, self-help groups, counselling service, complementary therapies and youth service	Tel: 0141 211 1932 www.taktent.org.uk
Tapping House Hospice, Norfolk	Holistic support	Tel: 01485 543163

Tavistock Cancer Support Group	Holistic support	Tel: 01822 613082
Wessex Cancer Help Centre	Holistic support	Tel: 01243 778516
Yorkshire Cancer Help Centre	Holistic support	Tel: 0113 216 8894

10.3 Support Groups by Type of Cancer

Beating Bowel Cancer	Information for bowel cancer sufferers	Tel: 0208 892 5256 www.bowelcancer.org
Bladder Cancer Web Cafe	Tests, treatments, support	www.blcwebcafe.org
Bowel Cancer Forum	Works to raise awareness of early warning signs of bowel cancer	Tel: 0207 381 4711
Brain Tumour Action	Support, information, counselling, research	www.braintumour action.org.uk
Brain Tumor Society	American Brain Tumour Society site. Excellent explanations and information on treatment options	www.tbts.org
Brain Tumour Society (UK)	Non-medical support site	www.ukbts.org.uk
Breakthrough Breast Cancer	Fighting breast cancer through research and awareness	www.breakthrough.org.uk

British Brain and Spine Foundation	Helpline provides information and support about neurological disorders for patients, carers and health professionals	Tel: 0808 808 1000 (Mon, Tue, Thu, Fri 9 a.m. – 1 p.m., Wed 10 a.m. – 6 p.m.)
British Colostomy Association	Information, advice and support from those who have experience of living with a colostomy	Tel: 0800 328 4257 www.bcass.org.uk
Colon Cancer Concern	Dedicated solely to colorectal cancer	www.coloncancer.org.uk
Disabled Living Foundation	Expert and impartial advice about specialist equipment	Tel: 0845 130 9177 (Mon-Fri 10 a.m. – 4 p.m.) www.dlf.org.uk
Eyecare Foundation	Information relating to all cancers affecting the eyes	www.eyecarefoundation .org
Hodgkin's Disease	Mailing list and information site	www.hodgkinsdisease.org
International Myeloma Foundation UK		www.myeloma.org.uk Tel: 0800 980 3332
Kidney Cancer UK	Kidney Cancer Association. Excellent resource and organization information	www.kcuk.org Tel: 024 7647 4993
Leukaemia CARE Society	The Leukaemia CARE Society, caring for sufferers of the leukaemias, Hodgkin's and other lymphomas, myelodysplasia, myeloproliferative disorders, myeloma and aplastic anaemia	Tel: 01905 330003 Careline: 0800 169 6680 www.leukaemiacare.org

Leukaemia Research Fund	Information about research currently underway for leukaemia	43 Great Ormond Street, London, WC1N 3JJ Tel: 0207 405 0101 www.lrf.org.uk
Liver Cancer Network	Based at Allegheny General Hospital. Provides information about treatment options	www.livercancer.com
Lymphoedema Support Network	Information, newsletters, telephone support – recorded message giving helplines	Tel: 0207 351 4480 www.lymphoedema.org
Lymphoma Association	Provides emotional support and information on a range of issues to anyone with lymphatic cancer and to their families, carers and friends	Helpline: 0808 808 5555 (Mon-Fri 9 a.m. – 5 p.m.) Tel: 01296 619400 www.lymphoma.org.uk
Lymphoma Information Network	Information on lymphoma, Hodgkin's disease and Non-Hodgkin's lymphoma	www.lymphomainfo.net
Mind over Matter	Increasing the awareness of testicular cancer, self-help and support, befriending	Tel: 01703 775 611
National Osteoporosis Society	Help and information for osteoporosis sufferers of all ages	Tel: 0845 4500 230
Neuroblastoma Society	Cancer of the nervous system: support groups and information	Tel: 01727 851818

Oesophageal Patients Association	Support, advice, visits, free leaflets for people with cancer affecting speech, larynx, vocal cords	Tel: 0121 704 9860
Oral Cancer Foundation	Oral cancer resources	www.oralcancer.org
Ovacome	UK-wide support group for all those concerned with ovarian cancer	www.ovacome.org.uk
Ovarian Cancer		Tel: 0207 600 5141
Pancreatic Cancer		Tel: 0121 449 0667 www.pancan.org
Pancreatic Cancer Online	Orthodox and alternative approaches to treatment	www.healthyfoundations .com/pancreatic
Prostate Cancer Charity	Information, self-help networks	Helpline: 0845 300 8883 www.prostate-cancer.org.uk
Prostate Cancer Support Association		www.prostatecancer support.co.uk
Prostate Cancer Support Group	For the West of England	Tel: 01761 411 580
Prostate Help Association	Information, newsletter, support network	Philip@prostatecancer. org.uk
(Prostate) Us Too! International	Large, independent, charitable network of education and support groups for men with prostate cancer and their families	www.ustoo.com

RareCancer.org	Difficult-to-find information on rare cancers	www.markmcc/RARE_CANCERS
Retinoblastoma Society	Information and support for people with eye and vision difficulties, research, publications	Tel: 0207 377 5578 Tel: 0207 600 3309 www.rbsociety.org.uk
Roy Castle Lung Cancer Foundation	Lung cancer nurses offering information, guidance and support to lung cancer patients and families	Helpline: 0800 358 7200 www.roycastle.org
Roy Castle Lung Cancer Foundation, Scotland		Tel: 0141 331 0580 email: glasgow@roycastle.liv.ac.uk
Sarcoma.net	Treatments, clinical trials in the US	www.sarcoma.net
Sarcoma Survivors	Support group, message board	www.sarcomasurvivors.com
Skin Cancer Foundation	Covers all types of skin cancer	www.skincare.org
Wessex Cancer Trust	Wessex Cancer Trust: home of the UK's only dedicated skin cancer helpline: 'Marc's Line', a phone line for men with cancer. Mutual support and self-help	Tel: 02380 772200 www.wessexcancer.org

10.4 Support Groups by Disability

| Ali's Dream | Childhood brain tumours | Tel: 0208 863 6068 |

Changing Faces	Counselling and social skills training workshops for people with facial disfigurements	Tel: 0207 706 4232 www.changingfaces.co.uk
Courage	National organization for radiotherapy damage support – mental and physical (non medical advice)	Tel: 0161 839 2927
Dial UK (Disablement Information & Advice Lines)	Information and advice on any disability	Tel: 01302 310 123 www.dialuk.org.uk
Laryngectomy Association of Ireland	Support Group	Tel: 00 353 1 668 1855
Let's Face It	Self-help group for those with facial disfigurement, Yateley, Hants	Tel: 01252 879630 www.letsfaceit.force9 .co.uk
National Association of Laryngectomee Clubs	Promotes welfare of laryngectomees within the British Isles	Tel: 0207 381 9993
Radiotherapy Injured Patients Support (RIPS)	Informal mutual support for those with radiotherapy damage	Tel: 01206 395 6106
Rage, London	Breast support and guidance to women who have sustained radiotherapy damage after treatment for breast cancer	Tel: 0208 460 7476
Rage, Manchester	National organization for radiotherapy damage support – mental and physical (non-medical advice)	Tel: 0161 839 2927

| Royal Association for Disability & Rehabilitation (RADAR) | Information on aids, equipment, access, holidays, mobility, leisure, campaigning for people with disability | Tel: 0207 250 3222 |
| Urostomy Association | Advice on appliances before and after surgery; also on practical problems | Tel: 01245 224 294 www.uagbi.org |

10.5 Support Groups by Gender, Religion, Ethnic or Minority Group

Black Network	A CancerLink support service for people affected by cancer from African-Caribbean, Asian and Chinese communities	Tel: 08088 080 000
Cancer Black Care	Addressing needs of black and ethnic minority patients	16 Dalston Lane, London E8 3AZ Tel: 020 7249 1097 www.cancerblackcare.org
Chai-Lifeline	Support, friendship and information for Jewish cancer patients and their families	Tel: 0208 202 2211 Helpline: 0208 202 4567
Gay & Lesbian Bereavement Project	Telephone helpline, same-sex difficulties, bereavement	Tel: 0208 455 8894
Gayscan	Information, self-help and support to gay men living with cancer, North Finchley, London	Tel: 0208 446 3896

Lesbian Network	A CancerLink support network for lesbians affected by cancer	Tel: 0800 132 905
London Lesbian and Gay Switchboard	Emotional support	Tel: 0207 837 7324
Women's Health	Can put you in touch with self-help support networks	Tel: 0845 125 5254

10.6 Support Groups for Children and Young Adults

ACT (Association for Children with Life-threatening or Terminal Conditions)	Information on support services for families whose children have life-threatening or terminal conditions	Tel: 0117 922 1566 www.act.org.uk
Cancer & Leukaemia in Childhood Trust (CLIC)	Support and advice for parents of children with Leukaemia and childhood cancer	Tel: 0117 311 2600 www.clic.uk.com
Captain Chemo Website	Animated cartoon site for children. Captain chemo takes them on an adventure as they learn about cancer treatments	www.royalmarsden .org/captchemo
CHIC	Children's cancer support group in Clwyd, North Wales	Tel: 01352 754 154
Christian Lewis Children's Cancer Care	Charity providing financial help for children and their families to improve quality of life. Information on respite care, local support groups, etc.	Tel: 01792 480500 www.childrens-cancer-care.org.uk

Compassionate Friends	Befriending for those who have lost a child. Bereavement self-help group	Tel: 0117 953 9639 www.tcf.org.uk
Family Funds	Some financial help for parents of chronically sick children. Help with bedding, clothing, etc.	Tel: 01904 621 115
Helen House Hospice	Hospice for children, offering short-term and terminal care	Tel: 01865 728 251
Help Adolescents with Cancer	Counselling, meetings and support for families and siblings of young people with cancer	Tel: 0161 688 6244 www.mwmsites.com/hawc
Rainbow Centre	Centre for children with cancer and life-threatening illness	Tel: 0117 985 3343
Rainbow House	Children's nursing, support, short-stays and holiday	Tel: 01372 453 309
Rainbow Trust	Provides carers and nursing for children with life-threatening disease	Tel: 01372 363 438 Tel: 01372 453 309
Sargent Cancer Care for Children	Provides financial assistance and practical help for parents of children with cancer. It can arrange short breaks for families and young people at specialist centres in Scotland and South London	www.sargent.org Tel: 0208 752 2800

Teenage Cancer Trust	20 specialist units to treat and care for adolescents suffering from cancer	Tel: 0207 387 1000 www.teencancer.org
Ulster Cancer Foundation	Support groups, helpline, counselling, rehabilitation support, information services, childhood and young adults' cancer support	Tel: 028 9066 3281 Helpline: 0800 783 3339 (Mon-Fri 9 a.m. – 5 p.m.) www.ulstercancer.org

10.7 Support Groups Offering Help with Sexuality Issues

Impotence Association	Advice and support for sufferers and their partners. Send SAE for further information	PO Box 10296, London SW17 9WH Helpline: 0208 767 7791 www.impotence.org.uk
Sexual & Personal Relationships of The Disabled (SPOD)	Association to aid the sexual and personal relationships of people with disabilities	286 Camden Road, London N7 0BJ Tel: 020 7607 8851 www.spod-uk.com
Sexual & Personal Relationships of The Disabled	Advice about personal relationships for the disabled	The Diorama, IA Peto Place, London NWl 4DT
Tantra	Classes and one-to-one help to develop sensuality and sexuality within a yogic framework	See self-help organizations

10.8 Support Groups to Help You Face Pain

| Pain Association Scotland | Chronic pain management, support groups, bereavement counselling | Tel: 0131 312 7955 |

10.9 Support Groups to Help You Face Death and Dying

| Natural Death Centre | Counselling, workshops, living wills, advice on alternative funerals | Tel: 0208 208 2853 www.naturaldeath.org.uk |
| Upaya Zen Center New Mexico | Offering a programme on being with the dying | Tel: 001 (505) 986-8518 www.upaya.org |

10.10 Support Groups Offering Care for the Carers

2Higher Ground	Registered charity offering seven hours of free coaching to carers, or former carers, of cancer patients. Qualified life coaches offer coaching, therapy, advocacy and career counselling, as required by the client	www.2higherground. org.uk
Action Cancer (Northern Ireland)	Full-time screening clinics for breast and cervical cancer. Workshops and information for men on detecting prostate and testicular cancer	Tel: 028 9080 3344 www.actioncancer.org
AQU	This website is dedicated to people who care for friends or	www.aqu.co.uk/carers

relatives with disabilities. It contains important factual information regarding benefits, and is of special use to those people who are not aware of the help that they are entitled to. There is some heartfelt information about coping with stress, including ways of identifying and removing it. This site will also enable people without direct experience to gain an insight into the lives of carers who so often go unseen. This is a time to appreciate the 8.5 million people who selflessly devote their time and energy to help others who are less fortunate than themselves

Carers' National Association	Information, advice and contacts for carers. Branches nationwide	Tel: 0207 490 8818
CarersNet	Official website of the Coalition of Carers in Scotland – an information network designed for carers, carer groups and organizations, and for people working with carers. Links to other useful carers' websites including Carers Online. **Carers Online** is a partnership between Carers UK, Devon, Surrey and West Sussex County Council's. These partners successfully applied for funding from the Government's Invest to Save (ITS)	www.carersnet.org.uk

Budget to design and develop an Internet site especially for carers. This Internet site will provide, to carers and professionals working with carers, information, advice and support, a communication tool and learning

Crossroads – Caring for the Carers	Trained care attendants to relieve the carer of an ill person	Tel: 01788 573 653 www.crossroads.org.uk
Crossroads (Northern Ireland)		Tel: 020 9181 4455 www.crossroadscare.co.uk
Crossroads (Scotland)	Respite care for carers across Scotland	Tel: 0141 226 3793 www.xroadsscot.fsnet. co.uk
Cruse – Bereavement Care	Individual and group bereavement counselling, advice and training	Tel: 0870 167 1677 www.crusebereavement care.org.uk
Cruse – Bereavement Care (Northern Ireland)		Tel: 028 9079 2419
Cruse – Bereavement Care (Scotland)		Tel: 01738 444178 E-mail: info@crusescot land.org.uk
Institute of Family Therapy	Counselling for recently-bereaved families and those with seriously-ill family members, London	Tel: 0207 391 9150 www.instituteoffamily therapy.org.uk
National Association of Bereavement Services	Helpline, information and local support services	Tel: 0207 247 1080

The National Strategy for Carers	The first ever by a Government in Britain – sets out what the Government has been doing, and what it is going to do. It offers practical help in ways which are needed, and which will work: carers will have better information, they will be better supported, they will be cared for better themselves. In **Caring about Carers** the Government made a commitment to provide details of the services or benefits affecting carers on the Internet. The Government feels that this site will be useful to carers, to carers' workers and voluntary organizations and others	www.carers.gov.uk
Partner Volunteer Service	Support for partners of people living with breast cancer	Tel: 0800 245 345
The Princess Royal Trust for Carers	National charity formed in 1991 at the initiative of Her Royal Highness The Princess Royal. The Trust exists to make it easier for carers to cope by providing information, support and practical help to carers. The national network of over 100 independently-managed Carers Centres across the UK currently reaches well over 100,000 carers a year. The Trust provides training and support for Carers Centres, as	www.carers.org

well as raising funds for development work. It also has a range of grant schemes for carers, including an Educational Bursary Scheme, a Carers' Relief Fund for carers in particular financial difficulties and a Young Carers Fund. To apply for funding under any of these schemes, carers should contact their nearest Carers Centre

| Sue Ryder Foundation | Nursing service, home visit, advice and bereavement counselling | Tel: 01787 280 252 |

11 Retreats, Spiritual Development and Holistic Holidays

11.1 Retreat Centres

Burrswood, Tunbridge Wells, Kent	Christian nursing home and retreat centre with healing	Tel: 01892 863637
The Findhorn Community, Scotland	Centre offering a wide range of excellent courses for personal growth and transformation	The Park, Findhorn, Forres IV36 3TZ Moray, Scotland Tel: 01309 690311 www.findhorn.org
Glastonbury N.F.S.H, Healing Centre	Healing service	8 Market Place, Glastonbury, BA6 9HW Tel: 01458 832 549

Kagyu Samye Ling Tibetan Centre	Courses, teaching either at the monastery itself or at the Purelands Retreat Centre	Kagyu Samye Ling Monastery and Tibetan Centre, Eskdalemuir, Langholm, Dumfriesshire DG13 0QL Scotland Tel: 013873 73232 www.samyeling.org
The Melangell Cancer Help Centre	Welsh Centre providing spiritual retreat for people with cancer	Tel: 01691 860408 www.st-melangell.org.uk
Music Passages	Retreats in idyllic settings	Jill Carlisle Tel: 01242 515389 E-mail: jill.carlisle@ virgin.net
Sacred Space Foundation	A charity providing peaceful guided retreats in the Lake District	Emmets Farm, Sparket, Dacre, Penrith, Cumbria CA11 0NA Tel: 01768 486868 www.sacredspace.org.uk
School of the Living Light	Recommended for spiritual development	Millslade Hall, Station Road, Ashcott, TA7 9QP Tel: 01458 211 047 www.schooloftheliving light.co.uk
The Tareth Centre	Recommended for spiritual development	10 St John's Square, Glastonbury, Somerset, BA6 9JL Tel: 01458 833929 E-mail: tarethway@tiscali.co.uk

11.2 Holistic Holidays

Magical Journey	Journeys in Peru, South Africa, Brazil, Tibet, Egypt and more	Tel: 00 2782 478 8743 www.travelperu.com E-mail: info@magical journey.org
Spirit of Life	Holistic and healing holidays	Henleaze Centre, 13 Harbury Road, Henleaze, Bristol BS9 3SN Tel: 0117 9738387 www.thespiritoflife.co.uk

12. Cancer Care and Practical Help: Nursing, Social, Financial, Insurance

12.1 Nursing Care

Association for Palliative Medicine	Palliative medicine – all cancers	Tel: 01703 672 888 www.palliative-medicine.org
Cancer Relief Macmillan	Home nursing service	Tel: 0207 351 7811
Helen House Hospice	Hospice for children, offering short-term and terminal care	Tel: 01865 728 251
Lyndon Hill Clinic, Reading	Nursing Home with complementary therapies run by Carole Eastman	Tel: 0118 940 1234
Macmillan CancerLine	Publishes directory of cancer support and care organizations	Freephone: 0808 808 2020, Monday to Friday, 9 a.m.

	in the UK, with telephone numbers addresses and website addresses; Macmillan CancerLine; can provide financial help and special nurses in hospital and in homes.	– 6 p.m. for information and emotional support for people living with cancer. www.macmillan.org.uk
Marie Curie Cancer Care	Day and night home-nursing service, education and research	Tel: 0207 599 7777 www.mariecurie.org.uk
Sue Ryder Foundation	Nursing service, home visit, advice and bereavement counselling	Tel: 01787 280 252
Teenage Cancer Trust	Have 20 specialist units to treat and care for adolescents suffering from cancer	Tel: 0207 387 1000 www.teencancer.org

12.2 Nursing Equipment

Red Cross Society	A range of services and aids relevant to cancer care, also escorts to hospital	Tel: 0207 235 5454 www.redcross.org.uk

12.3 Social, Financial and Insurance

Christian Lewis Childrens' Cancer Care	Charity providing financial help for children and their families to improve quality of life. Information on respite care, local support groups, etc.	Tel: 01792 480500 www.childrens-cancer-care.org.uk

Citizens' Advice Bureaux	For social and legal advice	Myddelton House, 115-123 Pentonville Road, London N1 9LZ No central phone number – look in your local phone book www.citizensadvice.org.uk www.adviceguide.org.uk (online advice)
Family Funds	Some financial help for parents of chronically sick children. Help with bedding, clothing, etc.	Tel: 01904 621 115
Macmillan CancerLine	Can provide financial help and special nurses in hospital and in homes. Also publishes directory of cancer support and care organizations in the UK, with telephone numbers, addresses and website addresses	Freephone: 0808 8082020, Mon-Fri 9 a.m. - 6 p.m. for information/ emotional support for people living with cancer. www.macmillan.org.uk
Malcolm Sargent Cancer Fund for Children	Financial assistance and practical help for parents of children with cancer	Tel: 0208 752 2800 www.sargent.org
Our Way Travel Insurance	For people with medical or physical disadvantages and for accompanying family and friends	Tel: 0208 313 3900 www.ourway.co.uk
Tenovus Centre	Cancer charity – free helpline, financial help, free publications, information and support, counselling service	Helpline: 0808 808 1010 www.tenovus.org.uk

12.4 Hospice

Helen House Hospice	Hospice for children offering short-term and terminal care	Tel: 01865 728 251
Hospice Information Centre	Directory of hospice and palliative care services	Tel: 0870 903 3903 www.hospice information.info

12.5 Political Cancer Patient Groups

National Alliance of Breast Cancer Organisations	Political patient body linking all those with an interest in breast cancer	www.nabco.org
Patients Association	Lobbying self-help group and forum for patients' concerns	Tel: 0208 423 9111 Helpline: 0845 608 4455

12.6 Cancer Services Management

The Cancer Tsar	Professor Mike Richards	Department of Oncology, St Thomas's Hospital, London SE1 7EH Tel: 020 7188 7188
The Cancer Plan		Department of Health, PO Box 777, London SE1 6XH Fax: 01623 724524
Cancer Services Managers	There is a CSM for each of the 40 NHS regions who can help you with any problems with your treatment	Contact your regional NHS Headquarters

12.7 Transport

Red Cross Society   A range of services and aids   Tel: 0207 235 5454
relevant to cancer care, also   www.redcross.org.uk
escort to hospital

13. Cancer Prevention

13.1 Genetic Cancer Screening

ICRF Family Cancer Clinics
Yorkshire Regional Genetics Service,
Department of Clinical Genetics,
St James' University Hospital,
Beckett Street,
Leeds LS9 7TF
Tel: 0113 283 7072

South Thames Regional Genetics Centre (East)
Division of Medical and Molecular Genetics,
5th, 7th and 8th Floors,
Guy's Tower,
Guy's Hospital,
St Thomas Street,
London SE1 9RT
Tel: 0207 955 4648/4649

Cancer Genetics Clinics
Churchill Hospital,
Headington,
Oxford OX1 7LJ
Tel: 01865 226048

13.2 Help to Eradicate Key Risk Factors

Obesity
The Obesity Resource Information Centre
Tel: 01454 616798 (a division of ASO)
www.aso.org.uk

The International Obesity Task Force
www.iotf.org

Weight Watchers
Tel: 0845 712 3000

Smoking
Quit line
Tel: 0800 002200

Alcoholism
Alcoholics Anonymous
Tel: 0117 926 5520

Mobile Phone Protection
R.A.D.A.R. Electromagnetic Stabiliser
Tel: 001 858 793 9230

13.3 Cancer Risk Factors

13.3a Environmental
Examples of chemicals in the environment known to disrupt the endocrine system are:

- DDT and its degradation products
- DEHP (Di(2-ethylhexyl) phtalate)
- Dicofol
- HCB (Hexo chlorobenzene)

- Kelthane
- Kepone
- Lindane and other hexo-chloro-cyclo-hexane congeners
- Methoxychlor
- Octa-chloro styrene
- Synthetic pyrethroids
- Triazine herbicides
- EBDC fungicides
- Certain PCB congeners
- 2,3,7,8 – TCDD and other dioxins
- 2,3,7,8 – TCDDF and other furans
- Cadmium
- Lead
- Mercury
- Tributyltin and other organo-tin compounds
- Alkyl phenols (non-biodegradable detergents and antioxidants present in modified polystyrene and PVCs)
- Styrene dimers and trimers

13.3b Household

Chemicals contained in household products which are carcinogenic or teratogenic (carcinogenic chemicals are those which affect the cells of the body whereas those classed as teratogenic have an effect on the 'germ' cells – which are the cells of the sperm and ovaries):

Chemical	Effect	Found In
Acetoxyphenylmercury	Teratogenic	Paints
Acid blue 9	Carcinogenic	Toilet bowl cleaners and deodorizers
Aluminium silicate	Some evidence of carginogenicity in the dry state	Some paints

Chemical	Effect	Found In
Artificial coal tar colours which contain lead and arsenic	Carcinogenic	Black and brown hair dyes
Benzene	Carcinogenic	Some adhesives
Bronopol	Breaks down to formaldehyde which is carcinogenic	Cosmetics
Cadmium	Carcinogenic, teratogenic	Some artists' oil colours
Cobalt	Carcinogenic	Some artists' oil colours
Crystalline silica	Carcinogenic in the dry state	Cleansers, cat litter, powdered flea control products
1,4-Dichlorobenzene (para-dichlorobenzene)	Carcinogenic	Moth repellents, toilet deodorizers
Dichlorvos (DDVP)	Carcinogenic, teratogenic	Some no-pest strips, flea collars and pet flea control products
Diethanolamine (DEA)	Reacts with nitrites to form nitrosamines, which are carcinogenic	Wide range of household cleaning products, cosmetics
Dioctyl phthalate	Carcinogenic	Adhesives and correction fluid
Ethoxylated alcohols	May be contaminated with 1,4-dioctane which is carcinogenic	Cosmetic products

Chemical	Effect	Found In
Formaldehyde	Carcinogenic	Some furniture polish, cleaners, waxes and a wide range of consumer items especially paints and related products
Hexachlorobenzene (HCB)	Carcinogenic	Some artists' oil colours
Hydramethylnon	Carcinogenic	Some home and garden pesticides
Lanolin	May be contaminated with DDT, dieldrin, lindane, diazinon and other pesticides. Carcinogenic	Cosmetics and body and hand creams
Lead	Carcinogenic	Some artists' oil paints
Medium aliphatic-hydrocarbons	Suggestive evidence of carcinogenicity	Some car waxes
Methoxychlor	Limited evidence of carcinogenicity	Some pet flea control products
Methyl chloride (dichloromethane)	Carcinogenic	Some paint strippers and spray paints
Morpholine	Reacts with nitrites to form carcinogenic nitrosamines	Some furniture polishes
Naled	Transformation products include dichloros, which is carcinogenic	Some pet flea control products

Chemical	Effect	Found In
Ortho phenylphenols	Probably carcinogenic	Some air fresheners and disinfectants
Padimat-O	Can cause the formation of carcinogenic nitrosamines	Sun screens and cosmetics
Permethrin	Carcinogenic	Some household and garden pesticides and pet flea control products
Petroleum distillates, hydrocarbons, process oils, solvents and spirits	May contain traces of benzene which is carcinogenic	Some furniture polish
Polychlorinated biphenyls (PCBs)	Carcinogenic, teratogenic	Some artists' oil paints
Propylene oxide	Carcinogenic	Some adhesives
Rotenone	Carcinogenic	Some pet flea control products
Sodium 2,4-Dichloro-phenoxyacetate	Carcinogenic	Herbicides in lawn care products
Sodium ortho-phenylphenol	Carcinogenic	Some bathroom cleaners
Solvent orange 3 dye, solvent red 4 dye, Blue 1, Green 3, D and C red 33, F, D and C yellow 5, F, D and C yellow 6	Carcinogenic	Some polishes, cosmetics

Chemical	Effect	Found In
Talc	Carcinogenic when inhaled	Cosmetics and some home and garden pesticides
Tetrachloroethylene (perchlorethylene)	Carcinogenic	Some spot removers
Tetrachlorvinphos	Carcinogenic	Some pet flea control products
Titanium dioxide	Limited evidence of carcinogenicity	Some paints and shoe polishes
Triethanolamine (TEA)	Can react with nitrites to form carcinogenic nitrosamines	Some liquid all-purpose cleaning products, metal polishes, spot removers and other household cleaning products and cosmetics
Trisodium nitrylotriacetate	Carcinogenic	Some bathroom cleaning products

13.3c Occupational cancer risk factors

Occupation	Likely Carcinogenic Agent	Site of Cancer Risk
Asbestos Workers Mining Shipyards Insulation Demolition Break Lining	Asbestos Fibre	Lung, Mesothelioma, Throat (Pharynx)
Brick & Ceramic Manufacture	Arsenic, Beryllium Chromium	Skin, Lung, Nose, Throat (Pharynx) and Liver

Occupation	Likely Carcinogenic Agent	Site of Cancer Risk
Cadmium Production Metal Workers Electro Plating Nuclear Plants	Cadmium	Lung and Prostate
Chemical Workers	Amino-biphenyl Benzene Benzidine Chloromethyl ether Cadmium Chromium 2-Naphthylamine	Leukaemia Pancreas Bladder Lung Prostate Throat (Pharynx)
Chromium and Alloy Production	Chromium and Chromium compounds	Lung, Nose and Throat (Pharynx)
Coal/Gas/Shale Oil Production/Coke Plant Workers	Aromatic hydro-carbons Coke-oven gases and vapours	Lung, Skin, Bladder and Pancreas
Copper Production Smelters, Electrolyses	2-Naphthylamine	Bladder and Pancreas
Dye Works	Aminebiphenyl Benzidine 2-Naphthylamine	Bladder and Pancreas
Electrical/Electronic Workers/Electricians Radio/TV repairers Telephone and Computer Mechanics	Electro Magnetic Fields (EMF), Beryllium	Leukaemia, Lymphoma, Brain and Bladder

Occupation	Likely Carcinogenic Agent	Site of Cancer Risk
Electro Platers/Electrolysis Workers	Cadmium 2-Naphthylamine	Prostate, Bladder and Pancreas
Farmers and Agricultural Workers	Ultra Violet Radiation Pesticides/Weed Killers	Skin, Lip, Lymphoma, Leukaemia, Prostate, Lung, Soft Tissue Sarcoma
Garage and Transport Workers	Diesel Exhaust	Lung
Glass Manufacture	Arsenic Chromium Compounds	Skin, Lung, Liver, Nose and Throat
Hairdressers	Hair Dyes	Bladder
Insulation Workers	Asbestos Fibre	Lung, Mesothelioma and (Pharynx) Throat
Leather and Shoe Workers	Benzene Isopropyl	Leukaemia and Sinuses
Nickel Production	Nickel 2-Naphthylamine	Nose, Bladder and Pancreas
Nuclear Plant/Nuclear Power Workers	Beryllium Cadmium	Bladder, Lung and Prostate
Office Workers	Tobacco Smoke	Lung and Throat (Pharynx)
Painters	Painting Materials Benzene	Lung and Leukaemia

Occupation	Likely Carcinogenic Agent	Site of Cancer Risk
Petroleum Workers	Arsenic Benzene Petroleum	Skin, Lung, Leukaemia, Gall Bladder and Bile Duct
Plastic Workers	Vinyl Chloride	Liver, Lymphoma and Lung
Radiologists/ Radiographers/Nurses	Ionising Radiation Cancer Drugs	Skin, Thyroid, Brain, Lung, Breast, Bone, Pancreas, Leukaemia and Myeloma
Rubber Tyre Manufacture	Asbestos Fibre Benzene Auramine 2-Naphthylamine	Lung, Mesothelioma, Leukaemia, Bladder, Pancreas, Gall Bladder and Bile Duct
Ship Yard Workers	Asbestos Fibre	Lung, Mesothelioma and Throat (Pharynx)
Steel Workers	Coke-Oven Gases and Vapours	Lung and Kidney
Tanners	Arsenic	Skin and Lung
Uranium Miners	Ionising Radiation Radon Gas	Skin, Thyroid, Brain, Lung, Breast, Bone, Pancreas, Leukaemia, Myeloma
Waiters/Bar Tenders	Tobacco Smoke	Lung and Throat (Pharynx)
Woodworkers Carpenters Furniture Makers Polishers and Finishers	Wood Dust Benzene	Nose, Sinuses, Throat (Pharynx) and Leukaemia

13.3d Known risk factors for specific cancers

Cancer of the Oesophagus (Gullet)

- Genetic inheritance
- Having a 'Barrett's oesophagus' – in this condition, there is reflux of the contents of the stomach into the gullet, which, over time, causes inflammation, scarring, narrowing or out-pouching
- Alcohol
- Smoking
- Smoked, pickled, cured and preserved foods
- Low intake of beta-carotene, vitamin C and vitamin E

Cancer of the Pancreas

- Genetic inheritance
- Occupational exposure of chemical workers and dye workers to nickel, copper and asbestos; uranium exposure in rubber workers; and radiation in radiologists and radiographers
- Chronic pancreatitis (inflammation of the pancreas). There is also a slightly increased risk in people with diabetes
- Smoking
- A diet high in fat and meat with low vegetable and fruit intake
- High alcohol consumption

Cancer of the Penis

- Papilloma virus (HPV) and genital wart virus (Herpes Simplex II)
- Having a narrowed foreskin with poor hygiene in the uncircumcised
- Unsafe anal sex, risking infection of the above viruses
- Occupational exposure in farmers to fertilisers, pesticides and weed killers
- Smoking

Cancer of the Bowel

- Genetic inheritance (15 per cent are inherited)
- High-calorie diet with excess fat and sugar, meat (especially red meat) and salt
- A diet low in vegetables, fruit, fibre, fish and calcium
- Overweight
- Inactivity

- High alcohol consumption (over 3 units a day for men and over 2 units a day for women) for 20 years
- Smoking (which is thought to account for 10 per cent of bowel cancers)

Breast Cancer
- Genetic inheritance (about 5 per cent of cases)
- Alcohol (more than 2 units per day)
- High hormone levels due to obesity, diet, HRT or the Pill (and possibly environmental oestrogen-mimicking substances called xeno-oestrogens)
- Physical inactivity
- Excessive radiation exposure to the chest
- High-calorie diet with excess meat and fat
- Obesity
- Low vegetable and fibre intake

Lung Cancer
- Smoking, which causes 85 per cent of lung cancers. About 1 in 5 people now living in developed countries will be killed by tobacco unless smoking habits change. This means 250 million people living in developed countries will die from smoking, which is the equivalent of the entire population of the United States. Most alarming is the increase in female deaths from smoking. Lung cancer has overtaken breast cancer as the major cause of death among women in Scotland and Northern England and this may soon be the case in the UK. In Britain, 100,000 people die every year because they smoke, 50,000 of which are due to cancer. This is the same as a jumbo jet crashing every day and killing all of the passengers on board.
- Chronic lung disease
- Excess chest radiation
- Passive smoking
- Asbestos (especially for those who smoke)
- Radon Gas. The average national level of radon gas in the country is 20 bequerels per cubic metre. At a level of 200 bq per cubic metre, the risk of lung cancer is 20 per cent higher. At 400 bq per cubic metre the increase is around 40 per cent. Radon is believed to be responsible for 5 per cent of lung cancers in Britain.
- Occupational exposure to nickel and chromium compounds and arsenic
- A diet low in vegetables

- A diet high in meat and fat

Prostate Cancer

Possible causes – though it should be noted that the causes of prostate cancer are still not well understood:

- High testosterone levels or high testosterone/oestrogen ratios
- High-fat diet
- Genetic inheritance
- Physical inactivity
- Smoking (which increases the testosterone/oestrogen ratio)
- Occupational exposure to pesticides in farmers, cadmium in battery and alloy workers and during electro-plating
- Obesity
- Physical inactivity
- A diet low in foods containing beta-carotene and vitamin E
- Low intake of green leafy vegetables
- Inadequate sunlight with resulting low levels of vitamin D
- Vasectomy at a young age
- Smoking

Melanoma

- Excessive sunlight (90 per cent of cases)
- Genetic inheritance (2 per cent of cases)
- Compromised immune function (with co-existing leukaemia or lymphoma or when using immune suppressant drugs e.g. after transplants)
- Radiation
- Multiple skin moles
- Use of sunbeds
- Chronic leg ulcers
- Occupational exposure to tar, asphalt, pitch, waxes, heavy oils (including shale oil) and arsenic
- A diet which is low in vitamin A, beta-carotene and vitamin C
- High fat intake

Cancer of the Uterus (Womb) and Ovaries

- Genetic inheritance – in association with hereditary non-polyposis colo-rectal cancer or breast/ovarian cancer syndrome
- Previous breast, colo-rectal, ovarian or uterine cancer
- Use of oestrogen-only HRT (this increases the risk of uterine cancer more than ovarian).
- Polycystic ovaries (PCOS)
- Use of fertility drugs (raises ovarian cancer risk)
- Tamoxifen, the oestrogen-blocking drug used to help prevent breast cancer or its recurrence, increases risk to the endometrium or lining of the womb (uterus)
- Long menstrual life with periods starting before 12 years and finishing after 50 years of age
- Not having children
- High blood pressure or diabetes
- A high-calorie and high-fat diet
- A diet low in vegetables, fruit and fish
- Overweight
- Physical inactivity
- Never having used the birth control pill

Stomach Cancer

Can be linked to:

- Family history
- Type A blood group (this increases the risk by 20 per cent)
- Infection with the bacteria *Helicobacter pylori*
- Previous surgical removal of part of the stomach (which can have an effect 15 to 40 years later)
- Pernicious anaemia where there is no normal stomach acid production
- All conditions which cause low stomach acid
- A diet low in vegetables, fruit and cereals, beta-carotene and vitamins C and E
- A diet high in pickled, salted or cured foods or foods preserved in nitrate – such as salami, sausages, hot dogs, smoked meat, smoked fish or pickled food (all of which cause production of carcinogenic nitrosamines in the bowel)
- Smoking

Anal Cancer
- Genetic inheritance
- The sexually-transmitted infection human papilloma virus (HPV)
- Anal and genital warts caused by genital herpes (Herpes Simplex II)
- Anal fissures and fistulas
- Anal intercourse
- Immuno-suppressive drugs
- Smoking (possibly)

Bladder Cancer
- Smoking
- Painkillers containing phenacetin (now withdrawn from sale)
- Bladder papilloma
- Artificial sweeteners (possibly)
- Excess coffee
- Recurrent bladder infections
- Radiation to the pelvis
- Occupational exposure to aromatic amines, paints, hairdressing products, printing products

Brain Tumours
- Genetic inheritance (in association with neuro-fibromatosis)
- Use of pesticides and insecticides
- Exposure to petro-chemicals (chemicals linked to the petroleum industry), rubber and vinyl chloride, electromagnetic fields in electrical and electronic workers, radiation in radiologists and radiographers, and uranium in uranium miners
- Head injuries where there is a slightly increased risk of meningioma
- Excessive dental X-rays (slight increased risk of meningioma and glioma)
- Nitrate-containing foods e.g. sausages and salamis
- Smoking (possibly)
- Possibly living or playing near to high-tension electricity wires for children due to low frequency electromagnetic fields

Gall Bladder Cancer

- Genetic inheritance where there is a tendency to cholesterol gallstones. Gallstones are more common with multiple pregnancies, obesity, high-calorie diet and diet low in fruit, vegetables and cereals
- Gallstones especially if they are big and the gall bladder wall is calcified
- Occupational exposure in the car manufacturing, petroleum, rubber and textile industries

Kidney Cancer

- Genetic inheritance in association with non-polyposis colo-rectal cancer syndrome
- Occupational exposure to leather, dyes, textile dyes, rubber, plastic, coke ovens, cadmium, asbestos, petroleum, tar and pitch products
- Phenacitin pain killers (now off the market)
- Some diuretics and anti hypertensive drugs and diet pills
- Kidney injury
- Radiation
- Long-term haemodialysis
- Large kidney stones
- Smoking
- Overweight

Leukaemias

- Genetic inheritance (very rarely.) This is higher in those with Down's Syndrome
- Occupational exposure in the chemical industry, shoe trade and uranium mining, exposure to the solvent benzene (also found in unleaded fuel), radiation and low-frequency EMFs in electrical and electronic industry workers and pesticides in farmers
- Previous radiation exposure from diagnostic X-rays or radiotherapy
- Chemotherapy with melphalan and chlorambucil
- The antibiotics chloramphenical and phenylbutazone
- Smoking (possibly)

Liver Cancer

- Alcohol intake (over 2-3 units per day)
- Smoking (possibly)
- Very rarely genetic inheritance

- Past Hepatitis B and Hepatitis C infection
- Aflatoxin exposure in tropical countries (especially Africa)
- Chronic liver disease e.g. liver cirrhosis
- Previous steroid use – especially androgenic anabolic steroids
- Possibly oral contraceptives
- Previous blood transfusion

Lymphomas

Hodgkin's Lymphoma:

- Genetic inheritance
- Occupational exposure in woodworkers, rubber workers, chemical workers (where there is exposure to tar and benzene)
- Tonsil removal
- Amphetamine usage
- (Possibly) use of the drug phenytoin in epilepsy
- Viral infection in glandular fever with Epstein Barr
- Immune deficiency

Non Hodgkin's Lymphoma:

- Genetic inheritance
- Occupational exposure to chloro-phenols, phenoxy-acids, asbestos, benzene, radiation, uranium, low-frequency EMFs, pesticides, herbicides and fertilizers
- Viral infection with Epstein Barr viruses and viruses associated with AIDS
- Poor immunity and suppressed immunity
- Immuno-suppressant drugs, especially after a kidney transplant
- Use of the drug phenytoin for epilepsy
- Radiation treatment

Mouth and Throat Cancer

- Occupational exposure to nickel, asbestos, and mustard gas (historically)
- Exposure to sunlight – especially on the lip
- Leucoplakia
- Radiation

- Infection with Epstein Barr virus
- Use of tobacco, snuff and marijuana
- Alcohol consumption
- Repeated irritation or abrasions in the mouth
- Diet low in Vitamin C, E and beta-carotene

Sarcomas (Cancers of the Bones or Connective Tissue)

- Genetic inheritance (rarely) in association with Von Recklinghausen's disease
- Occupational exposure to herbicides, wood preservatives, radiation and defoliants
- Paget's disease of the bone (where cartilage grows into the bone)
- Radiation and chemotherapy treatments
- HIV infection progressing to AIDS – Karposi's Sarcoma
- Metallic surgical implants
- Bullet and shrapnel fragments in the body in the connective tissue
- Smoking

Testicular Cancer

- Genetic inheritance (very rarely)
- Occupational exposure (as in the case of Vietnam veterans) to defoliants
- Undescended testicles
- Mumps orchitis (inflammation of the testicles due to mumps)
- Diethyl-stilbestrol use in mothers (banned since 1965)
- Synthetic oestrogens in food
- Sedentary lifestyle
- Tight trousers

Thyroid Cancer

- Genetic inheritance
- Occupational exposure in radiologists, radiographers, and uranium miners
- Excess alcohol consumption
- Pre-existing thyroid illness
- Radiation exposure. Since 1987, more than 1,000 children have developed cancer of the thyroid around the Chernobyl area due to exposure to radioactive iodine after the nuclear accident.

Vaginal and Vulval Cancer
- Maternal use of diethyl-stilbestrol (off the market since 1965)
- Infection with human papilloma virus (HPV) and genital herpes virus (Herpes Simplex II)
- Abnormalities in the skin or mucus membrane of the vulva or vagina
- Radiation treatment
- Extensive sex in the very young without adequate protection, due to sexually transmitted diseases
- Smoking

Cervical Cancer
- Infection with the human papilloma virus (HPV) and genital herpes virus (Herpes Simplex II)
- Abnormalities in the mucous membrane of the cervix (CIN 1, 2 and 3)
- Abnormalities in the mucous membrane of the vagina or skin of the vulva
- Unsafe sex
- Smoking
- A diet low in vegetables, fruit, beta-carotene, vitamin C and folic acid

14. Product Suppliers and Diagnostic Centres

14.1 Health Creation Products and Services

Health Creation is Dr Rosy Daniel's organization which produces interactive integrated medicine products into which she has distilled the learning of her 20-year career at the forefront of holistic cancer medicine. The products are supported by a telephone Mentor Service and Helpline. The Health Creation team also puts on seminars and runs a Health Creation consultancy service called Creation in Business for Health for those wishing to help prevent cancer and heart disease and achieve positive health in the workplace.

Health Creation supplies Dr Rosy Daniel and Jane Sen's products and services including: The Cancer Lifeline Kit in its entirety or as any of its 10 component parts:

1. The Cancer Lifeline Programme (for the newly diagnosed)
2. The Health Creation Programme (to create sustainable health once treatment is over)
3. The Carer's Guide
4. The Cancer Lifeline Recipe Cards by Jane Sen
5. *The Message of Hope* Video
6. *Cope Positively with Cancer Treatment* CD
7. *Images for Healing Cancer* CD
8. *Heal Yourself* CD
9. *The Frontier Cancer Medicine Guide*
10. *The Alternative Cancer Treatment Guide*

Health Creation Helpline: 0845 009 3366; Website: www.healthcreation.co.uk

Also from Health Creation:

- *Holistic Approach to Health* Video by Dr Rosy Daniel
- *The Cancer Prevention Book* by Dr Rosy Daniel
- *Eat to Beat Cancer* by Jane Sen and Rosy Daniel
- Jane Sen's three videos
- Health Creation Mentor Support
- Litmus paper to assess your pH
- The acid-free booklet 'Where's the Meat' by Gillian Gill

14.2 Vitamins, Minerals and Herbs

The Nutri-Centre, London

Dr Rosy Daniel's recommended supplier for all vitamins, herbs and homoeopathic medicines is the Nutri Centre, London, who do same-day dispatch from phone phone or email orders. They offer a 10 per cent discount on quotation of the reference: ZZ-RMD-001. They also have in-house nutritional consultants to answer your personal queries.

Tel: 020 7637 8436 (Quote reference: ZZ RMD 001 for a 10% discount given to friends of Health Creation)

Argyll Herbs

For Chest Herbs, Liver Herbs, Lymph Herbs, and Menopausal Formula. You may also get a phone consultation with herbalist Ute Brookman via this number. Ute is senior nutritional therapist and herbalist at the Bristol Cancer Help Centre.

Tel: 01984 624 911

Bristol Cancer Help Centre Shop

Louise Brackenbury Radiation Cream and *Radiation Remedy*

Tel: 0117 980 9504

Cankut Herbs

Sole UK distributor for Carctol herbs. Carctol must be obtained with a prescription from a prescribing doctor. See page 335 of this Directory for a list of prescribing doctors. Doctors wishing to prescribe Carctol should contact Cankut for a prescription pack

Tel: 0117 973 6052 www.newlifeayurvedic herbs.co.uk or www.carctolhome.com

Galen Homoeopathics	Homoeopathic and Flower remedies	Tel: 01305 263 996
Gerson Supplies	Supplier of Gerson medications and literature, Gerson Diet	Tel: 01525 875 739
Oasis Pure Water Limited, UK	Suppliers of Reverse Osmosis Water filters	Tel: 0845 1662 356
PC SPES – Botanics, US	At the time of printing, PC SPES is not available but this may change.	Tel: 00 1516 432 1758
Weleda, UK	Maker of iscador and supplier of homoeopathic remedies	Tel: 0115 944 8200

14.3 Orthodox Medicines

All Cures – an online pharmacy	NHS prescriptions sent post free, private prescriptions and OTC medicines postage to pay; can speak to the pharmacist. Complementary and alternative remedies plus complementary medicine information.	www.allcures.com

Bibliography

Alternative Guides and Medicine
Cancer – The Healthy Option, Terry Moule (Kyle Cathie Ltd)
The Definitive Guide to Cancer, John Diamond, William Lee and Burton Goldberg (Future Medicine)
Everything you Need to Help You Beat Cancer, Chris Woollams (Bath Press)
How to Prevent and Treat Cancer with Natural Medicine, Dr Michael Murray (Riverhead Books)
Options: The Alternative Cancer Therapy Book, Richard Walters
The Prostate Cancer Protection Plan, Robert Burns Arnot (Little, Brown)
What's the Alternative?, Chris Woollams (Bath Press)

Integrated Medicine
The Cancer Lifeline Kit, Dr Rosy Daniel (Health Creation)
Choices in Healing, Dr Michael Lerner (MIT Press)

Anti-Cancer Nutrition
The Breast Cancer Prevention and Recovery Diet, Suzannah Olivier (Michael Joseph)
Cancer and Its Nutritional Therapies, Dr Richard Passwater (Keats Publishing)
Health Defence, Dr Paul Clayton (Accelerated Learning Systems Ltd)
Eat to Beat Cancer, Dr Rosy Daniel and Jane Sen (Thorsons)
Natural Detox, Suzannah Olivier (Simon and Schuster)
Nutrition and Cancer: State of the Art Positive Health, Dr Sandra Goodman (Positive Health)
The Optimum Nutrition Bible, Patrick Holford (Piatkus)
Raw Foods, Leslie Kenton (Vermilion)
Say No to Cancer, Patrick Holford (Piatkus)
Your Life in Your Hands – Understanding, Preventing and Overcoming Breast Cancer, Professor Jane Plant (Virgin Publishing)

Healthy Recipes
The Cancer Lifeline Recipe Cards, Jane Sen (Health Creation)
Eastern Vegetarian Cookery, Madhur Jaffrey (Jonathan Cape)
Hom's Vegetarian Cookery, Ken Hom (BBC Books)
Italian Vegetarian Cookery, Paola Gann (Optima)

Leaves from Our Tuscan Garden, Janet Ross (Penguin)
More Healing Foods, Jane Sen (Thorsons)

Household Carcinogens
The Safe Shopper's Bible, David Steinman and Samuel Epstein (Macmillan)

Emotional and Spiritual Health
The Journey, Brandon Bays (Thorsons)
Life Lessons, Elizabeth Kubler-Ross and David Kessler (Simon and Schuster)
Molecules of Emotion, Candace Pert (Simon and Schuster)
Something More, Sarah Ban Breathnach (Transworld)

References

The supportive research is divided into the areas of:

- The effect of coping style, support, relaxation and visualization on cancer survival
- Nutrition and cancer
- Spiritual healing
- Complementary therapies
- The mind–body connection
- Exercise
- Massage

Research references for each alternative cancer medicine listed are given in Section 3.3.

The Effect of Coping Style, Support, Relaxation and Visualization on Cancer Survival

Fawzy, F. *et al.*, 'Malignant melanoma, effects of an early structured psychiatric intervention, and coping and affective state on recurrence and survival six years later', *Archives of General Psychiatry* 50 (1993): 681

Greer, S. *et al.*, 'Psychological response to breast cancer and 15 year outcome', *Lancet* 335 (1990): 49

Spiegel, D., 'Effect of psychosocial treatment on survival of patients with metastatic breast cancer', *Lancet* 2 (1989): 888

Walker, L. G., 'Psychological interventions, host defences and survival', *Advances in Mind–body Medicine* 15 (1999): 236–81

Walker, L. G., Ratcliffe, M. A. and Dawson, A. A., 'Relaxation and hypnotherapy: long-term effects on the survival of patients with lymphoma', *Psycho-oncology* 9 (2000): 355–56

Walker, L. G., Walker, M. B., Ogstonn, K., *et al.*, 'Psychological, clinical and pathological effects of relaxation training and guided imagery during primary chemotherapy', *British Journal of Cancer* 80 (1999): 262-8

Zachariae *et al.*, 'Effect of psychological intervention in the form of relaxation and guided imagery on cellular immune function in normal healthy subjects. An overview', *Psychotherapy and Psychosomatics* 54 (1990): 32

Walker, L. *et al.*, 'Guided imagery and relaxation therapy can modify host defences in women receiving treatment for locally advanced breast cancer', *British Journal of Surgery* 84, suppl 1 (1997)

Rider, M. *et al.*, 'Effect of immune system imagery on secretory IgA', *Biofeedback and Self Regulation* 15.4 (1990): 317

Cannici, J. *et al.*, 'Treatment of insomnia in cancer patients using muscle relaxation training (review)', *Journal of Behaviour Therapy and Experimental Psychiatry* 14.3 (1983): 251

Burish, T. *et al.*, 'Conditioned side-effects induced by cancer chemotherapy; prevention through behaviour treatment', *Journal of Consulting and Clinical Psychology* 55.1 (1987): 42

Spiegel, D., 'Can psychotherapy prolong cancer survival?', *Psychosomatics* 31.4 (1990): 361

Cain, E., 'Psychosocial benefits of a cancer support group', *Cancer* 57.1 (1986): 183

Fawzy, F. *et al.*, 'A structured psychiatric intervention for cancer patients. II. Changes over time in immunological measures', *Archives of General Psychiatry* 47.8 (1990): 729

Shrock, Dean, Palmer, Raymond F. and Taylor, Bonnie, 'Effects of a Psychosocial intervention on survival among patients with Stage 1 breast and prostate cancer: A matched case-control study', *Alternative Therapies in Health and Medicine* 5.3 (May 1999)

Nutrition and Cancer

Food, Nutrition and the Prevention of Cancer: A Global Perspective (World Cancer Research Fund and American Institute of Cancer Research, 1997)

Thorogood, M. *et al.*, 'Risk of death from cancer and ischaemic heart disease in meat and non-meat eaters', *British Medical Journal* 308 (1994): 6945

Holm *et al.*, 'Treatment failure and dietary habits in women with breast cancer', *Journal of the National Cancer Institute*, 85.1 (1993)

Cummings, J. and Bingham, S., 'Diet and the prevention of cancer', *British Medical Journal* 7171 (1998)

Plant, Professor J., *Your Life in Your Hands – Understanding, Preventing and Overcoming Breast Cancer* (Virgin Publishing)

Spiritual Healing

Dixon, M., 'Does "healing" benefit patients with chronic symptoms? A quasi-randomised trial in general practice', *Journal of the Royal Society of Medicine* 91.4 (1998): 183-8

Olson, K. and Hanson, J., 'Using reiki to manage pain; a preliminary report', *Cancer Prevention* 1.2 (1997): 108-13

Astin, J. A., Harkness, E., Ernst, E., 'The efficacy of distant healing; A systematic review of randomised trials', *Annals of Internal Medicine* 132: 900–903

Complementary Therapies

Cassileth, B. R., 'Alternative and complementary cancer medicine', *Journal of Clinical Oncology* 17.11 (1999): 44–52

Gray, R. *et al.*, 'Perspectives of cancer survivors interested in unconventional therapies', *Journal of Psychosocial Oncology* 15.3/4 (1997)

Seago, M. and Conn, C., 'Mind–Body Partnering for clinical practice', *Journal of Psychosocial Oncology* 14.4 (1996)

Turton, P., 'Complementary therapies and cancer', *Cancer Topics* 11.4 (2000): 16–19

Turton, P. and Cooke, H., 'Meeting the needs of people with cancer for support and self-management', *Complementary therapies in nursing and midwifery* 6 (2000): 130–7

The Mind–Body Connection

Barraclough, J. (ed), *Integrated Cancer Care – Holistic, Complementary and Creative Approaches* (Oxford University Press, 2001)

Lewis, C. E., Sullivan, C. and Barraclough, J. (eds), *The Psychoimmunology of Cancer – Mind and Body in the Fight for Survival* (Oxford University Press, 1994)

Martin, Paul, *The Sickening Mind* (Flamingo, 1997)

Pert, Candace, *Molecules of Emotion* (Simon and Schuster, 1997)

Watkins, Dr Alan (ed), *Mind–Body Medicine – A Clinicians Guide to Psychoneuroimmunology* (Churchill Livingstone, 1997)

Exercise

Mock, V. *et al.*, 'A nursing rehabilitation program for women with breast cancer receiving adjuvant chemotherapy', *Oncology Nursing Forum* 21.5 (1994): 899

Grossarth-Maticek R. *et al.*, 'Sport activity and personality as elements in preventing cancer and coronary heart disease', *Perceptual & Motor Skills* 71.1 (1990): 199–209

LaPerriere, A., Antoni, M., Schneiderman, N. *et al.*, 'Exercise intervention attenuate emotional distress and natural killer cell decrements following notification of positive serologic status for HIV-1' *Biofeedback Self-Regulation* 15 (1990): 229–42

Massage

Corner, J., Cawley, N. and Hildebrand, S., 'An evaluation of the use of massage and massage with the addition of essential oils for the well-being of patients', *International Journal of Palliative Nursing* 1 (1995): 57–63

Weinrich, S., 'The effect of massage on pain in cancer patients', *Applied Nursing Research* 3.4 (1990): 140

Ferrell-Torry, A. T. and Glick, O. J., 'The use of therapeutic massage as a nursing intervention to modify anxiety and the perception of cancer pain', *Cancer Nursing* 116.2 (1993): 93

Art and Music Therapy

Burns, S., Harbuz, M. S., Hucklebridge, F. and Bunt, L., 'A pilot study into the therapeutic effects of music therapy at a cancer help centre', *Alternative Therapies* 7.1 (2001): 48–56

Tsao, J., Gordon, T. F., Dileo, C. *et al.*, 'The effects of music and biological imagery on immune response', *The Centre for Frontier Sciences – Frontier Perspectives* 8.1 (1999): 26

Aldridge, D., 'The Music of the Body: Music Therapy in medical settings', *Advances* 9.1 (1993): 17

Beck, S., 'The therapeutic use of music for cancer related pain', *Oncology Nursing Forum* 1 18.8 (1991): 1327

Connell, C., *Something Understood: Art therapy in Cancer Care* (Wrexham Publications, 1998)

Please let us know of any other research papers in the area of integrated cancer medicine at:

The Cancer Directory,
77a Alma Road,
Clifton,
Bristol,
BS8 2DP

Glossary

Adjuvant treatment	Any treatment used in conjunction with another to enhance its activity
Aerobic exercise	Light exercise intended to increase oxygen consumption and to benefit the heart and lungs. Examples are swimming and jogging.
Alternative medicine or treatment	Therapy that can be used as an alternative to orthodox or conventional medicine
Benign tumour	A tumour that does not invade or destroy surrounding tissue. It will not spread to other parts of the body. It is non-cancerous.
Biopsy	Removal of a small piece of tissue for microscopic examination
Blood marker	Some cancers produce chemicals that find their way into the bloodstream. A simple blood test can monitor these chemicals and give doctors information about the size of the tumour and the effects of treatment. Also called a tumour marker.
Cancer	A malignant tumour arising from the abnormal and uncontrolled growth of cells, that then invades and destroys the surrounding tissue
Chemotherapy	The prevention or treatment of a disease using chemical medicines
Complementary medicine	Various different types of therapies that can be used alongside or as an adjunct to orthodox or conventional medicine
Computerized tomography (CT) scan	A form of X-ray examination in which cross-sections of the body are viewed in great detail

Conventional medicine	Modern medicine, as practised by most doctors in the NHS and privately
Diagnosis	The process of finding out the nature of a disorder by considering the patient's signs, symptoms and other tests when necessary
Essential fatty acids	Vital nutritional fats found in the oils of fruit, nuts, seeds, grains and fish
Gland	Another name for a Lymph node
Histology	Study of the structure of tissues
Histo-pathology	Combination of histology and pathology
Holistic medicine	Treating the patient as a whole. The person's physical, mental, spiritual, social and environmental background are all taken into account in diagnosis, therapy and self-help processes.
Hormone	Substance produced in one part of the body, that affects the structure or functioning of another part of the body
Hormone receptor	Some breast cancer cells have special receptors on their surfaces that bind a specific hormone. If present, the tumour is called hormone receptor positive. If positive the hormone can affect the way the tumour grows.
Lymph fluid	Fluid found in the lymphatic system. Resembles blood plasma.
Lymph gland	Another name for a Lymph node
Lymph node	Small branches off the lymphatic system, which is part of our immune system. Also known as lymph glands or just as glands.

Lymphatic system	Network of vessels that convey lymph fluid around the body. It is a major part of the immune system.
Lymphoedema	Build-up of lymph fluid in tissues, causing swelling and pain
Magnetic resonance imaging (MRI) scan	An examination in which a magnetic field and radio waves are used to produce images of the inside of the body
Malignant tumour	A tumour that invades surrounding tissue. It can spread to other parts of the body. It is cancerous.
Membrane	Thin layer of tissue surrounding the whole or part of an organ or body cavity
Metastases	Another name for a secondary tumour
Metastasis	The spread of cancer from one part of the body to another
Metastasize	The spreading of cancer cells from one part of the body to another
Mineral	Naturally occurring chemicals required in small amounts for healthy growth and development
Mucous membrane	Moist membrane lining many parts of the body
Oncologist	A doctor who specializes in the study and treatment of tumours
Oncology	The study and treatment of tumours
Orthodox medicine	Another name for conventional medicine
Palliative medicine	Treatment that gives temporary relief from the symptoms of a disease, but does not cure the disease
Pathology	The study of the nature and causes of disease

Pituitary gland	A small gland found in the brain that controls many processes in the body
Primary tumour	The initial site where cancer grows to form a tumour
Prognosis	Assessment of how the patient's disease will progress and what the outcome will be
Radiotherapy	The use of penetrating radiation to treat a disease
Secondary tumour	The primary tumour can spread to different parts of the body to form secondary tumours, also known as a metastases
Steroid	A group of chemical substances including hormones and anti-inflammatory agents
Tissue	Collection of cells in the body specialized to carry out a particular function
Tumour	An abnormal swelling in the body that may be malignant or benign
Tumour marker	A chemical produced by some cancers that can be used to check the size of a tumour and how it is responding to treatment
Vasoconstrictors	Type of drug that cause the blood vessels to narrow, reducing blood flow
Vitamin	Group of chemical substances required in small amounts for healthy growth and development

Index